Leading and Managing in Health & Social Care

Copyright: Dr Neil Wheeler 2014
Published and Printed by:
Createspace Publishing.
Slough, UK
ISBN-13: 978-1542795456
ISBN 10: 1542795451

CONTENTS

Chapter 1	Introduction	Page:	5
Chapter 2	Managing Time	Page:	13
Chapter 3	Managing Human Resources	Page:	51
Chapter 4	Managing Quality	Page:	151
Chapter 5	Managing Change	Page:	188
Chapter 6	Leadership	Page:	249
Chapter 7	The NHS	Page:	277
Chapter 8	Collaboration	Page:	291
Chapter 9	Managing Projects	Page:	308
Chapter 10	Managing Information	Page:	345
Chapter 11	Managing Financial Resources	Page:	384
Chapter 12	Marketing	Page:	425
Contributors		Page:	469
Index		Page:	470

Note: *This text is offered on the inventive new 'Createspace' Publishing platform for two reasons:*

1) *The costs to the reader are far lower than traditional publishing houses.*
2) *It is easy to update and improve the work; the text is continually under review. To this end the readers and the authors form a community to develop the work. As a reader, you are invited to email suggestions to nwheeler@brookes.ac.uk Contributions may be simple 'typo' alerts, additional references, new areas to cover, etc. All contributors are acknowledged in the print and E-Book versions, and this may be used as material to enhance a CV.*

Foreword by Julia Foster-Turner, Course Leader: MSc Management & Leadership

A challenge in reading about management and leadership is to translate ideas and theories from the written page into something useful in real situations. This particularly for those working in highly pressured, under resources and increasingly complex environments. Enhancing learning around leadership and managing is crucial for the resilience and sustainability of both organisations and the people who work within them.

Dr Wheeler's latest volume: *Leading and Managing in Health and Social Care* has done just that, creating an ideal balance between that practical 'know how' needed to function effectively and the concepts and theories that ultimately enable practitioners to make better informed choices about the management and leadership decisions they make and how these are carried out.

The content of this book is comprehensive, including sections on self-management, managing and leading people, information and finance, running projects, improving quality, marketing and managing change.

It incorporates and explains relevant policies, legislation and how all these fit with the current reformation of health and social care.

The language of this book is very accessible, jargon limited and chapters are structured consistently in three parts- introduction, theory and application, which help the reader to navigate their route through a topic and immediately locate their area of interest. Chapters are also free standing which means the reader does not have to trawl through numerous chapters to understand a particular subject.

Leading and Managing in Health and Social Care is valuable book for those studying management for the first time, as an undergraduate or newly qualitied practitioner. It is also a very useful volume for professionals wishing to refresh or advance their management/leadership knowledge.

Julia Foster-Turner MSc

Julia Foster-Turner is course leader for a number of Master's level management and leadership programmes. She has extensive experience of management and clinical work in the NHS and in the private sector.

Foreword by Brian Donnelly, Government Advisor and CEO of the UK independent standards body, CECOPS CIC.

Whether you consider management and leadership a science or an art becomes irrelevant when you find yourself working in a busy health and social care environment. I started out in the health sector intending to improve things, regardless of how difficult they said that would be. I was soon faced with the cold reality: urgent requests, pressure to integrate, not enough staff and constantly changing policies. There were demands to save money, increase performance and elevate quality - as well as doing the day job! I relied on 'survival instinct'. But 'survival instinct' isn't enough in health and social care; tools, skills and experience are crucial.

To help me in the workplace I embarked upon an MSc in health and social care management, which added even more pressure to my already busy agenda. I soon realised, however, that the topics I was being taught were actually 'tools' to help me in the workplace. Basic principles like time management, all of a sudden made sense, and applying my learning went a long way in easing the pressures I was experiencing.

My course lecturer at that time was Dr Neil Wheeler, and I am delighted to see his excellent and practical solutions for management and leadership set out in his latest contemporary book.

The health and social care sector in the UK employs around 3 million people; the sector needs good leaders and managers, especially in the current climate of increasing demand, static resource, and mounting pressure. *Leading & Managing in Health & Social Care* will help equip you with the skills to inspire your team.

Today, we are all talking about 'outcomes'. But without the right structure and processes in place, it is very difficult to achieve them. This book can help by laying the foundation and building blocks of both management and leadership.

There is currently a greater emphasis on 'integration' between health and social care, and it is great to see that this book links these sectors effectively.

Whether you are studying for a degree or using *Leading & Managing in Health & Social Care* in the workplace, this book will prove an invaluable resource. Although not all of its content will apply in every setting and on every occasion, I am confident that you will at some point in your career find that all of the principles set out in this book prove to be relevant to call upon.

Whilst the content of management books is often considered 'theoretical', I can testify that I have proved the value of the principles set out in this and Dr Wheeler's earlier texts through my own practical experience. I have also had the immense privilege of working professionally with Dr Wheeler on a number of projects, and I found his approach very much akin to what he sets out in this great resource!

Brian Donnelly MSc

Brian Donnelly is a leading thinker and strategist in the world of commissioning and providing disability equipment and assistive technology, and is one of the most respected individuals in this field of work. He has written extensively on this subject, including his new 'Code of Practice for Disability Equipment and Wheelchair Services'. Brian formerly worked as an advisor at government level and his work is known nationally and internationally. He has an MSc (with distinction) in health & social care. Brian is the founder and chief executive of the UK independent standards body, CECOPS CIC. He is also the designer of iCOPS®, the quality and performance management software tool.

Introduction

What is management?

Among the earliest UK attempts to define management is that of Fayol (1841–1925) who considered management to consist of six functions:

Forecasting, Planning, Organizing, Commanding, Coordinating and Controlling.

Since then writers have adapted Fayol's list but none entirely dispute it and it heavily influences current thinking.

However, Fayol is discussing management *processes*. Donabedian (1988) would encourage us to think about:

Structure, Process and Outcome.

This contribution is helpful; an organisation can only be well managed if we get the *structure* right, go through the right *processes* and achieve the right *outcomes*.

To practice management and leadership according to the Fayol model might be seen as overly focused on *process* without enough consideration of *outcome*. Indeed, this can be seen to explain some poor middle management practice. Junior managers and some administrators can create and enforce complex *processes* that have no discernible benefit in terms of *outcome*.

'*Command and Control*' management, which we will later associate with McGregor's Theory X (1960) and Transactional Leadership (Bass and Alvolio, 1994), can lead a manager to believe that if he/she has absolute control over the workers, then he/she is a good manager. However, it is possible to hold absolute *process* control through coercion and bullying without achieving any good *outcomes* at all. The manager who wants to know exactly what workers are doing and where they are at all times, is in control of *processes* and creates a workforce who are always at their desks. They may not, however, be achieving much in terms of *outcome*. The manager who establishes goals and targets and then allows a large degree of autonomy might achieve far more satisfactory *outcomes*.

Occasionally the desire to control people is an intrinsic personality trait not associated with work at all and it is important for a manager to avoid abusing his/her position to gratify this need.

Pursuing this *outcome* notion Mary Parker Follett (1868–1933) started a different line of thought when she defined management as "The art of *getting things done* through people". She described management as philosophy. This competing definition also remains topical and leads to an approach to management that is far more *outcome* focussed.

> **We will say that:**
> *'Management is whatever structure and processes it takes to produce the very best outputs from the finite resources available to us'.*

That may mean offering close supervision and coaching when working with novice workers, but no more than getting out of the way with highly motivated and experienced workers to allow them to do their job. In the Leadership Chapter, we will associate this with Transformational Leadership (Bass and Alvolio, 1994) and Contingency Management (Hersey & Blanchard, 1996).

Fayol's *process* list remains valuable in itemising the *processes* to be considered, but each needs to be tempered to achieve the very best *outcomes* in terms of activity levels and quality.

> Management needs to be more than just doing the things (*Processes*) managers do. It needs to focus those things on achieving *outcomes*. These ideas are developed in the chapter on Leadership.

Purpose

This text sets out to enable the reader to understand leadership and management in the specific arena of health and social care, and to come rapidly to the point where he/she can make a contribution to that and discharge clinical management duties with sensitivity. It is written for the benefit of those studying to become professionals or new managers in health and social care. It seeks, also, to assist those experienced health practitioners moving into management.

The text recognises that leadership and management are a responsibility of all professional people in health and social care as well as managers. The budget holder may imagine that he/she controls the spending of resources, but this is largely an illusion. In reality resources are committed by health and care professionals when they decide what care to give to clients and patients. Equally, leadership may appear to come from line managers but in reality patients, clients and colleagues are far more strongly influenced and inspired by health and care professionals than they are by line managers. For these reasons, the text assumes that all clinicians and care professionals need to understand and practice leadership and management just as do professional managers.

The text sets out all of the foundation management knowledge necessary for a sound understanding and safe practice in health and care management. The book acts as an introductory grounding for those studying health care management at a higher degree level, anticipating additional study in those areas selected for special expertise.

The text covers three general areas:
- How to manage oneself;
- How to manage organisations; and
- How to manage health and social care organisations.

It is concerned throughout with: *quality, leadership, collaboration and change.*

The text sets out to meet three discrete but related needs:

a) to provide sufficient management knowledge and understanding to enable the student to meet the requirements of an honours degree;
b) to provide management skills, knowledge and understanding sufficient to enable the clinician or manager to enter practice with a very high level of organisational proficiency.
c) to act as a source reference for professional practitioners and managers in practice and to support them as they progress in management.

The insights and the pragmatic guidance given, as well as being theoretically grounded, have all been tested in the work-place. Each recommendation is capable of being achieved by all readers, albeit that they are the ideal. It is recognised that not every reader will achieve on all of the recommendations because of local circumstances and personal priorities. None-the-less, the text un-apologetically sets out the ideal as the recommended course of action. The ideal should always be the goal.

The text is based upon extensive experience and research regarding the requirements of the health and care professions for management knowledge and the content reflects that. It is understood that health and social care can never be considered simply as a business, but there are business principles able to improve efficiency and effectiveness that may be productively applied in these settings. These disciplines are described in their original language and adapted, where necessary to fit the setting. Terms such as "Productivity", "Value for money" and "Efficiency" are used throughout the text because they are essential if care is to be maximised although it is understood that they may be interpreted in different ways in some health and care settings.

In post-modern management, progressively more emphasis is placed upon individual autonomy, with employees of a high calibre and high educational attainment having significant scope to make their own decisions about their strategic aims and immediate objectives. If these aims are dynamically aligned with those of the organisation, achievement for the organisation is also achievement for the individual. The individual is expected to supply much of his/her own direction and motivation and contribute to achievement of the corporate aims without the direct and detailed instruction (micro-management) that was deemed necessary by in past decades. This is particularly evident in the health and social care industries where most professions have been elevated to graduate entry. Achievement in this setting requires high levels of organisational understanding. There are certain specific skills and knowledge required in health and care enterprises and a raft of generic skills. Together, these form the content of the text.

It is hoped that the student will make significant use of the text during undergraduate training and thereafter make reference to the text as issues e.g. time management or the distinction between full and marginal costing arise in the early years of practice.

Structure

The text is organised for the convenience of the reader, and recognises that health & social care students and practitioners are under increasing time pressure. Consequently, it has been written to enable the greatest return for the reader for the time invested, thus enabling you to be efficient in your research and studies. The book may be read for theoretical understanding and/or for clear instruction on how to perform management in health and social care, or for a rich combination of both. I.e. a blending of theory and practice.

Each chapter stands alone. Where there is some building upon notions illuminated in earlier chapters these are clearly identified with a section reference.

Each chapter appears in three parts:

Part 1 The Introduction: sets the scene for the topic area.

Part 2 The Theoretical Framework, supplies essential management knowledge for professional and managerial practice,

Part 3 The Practice, or How You Might Do It, supplies pragmatic guidance about the practice of management in health care.

These sections 2 and 3 may be equated to: Methodology - the science of what is done and Method: what is done. The text thereby meets the dual need for knowledge and practical ability.

Where appropriate, parts three of each chapter will also apply principles developed for management of organisations to management of oneself. This will enable the reader to benefit personally both in the work setting and in other aspects of a well-rounded life. For example, the discipline of marketing described for application to a large corporation, such as an NHS Trust, may equally be applied to marketing yourself, and maximising your career achievements, or even marketing a good diet to your children.

Case Examples

Where it is considered helpful, the points made are illustrated with brief case examples. These are manufactured specifically to fit each point to be made, from extensive experience of functional and general management. The examples are not, however, direct histories and any similarity to individual events is purely coincidental.

Reading Guidance

Although there would be considerable benefit gained from reading a chapter in its entirety, the text is set out to make it easy to read any one of the above sections individually. Therefore, for example, the section "The Practice" sets out to carry the necessary information to ensure good performance. The section "A Theoretical framework" carries the theoretical notions that underpin these ideas. You may choose to skip between sections in order to gain a robust understanding.

In reading this text, as with any textbook you might usefully consider the following advice:

a) Decide in advance, what you want to gain by reading the piece. That makes it easier to know when you have succeeded,
b) Note from each piece a short quotation, which encapsulates the point made (and may support your own writing).
c) File the reference in two or three key areas in a comprehensive lifelong filing system (see The Management of Information). This should include all information necessary to enable the piece to be used as a reference in a future paper.
d) The reading lists are intended for selective attention, according to the reader's areas of interest and need, not to be pursued slavishly.

e) Writers selected for chapter references are personally known to the author and/or are well-recognised authorities. Students are commended to other works of these writers.

Chapter References

Bass, B.M., & Avolio, B.J., (Eds.). (1994). *Improving organizational effectiveness through transformational leadership.* Thousand Oaks, CA: Sage Publications.

Donabedian, A. (1988). "The quality of care: How can it be assessed?". *JAMA* **121** (11): 1145–1150.

Hersey, P., & Blanchard K.H. (1996) *Management of Organizational Behaviour.* Englewood Cliffs NJ: Prentice Hall.

McGregor, D. (1960) *The Human Side of Enterprise.* New York: McGraw Hill.

Fayol, H. (1916) The administrative theory in the state. Papers on the science of administration *Journal of the institute of public administration.* 21 (3) 101 - 104

Managing Time

Introduction

This chapter addresses, in *The Theoretical Framework*, the notion of actively managing your time and the importance of that notion to: - 1) the individual, 2) the patient/client and 3) the employer. In part two, it gives pragmatic instruction on how to manage time to the best advantage of all concerned.

Efficiency

Time is a finite resource, and the effectiveness of the individual is largely a matter of the efficiency with which his/her time is deployed. All full-time employees have the same amount of time to commit, but their value to the employer depends upon the amount and quality of productivity that they can achieve with that resource (Clayton, 2010).

It is not enough to work hard and long. It is only useful to produce results (products, services, service user benefit, etc).

Efficiency = output /input = value/costs

Efficiency = the amount of benefit for service users that you achieve for a day's work.

The employee needs to minimise his/her costs and maximise his/her productivity in order to maximise efficiency. It is possible to be very busy, working hard and long - even to the detriment of one's health, and yet to produce output of very low value, because the work produced, although high volume is of low utility. Alternatively, the employee can achieve a constant, manageable and healthy work-rate applied to high value activities and have a very high value output when measured in terms of benefit to patients/clients. An important distinction, therefore, is that between volume of work done and value of work done. This achievement requires examination of the work that presents and selection of the essential and most productive tasks in order to ensure that time is used to the greatest benefit. This principle is the same whether the value to be maximised is profit earned or patients/clients treated or even leisure time enjoyed. Regardless of the currency considered, to maximise the value of the work achieved is essential.

The purpose of time management is to achieve the most productivity with the available time. However, although it is possible to define high reward in relation to business productivity, it might equally be used to mean the work, which the individual will find most rewarding (Clayton, 2010). Therefore the benefit to be maximised is not just that that to the employer & client/patient, but also to the individual. It is foolish to waste leisure time on a task that delivers low personal reward when a more rewarding activity is waiting, just as it is foolish to produce low value productivity when highly productive tasks go undone. The discipline of good time management may be applied to all aspects of life. This self-evident fact is not always translated into action. The following chapter discusses areas where the individual can re-conceptualise practice to be more effective and then progresses to section two identifying mechanisms that might be useful in making the most of the time available.

This subject is chosen for chapter one of the text to reflect the importance of the material and to recognise that time management practice underpins all management behaviour, including study.

Apply time management ideas to reading this book. Be efficient - get the maximum benefit for the minimum input.

The Theoretical Framework

Deadlines

Good time management enables workloads to be made even, reducing peaks and troughs and ensuring that deadlines are achieved in good time without last minute anxiety. "All Night-ers" routinely result in unnecessary failure to achieve the best results.

It may be that immediate time pressure is a convenient motivator and it is easier to work reactively to impending deadlines, but this is a risky strategy. Last minute strategies routinely result in unnecessary failure to achieve because, for example, illness interferes with work during the final week before a deadline. One week of illness may, in reality, be a pretty poor excuse when a task has been ongoing for six months. Work completed after midnight will be of relatively poor quality and late papers are often not proof read.

It may be argued that high workloads result in work pushed the last possible moment. In reality, again, this is a false premise. It takes no longer to perform a task ahead of a deadline than it does at the last minute. On the contrary, work may be lighter when addressed in advance of a deadline because more can be delegated and advantage can be taken of pre-existing work or colleague ideas rather than always beginning from first principles.

If a major task (University Thesis?) has a deadline 12-months hence then workloads are difficult to schedule. Use a time line or CPA (see below) to create staging deadlines along the way. Major tasks are undertaken by Project Management tools which usually amount to no more than creating sophisticated staging deadlines (Reid & Williams 2011). See Chapter 11 Project Management.

Waiting lists/Waiting times

It takes no more time to perform a task when it is requested than to perform it six months later. Therefore, waiting lists do not ease a workload. If a waiting list is roughly static, then the volume of work coming in is the same as the volume of work being performed. If more work was coming in than the service could perform, then the waiting list would be expanding, and *vice versa*. The static waiting list, which is damaging the reputation of the department, is unnecessary, being simply a reflection of an accumulation of work at some time in the past not being addressed. In the NHS, waiting list initiatives are made periodically to remove these lists and allow departments to respond to demand without unnecessary delay. This type of initiative is also appropriate for the individual. These are explained below.

Anecdotally, a manager may comment that he/she "comes up with a waiting list when she wants one, although generally he/she considers that good management results in very little waiting". In fact, waiting can be used deliberately for a number of reasons:

Queuing Theory

Queues are necessary to smooth the activity level of employees. If enough staff were employed to eliminate all waiting, then there would be periods of idleness at times of low demand. Therefore even in the most customer friendly situation, some waiting will be involved at peak times and then resolved during quiet times. The queue only becomes dysfunctional when it is not cleared during the quiet periods. A standing, year round delay of x-months frequently indicates poor management.

The individual, in the same way, might at a busier time accumulate a pile of work waiting for attention that will be cleared when the workload is in a lighter phase. However, if the clearance does not happen, then the queue has become dysfunctional and the overall relationship between workload and resource needs to be re-examined. Note that this is not always a matter of demanding more resources. Commonly it is an exercise of reshaping and reprioritising expectations. I.e. workload and resources should both be considered in order to repair the balance between them.

Queuing theory suggests that to some extent queues are self-limiting. When a queue is at a certain length then those desiring a service or product will not be willing to wait and will therefore chose not to consume, or will chose a substitute service such as private care. This may be used as a discrete method of rationing and it may be said that, in the NHS, waiting lists cannot be eliminated because removing the rationing influence of waiting lists would result in a dramatic increase in demand.

Occasionally, an individual may use the rationing effect of a waiting time for services to control his/her workload *(one prefers to work a willing horse)*. A worker might claim to be unable to respond quickly to manager demands as a strategy to reduce the demands being made. He/she might stop delivering in order to stem demand. This strategy carries a risk in terms of gaining a reputation for refusal to perform. However, if time will not allow success, then it is better to refuse a task than to accept it and then fail to deliver.

A manager who wishes to appear to be extremely busy and productive when bidding for additional resources occasionally engineers a waiting time for services. This strategy might be adopted by the individual, but with caution.

Reactive or Proactive?

At any particular moment, individuals may be operating reactively or proactively (Lambley,2009). When reactive, they are solving problems and performing tasks as they present themselves; when proactive they can consider in advance those tasks that might be done and choosing those which will deliver the highest value results and choosing the most efficient time to perform them. Proactive time managers, therefore, select high value activities and allocate them to particular time slots where they can be best achieved. Reactive managers, however, perform tasks as they present regardless of whether they represent the best use of time.

Management, at all levels, involves a significant amount of problem solving. It is possible to find solutions to emergent problems and maintain fluent running of the organisation, with a reactive approach. However, if a sense of strategic direction is in place through a proactive management style, then the solutions found, in addition to solving problems, also help move the organisation towards its longer-term goals.

Reactive use of time leads the individual to feel frenetically busy and even out of control, and yet results in him/her reaching the end of each week without achieving those tasks which he/she considers to be the top priority. This is a stressful and frustrating experience and the high level of activity does not deliver commensurately high productivity. Proactive management of a schedule will result in the individual being in control of his/her time and achieving that which he/she considers to be of the highest potential benefit (Covey, 2007).

Reactive	*Proactive*
Frenetically busy	Controlled work load
Stressful and unrewarding	Reduced stress and increased satisfaction
External control of priorities	
High/medium/low value tasks achieved	Personal control of priorities
Work done as it arises	High value tasks achieved
Short term solutions to immediate problems that ignore long term plans	Work done at the most effective and efficient time
	Solutions to immediate problems also advance long term plans

> **Case example**
>
> *A nurse is beside a river when he notices a drowning man floating down the river. Naturally he leaps in and rescues the man, giving life support on the river bank. His patient is recovering nicely when a second man is seen in the same predicament, so the story repeats.* This is reactive practice.
>
> *There is another drowning man and then another, and another. At what point does the nurse stop rescuing people and go upstream to deal with the person who is throwing them in?* That would be proactive practice.
>
> *This highlights a very common dilemma. To get in control and become proactive is essential but can require us to back off from our current problem solving behaviour which is essential but not so easy.*

Parkinson's Law

Parkinson's Law, (Parkinson,1955) was coined with a degree of humour but proves to be strikingly accurate. The "Law" includes the notion that *the task will expand to fill the time available*. Thus, however much time you allow for a task, that time will be consumed. Meetings allowed a full morning would consume a full morning, albeit that most of the agenda is covered in the final ½ hour. The same meeting given a shorter time window will also complete its agenda - particularly if scheduling puts lunch at the end of the meeting. Pressure will be felt to finish on time and eat, with the consequence that business is achieved in the time available. Thus, the "Law" *the task will expand to fill the time available* is reversible. Many tasks will shrink to fit into the time available.

Most attention goes to the early agenda items when there is a feeling of freedom and as the deadline for the close of the meeting moves nearer, items receive progressively less attention. Experienced meeting practitioners exploit this phenomenon to the full. When they want to receive detailed attention for their matter, they ensure that their item appears early in a meeting agenda, and if they want their question to be agreed *'on the nod'*, they will seek to appear at the end of an exhausting agenda.

The knowledge of the amount to be done and the time available operates at a semi-conscious level in most people to enable them to budget time and achieve their goals. Thus if a workload increases or decreases it will still, generally, be completed in the time available. Thus is Parkinson's Law sustained. By the same token, if the time available increases or decreases the work will still (just) be done. Many people are 'so busy' that they routinely work during their days off just to get it all done – and they do (just) get it all done. Generally, they find that if they tell themselves that Saturday and Sunday are 'off limits' except in a dire emergency, they find that the work can still (just) be done. The task will frequently expand or contract to consume the time that you decide to give it.

This practice breaks down, of course, when the workload is too great or when a novice practitioner fails to accurately estimate the time demands of the tasks before him/her. This is seen ever more frequently in health and social care settings, and may result in reduced reputation and self-esteem leading to *'burn out'* At this point active management of time becomes crucial. Don't take on what cannot be achieved. It is better to be seen as sometimes saying 'No' than as someone who says, 'Yes', and then does not deliver.

Routine and exceptional strategies

If it is implicitly accepted that the working time extends until late in the evening or into the weekend, then Parkinson's Law states that the workload will expand to fill that time. If, alternatively, an explicit limit is set to the time available for work, then the workload will tend to fit within that time. Accepting that a good clinician or manager is one who lives a well-balanced life requires that adequate time be protected for non-work activities.

Occasionally, however, there is an exceptional reason for working beyond the working week, and this is expected of the health care professional or manager (Reid & Williams 2011). In such circumstances, an employee will work evenings and/or weekends to complete a special task. To be available for such effort might be seen as essential in many jobs. However, when this exceptional strategy is happening routinely, leading to extended periods of evening and/or weekend working, than work load and time management needs to be reviewed using the strategies explained below in "The Practice". This means that to occasionally take work home is normal, but to routinely do so is an indicator of poor management. For many people, drift will occur, leading to a gradual expansion in the working week and the exercise of workload and time management review will be needed on a regular basis.

Managing a diary

Well-managed appointment diaries will contribute to making a sound plan for getting the most from the available time (Reid & Williams 2011). A diary will show meeting start times and the maximum probable duration. The diary should also show the time needed for travelling between meetings and recovery, natural breaks, collection of papers/briefing for the next meeting, etc. If these transition times are not protected, then contribution at each meeting will be significantly impaired. It is generally better to be occasionally unavailable for a meeting than to earn a reputation for high attendance but poor time keeping and badly briefed contributions.

Meetings serve the purpose of communication and decision-making, but rarely produce anything. If a high number of meetings are to be attended, it will be necessary to protect time to act on the decisions made and the information gained. If this is not the case then it is difficult to see the justification for attendance. The diary must show a sufficient amount of time protected for action based upon meeting decisions. In some cases, it will be necessary to mark out slots for work, thus making these times unavailable for meetings. Failure to do so can result in a diary being filled with meetings leaving no time for resultant work. This gives a false impression of the work that can be carried out. The result is that the individual uses all work time for meetings and then either fails to deliver on consequential tasks or carries out these tasks outside of working hours. If this occurs then poor diary management has resulted in acceptance of a workload that is not achievable within the paid week. This is acceptable in emergencies, as above, but will lead to failure if it continues indefinitely. Corrective action is taken by altering diary management practice to show enough time free from meetings to allow action to be taken on meeting decisions. Whenever a meeting booking is accepted, the diary is immediately marked out with sufficient time to prepare, travel to & from and act on the conclusions, in addition to the full duration of the meeting itself.

Clinicians not involved in such a high meeting load will find that the same difficulty arises when the diary is filled with direct client contact. This leads to associated work being performed outside of working hours. If this is the case then, again, the solution is to adjust diary management practice to allow non-contact tasks to be performed. It is generally considered that if a clinician can achieve 50% of his/her time in direct patient contact, he/she is achieving very well.

Diary example

	Mon	Tues	Wed	Thurs
8.00am	Preparation	Keep free to act on	Preparation	Keep free to act on
9.00am	Meeting A	meetings A & B	Meeting D	Meetings
10.00am	⇓ ⇓	⇓ ⇓	⇓ ⇓	⇓ ⇓
11.00am	⇓ ⇓	⇓ ⇓	⇓ ⇓	⇓ ⇓
12.00	Return to base	Preparation	⇓ ⇓	⇓ ⇓
1.00pm	⇓ ⇓	Meeting C	⇓ ⇓	⇓ ⇓
2.00pm	Preparation	⇓ ⇓	⇓ ⇓	⇓ ⇓
3.00pm	Meeting B	⇓ ⇓	⇓ ⇓	⇓ ⇓
4.00pm	⇓ ⇓	⇓ ⇓	⇓ ⇓	⇓ ⇓
5.00pm	⇓ ⇓	Return to base	Return to base	⇓ ⇓

This weekly schedule shows: - time allocated to meetings time to move between locations and time to act on meeting decisions. Although only half of the week is scheduled for meetings, the week is fully committed and requests for attendance at further meetings will be declined because the schedule is full.

Realistic Goal Setting

In the final instance, Parkinson's Law notwithstanding, time is constrained and there is a finite amount of work, which is going to be achieved (Reid & Williams 2011). The individual who accepts only achievable work onto his/her workload will have the experience of success and earn a reputation for delivering the goods. The individual who, through good-nature, allows more onto the task list than is ultimately achievable will know failure and earn a reputation for letting people down, in spite of the fact that both individuals have performed to the same level. Therefore in good time management, the ability to say "No" is essential and, paradoxically, will earn a reputation for achievement whereas always saying, "Yes" will not. Good nature takes workers a long way in health and social care, but saying 'Yes' and then failing, is not a kindness. Better to take the assertive route and say 'I Can't'.

In Summary

It is critical to control time rather than be controlled by time, to make time deliver that which is the greatest priority to the individual rather than to someone else and to maintain equilibrium in a very turbulent environment.

The Practice

or how you might go about it

Examining and revising the management of available time will bring you a sudden improvement in productivity reputation and job satisfaction. The exercise requires a forceful period of 'standing back', which is difficult because when it is needed is when it is most difficult to achieve. The cartoon might say, *"When I have time, I am going to get organised"*. However, the exercise has a payback time measurable in days and within weeks, the 'time profit' is significant.

The time management revision exercise is one that you should repeat throughout your career. Time management cannot be 'got right'. Objective analysis sets you up for a period, but drift immediately sets in and the exercise requires repeating on a regular basis. In time you will learn to notice when the exercise needs to be repeated. However, as a guide it is appropriate to see a time management review as twice yearly event.

Conscious insight into time usage is an essential precursor to improved time management. There follow suggestions for a practical approach, firstly to you give insight into current time usage and, secondly to improve your use of time.

Time use analysis

Gaining an explicit picture of how you are using your time is the first step to improving that use. It may be a base line against which you will make improvements, or it may be a diagnostic tool to see where time is wasted, but it essential that any concern about time efficiency be based upon an assessment of the present situation. There are a number of approaches to assessing your time usage.

Descriptive diary

A diary of your day's activities, completed at least hourly, describing what you have done over that last hour will capture all of your activity. This can then be analysed after a period of perhaps a week and you will gain a detailed picture of where the time goes.

This is a very rich form of data and allows all activity to be accurately recognised. This device has the advantage of spotting time usage that you could not predict. However, it will be a very time consuming exercise. Although there is certain to be a swift payback after which time you will have gained at least as much as you lost, you may still feel that the exercise cannot be afforded in the short run.

Time Log

After a predetermined interval throughout your working day you stop work and tick the box that best corresponds to the activity that you have been doing during that period. This requires you to categorise all the possible activities in advance. Since the ticking boxes exercise is very quick, the intervals can be very short. It is common practice to carry some kind of alarm that will alert you to the passage of another time interval. Intervals may be as short as ¼ hour or as long as an hour. The defining factor is how quickly you change activities. What is the longest interval you can choose and be confident that it will have been spent on just one main activity? The log can then be quickly analysed and data collated about the aggregate hours spent on each type of activity. You must ask whether the items you spend most time performing are your highest priority. If they are not, then why are you giving them so much time? Sometimes several definitions are possible. Should you call getting an unnecessary telephone call: an *interruption*, or a *telephone call*, or *client related work*? The solution to this lies in setting the exercise up very thoughtfully. Select categories for yourself that will have most meaning to your work, or your life.

Ask yourself:

1) whether you really want to allocate your time to those five most popular categories in your log?

2) does your allocation of time match your stated priorities?

3) that last thing I did, which of my priorities does it address? if none of them, then why did I do it?

4) how would you stop things taking up your time when they do not benefit you or your job?

5) are there regular offenders that eat into your time unproductively?

Time Sampling

As a still cheaper option, it is possible to take a sample, either at random which requires an assistant to say "Now!" to you periodically during the day, or regularly which requires an alarm to go off at pre-set intervals. When the call comes, note down what you were doing during the previous ¼ hour. This involves less data collection and analysis, but delivers less complete information. Time sampling might be done as an intermittent diary entry log or by placing the relevant activity into one of a range of pre-set categories in a time log. You might make this sampling exercise more representatives by considering a diagonal slice. Week one Monday, week two Tuesday, etc will give you a picture of each weekday but over a period of five weeks so that monthly patterns are also reflected.

Whatever your method of collecting activity information, you will wind up with a statement of where you are deploying your time and you can compare that with your list of priorities. Are you spending the greatest amount of time on top priority tasks, or are you being drawn into spending time on tasks that you do not consider to be if optimum importance? If the latter, then you must better control your choice of activity.

Prioritising

Having measured your actual use of time, it is necessary to decide your ideal use of time. All potential tasks need to be captured onto some sort of list and you need to decide, seeing them together, what is the most important (Covey, 2007)..

First, make a list.

It is necessary for you to record emergent work as it arises, in order to remove it from your active memory. Just as a computer slows down when its Random Access Memory (RAM) is over extended, so you will observe that your own mental processes are impaired by having to hold a long list of duties in your head. Talking to colleagues who have "A lot on their mind" you will note that their speech and responses are slowed. Record your emergent tasks and then let them go. You will address them later along with tasks that have arisen from other sources and then you will decide on their importance and urgency thereby deciding which to do and when. In order to do this you will need to carry around a suitable "To-Do" list. This will have a section for the tasks you are carrying out today and another for the tasks that you are collecting for later consideration. This list must be in one place only. Avoid having a plethora of scraps of paper and sticky yellow notes. One clinician made this list on the inside of her uniform hem. It worked acceptably until she sent her "notes" to the cleaner and lost everything. The method recommended is to designate one section of your Personal Organiser "*Today's To-Do*" and another section "*New Tasks*". You can then keep to your planed priorities and consider new tasks alongside tasks arising through other channels in order to set new priorities.

Second, establish priorities

Potential tasks present themselves by an array of routes, and it you must learn to rapidly sift and categorise them. Generally, it is possible to designate any task importance either:

"A" 'essential', "C" 'non-essential' or "B" 'maybe'

"A" tasks need storing, and attending to as soon as is possible. These are the tasks that you will put onto your *"Today's To-Do"* list. Chose a time for them to be done that will allow you to meet deadlines and to do the task when it can be done to the best effect for the least effort. I.e. essential case notes, or meeting records are most easily made if they are done immediately after the event, not put off until your memory is challenged. However, telephone calls may be best performed in batches, when you have desk time and interruptions can be controlled.

"C" tasks do not need doing. This does not mean that they can be put aside for doing later. If they do not merit doing now, then they will not merit doing later unless the priority changes and then they become "A" tasks. These "C" tasks are stored for a period because they may become important later as a result of developments. A client situation may change or your manager may follow up the task. Either of these developments could re-designate a task from "C" to "A". At this time, the papers are retrieved and the task joins the "A" list for attention as soon as desirable. If you feel that a task must be done, but can be left until later, then the task is no less important, only less urgent. Any task that is essential, regardless of time frame is an "A" task.

Tasks are in the "B" category because of your indecision. You must carefully re-considered and re-categorise these tasks. Thus, everything either goes into an "A" pile, for attention or a "C" category for storing in case they later develop into something important. As you get better at prioritisation, the B pile will disappear. Only in the very rare event that all work in the "A" pile has been completed, without exception, should a task from the "C" pile be addressed. If a task has been put into the "C" category but your feeling is that it must be done eventually, it has been wrongly categorised. Perhaps it was important but not urgent - see "Urgency/Importance" below. This can be seen as a way of validating the categorisation process. If the lists feel right, then the process is working. If the feeling is that the "C" pile cannot be comfortably ignored, then the categorising needs further work. Periodically the contents of your "C" pile can be transferred to a waste bin for disposal, or if you are very unconfident, they can be filed away - the further away the better.

Beware the medium through which the task has emerged

It is important to ensure that you categorise tasks according to content rather than medium. Many people feel disposed to attend to requests received verbally or by telephone and allow tasks received by Email or paper mail, to fall behind, which often means to be left undone by default. It is not unusual to find "C" tasks being completed in preference to "A" tasks, simply because they came by telephone rather than by email or letter. This is a waste of the time resource because a low reward task has been performed in preference to a high reward task that came by another route.

Note, however, that you can exploit this phenomenon in trying to get colleagues to give priority to your "A" tasks. If your task is not their priority, they should not do it, but you can exploit this common mistake and get their help. Do they respond best to written, spoken, electronic messages? If you want a colleague to give high priority to your work be thoughtful about the channel through which you transmit it.

Ensure that it is *your* Priority

If another person passes a task to you, then they will have assessed it as important but only to them and their priority list may not match yours. It is essential to assess potential tasks according to priority against your own objectives. It is important not to allow your priorities to be distorted by those of others. Inevitably the priorities of your manager will influence yours, and in a perfectly managed organisation the priorities of the whole guide those of the individual with the consequence that priority conflict cannot happen. Where priorities do not match, however, it is necessary to negotiate compromise rather than letting your personal priorities be deflected by those of an assertive colleague. If you simply decide not to perform tasks passed to you by a colleague, because they are not your priority, then it is essential to be explicit about this reality, saying "No" because the alternative is to appear to fail to deliver.

It is a manager's task to ensure that individuals' goals are well aligned with each other and those of the organisation. See chapter: Managing People.

Urgency/importance

All tasks can be placed on two continua:

Urgent <===================> Non-urgent

and

Important <================> Unimportant

Seeing these together allows a grid to be composed:

	Urgent	Non-urgent
Important	Task V	Task W Task X
Unimportant	Task y	Task Z

The Urgency/important grid, Tasks v, w & x are important and should be categorised "A" and be performed. Broadly, they would be performed in order of urgency i.e. v, w and then x. **Task y is a trap**. Urgency, which simply means that the task must be done very soon if it is to be done at all, can lead to *immediate action* where *no action* was the better response. This means that an unimportant task has taken priority over an important task simply because it is time bound. Tasks: y and z should be categorised "C" (unimportant) and the swiftness with which they would have been done is therefore irrelevant because they are not to be done at all. This urgency trick is often used to pressure others into performing a task that they would otherwise call unimportant. A questionnaire with a deadline, for example, is more likely to be returned than one without. The sense of urgency is mistaken for importance. The thought is, "I had better do this now because it is urgent", rather than "Should I be doing this at all?" Consider only whether a task will deliver you sufficient benefit to warrant your time. If the answer is "Yes", then do it. If the answer is "No", then do not do it. Do the "Yes" or "A" tasks in the order of urgency, making adjustments for the time at which they may be most efficiently done, but not risking failure to meet the deadline.

Jobs for today

Because it is not sensible to make prioritising decisions whenever a time slot arises, you will need to make a list. You can devise your daily To-Do list either early morning or last thing in the previous day as you like. The important thing is that it is done. Look at the list of "A" tasks and select those that can realistically be achieved in the time available. Always select the highest priority. There is a temptation to select the tasks that neatly fit the time, even if that means performing the odd "C" task because it fits and there are no "A" tasks that can be completed in that time. You must steel yourself to address "A" tasks first and probably only. This requires that major tasks are broken down into manageable components and one of these A task components is handled in the available small time slot, rather than addressing a "C" task that happens to be conveniently sized.

Prioritising: conclusion

So, whenever a potential task comes to your attention, it goes onto a list. Daily, the list is examined and the first question is "Am I going to do this at all?" This is essential, whether the task came by letter, over coffee or by any other means, and whether the task is tightly time bound or not. If the answer is "No", then a record of the task joins the "C" pile in a remote part of the office just in case it becomes important later. If the answer is "Yes" then the task joins the "A" pile and is performed with the priority deriving from its deadline at a time when it can be performed most efficiently and well. Time pressures on a task or the direct approach from the supplicant must not distort this decision process.

Junk mail, of course, is thrown away immediately it leaves the envelope.

Perform in the present

Once you have prioritised your jobs and are working through a plan, focus on fulfilling the plan. Do not concern yourself about what you are not doing. When the prioritisation is done, then the plan is made and you should focus single-mindedly on achieving the best results. This attention to the present will allow you to perform each task to the best of your ability and achieve the best outcome. If you perform tasks with a part of your attention elsewhere, considering the things you are not doing right now, then your performance will be impaired. The benefit of the planning and decision process is that the decisions are made and your responsibility, now, is to carry out those tasks to your very best ability not to worry more about the prioritisation process. Other important tasks will be elsewhere and they should be considered in their turn with equal dedication, but not allowed to impair your immediate performance.

Focus on performing the current task as well as possible without also reliving guilt about an earlier failure or rehearsing anxiety about a future challenge. There are lessons to be learned from failure, and that should happen, but once the lesson is learned through sensible reflection, it is important to release it and focus on the current task. This attention to the present can be very liberating experience and will result in better enjoyment of life and improved performance.

This principle should be applied to all facets of your life. If you have decided to spend an hour out of a busy day with your mother, children, friends, lover, etc, then do so whole-heartedly, enjoy it and ensure that they do too. Do not allow it to be impaired by having your attention distracted by other tasks. Recreation is necessary for health and consequent work productivity. However, many of us feel uncomfortable about leisure or holidays and approach them with diminished energy, thereby deriving impaired (inefficient) benefit. Once you have made the decision, this is the most important way to spend that piece of time, then that decision is made and you should not revisit it or fret about the things that you are not doing. Opportunity cost tells us that there are always other things that could have been done. One activity is always at the expense of another. However, once the top priority has been chosen then that is the best use of your time and the other possibilities must be released. When you have made a decision in favour of an activity, pursue it with single-minded attention, maximise the benefit gained and enjoy the liberating effect of focussing on the present.

Strategy and Goals

In order to decide your priories it is essential to have an explicit understanding of your desired achievements. This will require you to have carefully considered and well expressed strategic and operational goals.

Strategic Goals (Aims)

Strategic goals are your long-term intentions (Clayton, 2010). This short list is a clear statement of what is to be achieved by performing your job over a defined period, and what you want to make of your position. Additionally, the strategic goals will include your individual development intentions and aspirations for your career as a result of achievements in the post. These goals must be discussed in detail with your family, manager and colleagues, so that they are agreed and understood.

Operational Goals (Objectives)

These are your short-term targets, and eventually they will add up to achievement of your long-term goals (Clayton, 2010). They may be in relation to problems that present themselves, or routine work opportunities. For each area of involvement, it is important to be conscious of the planned outcome and to ensure that all activity undertaken will advance your goals. Indeed they must not just advance your goals, but must advance them and more than would any alternative activity. Without this focus on goals, it is difficult to assess the importance of a possible task. It becomes easy to perform tasks that are generally a good idea, but which will not deliver the greatest possible benefit for you. This results in always being very busy and constructive, but without having the best possible quantity and quality output.

In achieving short-term goals, there may be a wide range of possible routes. Strategic objectives are achieved by careful choice of the routes by which we achieve operational objectives. If there are a number of ways to achieve a short-term goal, pick one that also constitutes a step towards achievement of a long-term goal (Aim).

Case Example

Basic grade occupational therapist (OT) in a District General Hospital (DGH)

Strategic goals:

1) to reduce the average length of stay of patients following hospitalisation.
2) to reduce the average readmission rates of patients
3) to gain experience and reputation necessary to enable promotion into a senior community-based position

Operational Goals:

1. to assess and facilitate personal independence in daily living skills in each referred patient

> 2. to facilitate safe return home for each referred patient.
>
> The patient presents with a request for a device to assist with dressing, which activity of daily living has become difficult.
>
> A device could simply be issued, thus satisfying the immediate demand. However, consideration of the operational goals would lead to the exploration of the problem to identify the cause. This would enable the OT to spot and resolve related difficulties that might otherwise impede independence and discharge.
>
> A number of solutions might offer themselves to the dressing problem, but the OT will prefer the one that delivers the best step towards achieving strategic goals 1, 2 and 3. I.e. the intervention must ensure swiftest possible discharge combined with lowest possible likelihood of readmission and constitute good experience for a potential Community Occupational Therapist.
>
> In this case the OT made an assessment of the home setting to know exactly what the patients would require on discharge and what would be required to ensure safe continuance at home. All of the strategic goals were thus addressed.
>
> Prioritising, within an explicit framework of goals, focuses effort and results in greater achievement without greater effort.

This is what was meant by the popular expression of the 1980s,

"Work smarter, not harder". (Lakin 1978).

The slogan is trite, but the notion is correct. Another useful slogan might take the form of a question on a poster on your wall:

"Which of my objectives were advanced by that last task?"

If the answer is "None" then ask yourself why you did it. If it was a necessary task, then the objective list is incomplete. If it was an unnecessary task then: ***Don't do it again!***

Delegation

If a task is to be done, by the above criteria, then the next thought is "By whom?" Delegation to another is not to be seen as shifting the load. Making one person busier in order to make another less busy will not benefit the organisation. However, if another person can do a task: better, quicker or cheaper than you, then delegation is appropriate. Frequently, delegation is to a subordinate. If that person can perform a task as well as you, then he/she will do so at a lower hourly cost, therefore increasing the efficiency of the organisation. In the case of administrative staff, it is usually the case that a good secretary can type a large document in less time than a clinician, to a superior standard and on a lower salary. In this case, delegation is a three-fold winner. Additionally delegation may be practised to protect the time of hard to recruit specialists such as clinicians by passing generic work to easy to recruit generalist employees.

If no staff time is available at the grade to which you would like to delegate, then this is a sign that the "Skill Mix is not correct. See The Management of People. The NHS had a history of favouring expensive, qualified staff, over unqualified assistants and secretaries and this impeded delegation. In recent years, this has changed and the popular press disapproves. However, it can often improve patient care to increase the available time of less expensive employees such as HCAs and secretarial support even at the expense of a reduction in more expensive qualified clinicians.

If a task is not important enough to be done, then it cannot be delegated!

There is a temptation to delegate a task that is difficult to categorise between "A"& "C". We do not think that a task is important enough to do personally but, not liking to refuse, we pass it to someone else. If it does not need doing, then it cannot be delegated. If the decision is that a task does not warrant doing by all objective criteria, but none the less, it feels wrong to leave it undone, then this is a cue to reconsider the criteria. If, however, genuine "C" tasks are delegated because the manager does not like to say "No" then the organisation rapidly degenerates into a "C" Task organisation, and the reduced cost of the labour employed is counteracted by the low value of the output. *In delegating there is a sequence:*

a) Ensure that the task is really necessary - "A" not "C"
b) Identify any essential skills needed to perform the task.
c) Select the lowest point in the organisation at which the task could be satisfactorily performed. Identify an individual who is suitable and has time. Identify the protocols for passing work to that individual.
d) Set the objectives for the task.
e) Communicate the task, with context, parameters, standards for success, monitoring arrangements, time-frame.
f) Brief colleagues in the organisation that the task is delegated, and confer any necessary authority.
g) Monitor, directly if necessary, but by exception reporting if possible (i.e. require a report back only if the task is not proceeding according to plan. Otherwise get out of their way!). Offer support when requested. Respect a subordinate's autonomy and ability to say when they need help. This allows a complete freeing of your time.
h) Evaluate, and recognise the achievement. The small cog in any machine may be just as important as the large cog. The subordinate can be just as crucial to success as the manager.
i) Consider whether this delegation points to the need for permanent change in processes and responsibilities.

Note: temporary or permanent delegation might alter Job Descriptions and/or Grades.

Delegation conclusion

Only delegate tasks that are justified within the organisations resources and priorities

Delegate to an officer who can perform mere effectively or efficiently than yourself;

Tell everyone who needs to know;

Delegate authority;

Monitor as much as is necessary;

Feedback, recognise and reward;

Consider whether the delegation can become a permanent change in routine and practice.

Use every moment

There are periods in the day that are traditionally wasted (Covey, 2007). When tasks are identified and prioritised, some can be allocated to non-traditional work times. Reading reports should be possible on train journeys, when outside an office waiting for an appointment, etc, providing that the need for confidentiality is remembered. This is only possible, however, if you keep a few such reports with you for such eventualities. Always ensure that you have pen, paper, highlighter, etc at hand, so that these opportunities can be fully exploited even when they arise unexpectedly. Therefore, if there is a risk that you will be kept waiting by someone, take some work to do, and always have some work on hand for the time when you are kept waiting unexpectedly.

Handle paper only once

Time is wasted by repeatedly reading a message that contains a job and setting it aside to do at some future time. Once tasks are categorised, then try to only pick up the document again when you are going to deal with it. Decide immediately who it goes on to, what the reply is, what the job will be etc. Then the message can be filed or thrown. It is often quicker and clearer to write a reply onto a letter and send it straight back. You may like to photocopy the message, with reply, for your records. Encourage colleagues to write an immediate reply to you about your queries by putting a reply section on the bottom of memos and letters. Email makes this a little less common but there are many cases in H&S Care when paper is essential.

Break up tasks into manageable slices.

Q: "How do you eat an elephant?" A: "One slice at a time." How do you address a huge task when your desk time is never more than ½ hour. The answer is to break the major task into manageable small ½ hour tasks. Perhaps a major task cannot be scheduled, but a string of small ones always can. This is also a good approach to a task that is too daunting to begin. See the task as a sequence of small steps and set out on the first step. Thus address the daunting "A" not the unthreatening "C".

Case Examples

Major task: Go through the files and remove records for all those clients who have not been active in the last two years

Smaller task: Deal with surnames: A & B

Without this active dis-aggregation, the task will be left until a full day can be committed, and this may not be soon. The minor (but "A") task can be scheduled into any normal day.

Major task: Revise skills mix for the ward you manage

Smaller task: Ask staff to complete a Time Audit for a Day/Week.

Spring-cleaning is, for most people, a daunting task, but to clean and organise the kitchen cupboards can be motivating and rewarding. The rest of the kitchen and the Lounge can then be scheduled for other days, and the kitchen success will help you motivate yourself for the next room.

Therefore:

Major task: Spring-clean your home

Smaller task: Clean and organise the kitchen cupboards Or even just one, to start with!

Note:

Many "A" tasks can be overwhelming, and you might never reach the situation in which you can address them. This leads to inaction and demoralisation, because you know that a really important task is not being addressed. You then attempt to feel better by working relentlessly on "C" tasks. The result is that you are exhausted, unproductive and still anxious about failure to address the real task. (EG you clean your desk or kitchen when you should be starting your university dissertation). This is a good way to achieve "Burnout". Breaking up of a task allows you to feel good about each step of achievement, and this periodic reward is essential to help maintain your moral and motivation. Breaking up huge "A" tasks into manageable small "A" tasks is therapeutic and ensures that you are highly productive by spending all of your time on "A" tasks.

Interruptions

Being interrupted in your work is very inefficient. If you are working on a task and a colleague enters your office for a five-minute query then you are likely to lose up to ½ hour's productivity in giving that five-minute attention. You may spend ten minutes in moving your attention to the new subject and coming to grips with the matter, five minutes of productivity, five minutes receiving gratitude/pleasantries, and ten minutes recovering your position on the task upon which you were working. Thus, you have lost ½ hour to achieve 5 minutes' productivity.

Avoid interruptions however you can. Often, work can be performed at home or away from the workstation, thus making you unavailable for interruption. The telephone can be transferred to a colleague or answer service. If you do not want to be interrupted at your workstation then you might have a "Do not disturb" sign. However, you may feel that this is very negative. To turn the position to a positive one, publish "Office Hours" when you are always available to deal with colleagues, receive telephone calls, and encourage enquiries at this time. This will make you appear very welcoming and save a lot of time in the abortive calls and visits, which arise when your colleagues do not know when would be a good time to call you.

Make maximum use of breaks.

Breaks in the working day are very constructive and result in a net increase in productivity. Being in a position to break for lunch and even Tea/Coffee on most days, can be seen as an indicator of good organisation and time management. Too busy for lunch just means badly organized. Productivity is better when you are refreshed, but the value of breaks is far greater than that. It is during your breaks that you will have freewheeling thoughts about your work and will recognise alternative, more efficient ways in which tasks may be achieved. Additionally, during informal conversation over lunch much fortuitous communication can occur that can save many hours of unnecessary work.

When you are having a break, focus whole-heartedly on that break. Do not do it with guilt or anxiety about what you are not doing. If you feel guilty about work not done, then you will still not be doing it, and you will also diminish the benefit you could gain from the break.

Meetings

Meetings consume a great deal of time. This time may be time well spent. However, some meeting time may be committed to material from which you will not benefit. Challenge the need to attend all meetings. If attendance is indicated, check whether you need to attend for the full meeting or whether you can attend only for selected items. Do not feel slighted by being allowed to attend a meeting for one item only, it simply means that you are too busy to sit through a full meeting of unproven importance. When running a meeting, there are a number of requirements on you as chair- see Management of People. Concerning time management, as chair of a meeting you have a duty to constrain discussion to the point that time committed is justified by the achievement. A two-hour meeting with twenty attendees costs the organisation the equivalent of one weeks' salary. One weekly meeting with twenty members, therefore, consumes the equivalent of a full time employee. Are you sure that each meeting is worth that?

Making effort count twice

With many activities, there is the opportunity to benefit from synergy. A task, once completed, may be utilised for various other benefits. The case report written for the referring General Practitioner might, with only a little additional work, become a teaching resource for your student, or the focus of a journal article. It will be far less time consuming to write the teaching resource or journal paper immediately after completing the case report than it would be to recall the information later.

Time & motion analysis

Time and motion analysis became fashionable and then unfashionable in the 1950/60/70s. However, it is still with us under the trendier title of 'Lean Thinking'. (Cleaner Workplaces, 2014)

Although a sophisticated analysis is infrequently thought appropriate, the principle of performing routine tasks efficiently remains valid. Consider those tasks that you perform repeatedly, which consume a significant part of your working week. Review how you go about those tasks and consider whether they could be performed in less time, if the circumstances were altered. Alterations might involve changing the location of the task, the time of day of the task, the order in which tasks are performed, the location of equipment stores, etc in order to enable the task to be performed in less time. This principle is evident in the location of ward-based stores. If storage of dressings and other consumable materials is as close as possible to the areas in which they are to be used, then time and energy in collection will be minimised. At home, if your dishwasher is close to your crockery cupboard, then the task of emptying it is far more quickly performed. If it cannot be close, then use a trolley and make a single journey. Do not carry a few plates over again and again. These examples are small, but clearly correct. Look at where your time is spent, and ask whether improved Time and Motion practices could reduce the time they take. If one task takes on average ten hours a week, eg filing, and you could reduce this by 20% by moving the filing cabinets, then this one-off reorganisation will net two hours benefit per week with the benefit recurring indefinitely.

Systematising routine tasks

Time is expended on the process of deciding how to respond to situations. It is wasteful to respond in less than the most efficient manner. Therefore, take time to set up systematic ways of performing routine tasks. This will save future thinking time, ensure time efficiency and, additionally, reduce time consuming errors. (Ackoff, 2010)

Form letters

Create letters that with minimal tailoring can be used in bulk situations. This considerably reduces time use and, also, ensures that all letters cover all necessary aspects of the matter in hand and are easily read because they are always in the same format.

When replying to a memo or letter, it is frequently possible to write a response on the received memo and return it. This saves a preamble reminding the recipient of his/her letter and saves typing. If a permanent record of both pieces of correspondence is required, then photocopy the document with your reply written on. You can save further time by encouraging colleagues to write on and return your letters and memos, by having a "Reply" section at the foot. This saves you time in reading letters and makes it more likely that you will receive your reply by return of post.

Setting standards

Tasks must be performed to the standard necessary for success. To perform to a lower standard is unacceptable, but to perform to a higher standard is to use resources wastefully. To produce ten results to the required standard is often better than to produce eight results far more than the required standard. Therefore decide what standard is necessary and ensure achievement of that standard. Do not strive for excellence unless that excellence will make a substantial difference. Excellence will consume time and thereby reduce your volume of output. You can perform more tasks if you perform them to the required standard than if you perform each to a level more than the required standard. However, poor quality is not at all efficient, so you will need to allow a safe margin for error in quality to ensure that you always meet the required standard. Additionally, you must continually improve quality in order to remain acceptable. However to reduce responsiveness and reliability in order to achieve excellence is not good quality.

Biorhythms

Recognise your most and least productive times of the day/week/year. Most people know that they are capable of greater achievement in the morning or in the afternoon. If you work best in the morning, then apply this period to your most demanding tasks, and during the afternoon, if this is a poor time for you, perform the routine tasks that require less of your focused attention. If you spend the morning getting the routine work out of the way so that you can have a good run at the difficult tasks after lunch, then you have used your most creative time on routine tasks and are left with the difficult work when you are least equipped to manage it. If you can barely stay awake after lunch, do not schedule desk tasks for that time. Rather make that a time for individual meetings where the other person will offer enough interest to keep you alert. However, do not fall asleep in company! Power napping may be preferable to public poor performance, and is best done alone!

Do not present for work if you are not fit

As a final thought, although you are urged to make the very best of every minute, there are times when you are sufficiently unwell or distracted to be unable to perform to an acceptable standard. On such occasions, your efforts might do more harm than good. It is better not to attend for work, than to attend and perform so badly as to damage your reputation and create a huge workload in correcting your mistakes. Therefore, if you are going to perform work of negative net value to you, then do not present for work.

Conclusion

How much value you achieve in exchange for your time, is the only measure of the efficiency of your work.

Efficiency = Output/Input = value/cost

Make every moment of your time deliver as much of the most valuable output as you can. Perform only the most valuable tasks, perform them as efficiently as possible and use all of the above tactics to maximise your efficiency. Consider your life holistically, so that you achieve the most for your employer, your family and yourself. It is easy to be angry with others about your diverted priorities but in the final analysis, how you use your time is your direct responsibility and that of nobody else. Your failures are your fault and if these suggestions are followed then your successes will be entirely to your credit.

References

Ackoff,R.L. (2010) *Systems thinking for curious managers* Axminster: Triarchy Press.

Babauta, I. (2009) *The power of less the 6 essential productivity principles.* London: Hay House

Clayton,M. (2010) *Brilliant time management* Harlow: Pearson.

Cleaner workplaces (2014) 7 lean principles www.kcprofessional.co.uk/lean-e-book *(Free to download)*

Covey,S. (2007) *The seven habits of successful people* London: Simon and Schuster

Lakein, A. (1997) *Give Me a Moment and I'll Change Your Life: Tools for Moment Management* Kansas City: Andrews & McMeel

Lakein, A.(1984) *How to get control of your time and your life* Aldershot : Gower

Lambley,A. (2009).*Proactive practice in SW practice*, Exeter: Learning Matters Ltd.

Mackenzie,R,A. (1981) - *About time! : A woman's guide to time management* - New York; London

Oncken, W.(1984) *Managing management time : who's got the monkey.* - London: Prentice-Hall,

Parkinson,C.N. (1995) *Parkinson's Law* The economist.

Reid,M. & Williams,K. (2011) *Time Management.* New York: Palgrave.

Managing People (Human Resources)

Introduction

Health care providers in the public or independent sector are Human Resource focused institutions with a collective direct and indirect workforce exceeding one million people. The efficiency and effectiveness with which these resources are deployed is the critical factor in determining organisational success (Griffiths,1984).

This chapter addresses the selection development, management and accountability of staff and identifies the players. It addresses how the individual manages others and how the individual managers him/herself to his/her best advantage and to that of the organisation.

The Theoretical Framework provides the necessary information and *The Practice* provides pragmatic guidance for successful practice.

The Theoretical Framework

The rise and fall of Line Management

Traditionally, the NHS was managed along military lines, with a continuous chain of command all of the way from the government Department of Health (DoH) to the clinician alongside the patient. This is line management (CIPD,2014). This involved very deep pyramid shaped organisation charts with strict accountability Managers held a span of control in which, generally, fewer than ten people reported directly to any individual. This ensured close supervision and firm control. Arguably, however, this control was unnecessary for self-motivating people such as health care professionals, and it has become ever less necessary as the academic level of attainment has drifted upwards. Simultaneously, the autonomy of clinicians and managers has been greatly increased.

Since the NHS reforms of 1990 "The NHS and Community Care Act" there has been a trend towards flatter structures in which many people can report to one manager. This is achieved by making the individual more responsible for his/her own actions and less reliant on direct supervision Managers and clinicians have a set of objectives to achieve for the organisation, these objectives encapsulate the job, and the individual is given some licence regarding how to achieve them. The task of the manager becomes strategic planning and negotiating objectives with development opportunities to facilitate individual achievement. Additionally, individuals may break away from line relationships by becoming members of client or task focused teams Bratton& Gold (2012). These teams may be semi-permanent or transient, depending on the nature of the tasks to be undertaken.

Periodically, there is a small resurgence of traditional close supervision. In most cases it is decried as 'micro-management', but occasionally has benefit over short periods to improve quality in areas such as infection control (Frances,2013).

Outsourcing and Tendering

In many situations, the need to manage subordinate staff has been eliminated entirely by buying services in from a specialised service provider. Early examples of this were cleaning and hospital grounds maintenance services. These services were bought in, subject to tender, from professional cleaning and gardening organisations. There were benefits and dis-benefits in this practice, but the eventual cost savings were sufficient for the practice to be continued and extended to other services. Now, a wide range of support services can be out-sourced in this manner. The process is even applied to some of the more peripheral clinical services such as the Nurse Bank.

Where an existing direct labour team wanted to continue to deliver services but on a contract basis, they had the right to compete as an "In-house" tendering organisation bidding for the work on an level footing with external tenderers. These in-house teams also tendered for business with other health and care providers and a complex picture of provision emerged. Occasionally, a department chose to buy the hardware from the employer, take over contracts of employment for the staff and become independent traders. This was known as a Management Buy Out This has been made more feasible by the creation of Social Enterprise Organisations (GOV.UK,2013)

As management of the service was devolved to NHS Trusts, which are a group of hospitals at most, it became uneconomic for them to employ technical experts such as Engineers and Lawyers. Consequently, these services, also, are commonly acquired by retainer contract with private sector engineering and law firms. The same model has been used to employ management consultants to help NHS Trusts to achieve a wide range of short-term projects. Therefore, a NHS Trust has come to employ three categories of employee. These are:

1) A core of directly employed clinical and managerial staff that is of high calibre and have a high level of commitment to the organisation.
2) A large number of non-professional staff who are employed indirectly through contracts with other organisations at market controlled costs.
3) A small number of highly technical individuals contracted to supply specialised services.

Managing supply and demand

Many of the NHS professions experienced long term staff shortages standing at ten percent and more. This periodically becomes worse during demographic downturn periods. There could be periods when the output of young adults from schools and universities cannot satisfy industry's needs. The result is a miss-match between supply and demand. Traditionally, this shortage has been met by recruitment that is more aggressive, leading to leapfrogging among salaries and inflation, but not resolving the difficulty. Seeing the problem as a two-sided mismatch where demand exceeds supply and then addressing both sides of the equation leads to some more creative solutions (Bratton& Gold, 2012).

Demand > Supply

The mismatch is corrected by increasing supply and/or decreasing demand. Each of these may be addressed tactically (Short term measures) or strategically (Long term measures).

Short term measures for reducing demand for permanent staff include: relying on bank/agency staff, increasing overtime working, reducing quality and reducing output.

Short term measures for increasing supply of staff include: intensifying recruitment, increasing salaries, relaxing recruitment standards (Bratton& Gold, 2012).

Long term measures for reducing demand for staff include: re-deploying staff, altering skill mix issues, increasing mechanisation, improving training improving staff efficiency, improving employee retention, harnessing the power of users and carers.

Long term measures for increasing supply of staff include: removing inappropriate discrimination and stereotyping, improving local status as an employer, building relationships with universities, schools and other educators, optimising employment packages (Bratton& Gold, 2012).

It can be seen that the long term measures will resolve the problem and also improve the performance of the organisation while the short term measure will resolve the problem but detract from organisational performance. Short-termism may be necessary to overcome acute difficulties, but for the overall health of the organisation it is the long-term strategies that are required. A dependence on short-term responses, sustained over an extended period will result in deterioration to the point where continuing viability may not be possible. Ideally, as in all planning, short term responses to difficulties will be chosen that are compatible with the long-term strategic intentions.

Periodically, as a transient effect of recession, resources for health and social care are constrained, services are diminished and supply and demand of healthcare staff moves away from its long term pattern.

The Human Resource (Personnel) Department

Most NHS Trusts employ professional people in the field of Human Resources (HR), who perform three distinct functions:

The largest part of a HR service is working with managers to ensure that recruitment, supervision training and employment termination is conducted by line managers to the organisation's greatest advantage.

Many HR departments also act as Organisation Development (OD) facilitators. In this, they are supporting the management of change and seeking to achieve a highly skilled, efficient and well-motivated workforce as part of a healthy organisation

The final and often smallest part of a HR service is attention to the welfare of the employees. This is important to an employer, as a route to gaining maximum performance and minimising casual absenteeism. Additionally, a reputation for care and attention to employee welfare can make a significant, and cost-effective contribution to recruitment and retention of staff. (Torrington, Hall, Taylor & Atkinson 2014)

The Employment Lifecycle

Employment requires: workforce planning, recruitment and selection, choosing and applying a form of contract, initial and continuous staff development, continuing appraisal and termination.

Recruitment & Selection

Attracting and employing the right combination of staff is one of the most important functions of a manager and the area where the most expensive mistakes are to be made. In appointing an individual, a junior manager may be committing a NHS Trust to spend between £10,000 and £1M. Few other expenditures of this magnitude are devolved to junior managers without complex caveats and fail-safe mechanisms. It is essential to perform this task well. It is necessary to be explicit about the responsibilities of the post, the consequent candidate qualities required and the means by which these qualities will be evaluated. A clear statement is required of the standard to be accepted, in order to be assured that the best candidate is also a satisfactory candidate. 'The best of a bad bunch' will make an unsatisfactory appointment. The requirements must be assessed objectively and an appointment only made when successful performance can be assured. Once a number of candidates have been demonstrated to be each of them satisfactory, then the best of this group should be appointed without consideration of race, gender, age or other irrelevant qualities. In an environment of uneven skill supply, objectivity is particularly important in order to counter pressure to make an appointment at all costs.

It is not, however, expected that a newly appointed post holder will commence a position able to perform all aspects of the job to the level ultimately required. In the case of promotion or transfer to a new field, a period of induction and development is anticipated. In this case, the task of the selection panel is to choose the candidate who has the aptitude for the task and learning skills necessary to come up to speed in the time available. A choice often exists between a candidate who already has the desired skills, but demonstrates limited inclination to develop, and a candidate who would need to learn new skills in order to perform, but shows aptitude for the position and enthusiasm to learn. The decision in this case may depend on the time available to the service before full performance is required. If time can be allowed for extensive induction, then the candidate with aptitude is preferable. However, if immediate performance were essential, then a different decision would be made. This highlights the benefit of succession planning in order to avoid the need for hasty appointments or choice of a capable employee over an employee with potential. It may be that a newly appointed executive will spend up to two years growing to peak performance in the position, three years performing at peak, and up to two more years satisfactorily coasting before he/she should seek new challenges. This period may be extended if dramatic in-post changes cause an employee to be addressing entirely new challenges within an existing position.

The pressure to appoint in health care is great, since during periods of staff vacancy patients and clients will go untreated. Cover of a vacant post by colleagues is possible only for short periods. If long-term colleague cover is practical, then what was that person doing during periods of full staffing? However, to be rushed into a doubtful appointment because of a patient waiting list is to risk a mistake that could take many months to correct. Leaving work undone because of difficulty in recruiting is not good management either, and may jeopardise a contract or the quality of services. If a position proves difficult to fill, then it is good practice to appoint a support worker or member of another, more plentiful, profession on a fixed term contract who can give best-next treatment for a limited period during which time a more careful recruitment exercise can be conducted. (Torrington, Hall, Taylor, & Atkinson 2014)

Types of HR Contract

Where direct employment remains the favoured option e.g. with clinicians and service managers, a number of options are available.

Many staff members have *substantive contracts (*permanent) that confer the possibility of employment for life, subject to acceptable performance.

Alternatively, as with the General Management scheme, staff may be awarded *rolling three-year contracts*, with the option of extension at the end of each year. Thus, managers always have two or three years of a contract to run. However, this distinction has proven to have limited impact. Where performance is satisfactory, contracts can be expected to be renewed indefinitely, and not to do so would constitute dismissal, which is potentially subject to the same protection as substantive contracts Where performance is unsatisfactory, individuals are required to leave at very short notice, with due compensation and the two/three years remaining in their contract becomes irrelevant. This type of contract has been explored for the employment of some clinician staff, but the belief that it gives the employee no tenure is not proven. Many Trusts have ceased to use this contract even for General Managers.

A truly *fixed term contract* may be used when tasks required will discontinue at the end of the contract period. This device is commonly used for finite development projects, and a cadre of worker has emerged who chain these fixed term positions in order to build a varied career and rich profile. However, it is common practice for staff to achieve career security by seeking the next job before the current contract ends. This often results in staff leaving before the task is satisfactorily completed.

Some attempts have been made to employ clinicians on short-term contracts in order to retain staffing flexibility. However, these schemes remain rare because they are difficult to recruit to and, unless the job can be demonstrated to have truly ended, then failure to extend this fixed term contract constitutes dismissal and the employee may yet be protected under employment law and nothing has been gained. The expiry of a fixed-term contract without renewal amounts to a dismissal in law. (ACAS,2014)

Equal Opportunities

In all industries, you must endeavour to recruit a workforce that reflects the population. This is captured in the NHS Constitution showing rights for patients and staff.

This imperative is enshrined in the following legislation:

Disabled Persons (Employment) Acts (1944 & 1958)

This Act requires large employers (more than twenty employees) to employ a minimum of 3% of their workforce from people registered as disabled. They are also required to designate some posts as exclusively for people with disabilities and record their efforts in this direction. The legislation is difficult to enforce, but gives a guide to good practice that is appropriate to follow.

The Disability Discrimination Act (1995)

The Disability Discrimination Act (DDA) 1995 aims to end the discrimination that continued to face many people with disabilities. This Act has been significantly extended to give people with disabilities rights in the areas of: employment, education, access to goods, facilities and services, buying or renting land or property and functions of public bodies such as issuing of licences

The Equality Act (2010)

It's against the law for employers to discriminate because of a disability. The Equality Act 2010 protects covers areas including: application forms, interview arrangements, aptitude or proficiency tests, job offers, terms of employment, including pay, promotion, transfer and training opportunities, dismissal or redundancy, discipline and grievances.

An employer has to make 'reasonable adjustments' to avoid candidates being put at a disadvantage compared to non-disabled people in the workplace. For example, adjusting working hours or providing a special piece of equipment to help you do the job.

The word 'reasonable' can be problematic, in this context, but many employers seek to obey the spirit of the legislation and a growing body of case law serves to clarify what can be expected.

Rehabilitation of Offenders Act (1974)

This legislation allows offenders to deem their offence "spent" and therefore not declare it when seeking employment. However, this legislation has no impact on the Health and Care industries as they are, generally, exempt and may require full disclosure from all candidates. For details see, "The Home Office Guide to the Rehabilitation of Offenders Act" (HMSO 1974

For some positions, such as those involving access to children and other vulnerable clients, employers are required to obtain hard copies of Police records for candidates before appointment. As there is no authority for these to be obtained in other situations, much relies on the candidate's honesty. As police records become more available to the people to whom they apply, employers are beginning to require that a transcript be obtained and presented by the candidate as a part of the application process.

Sex Discrimination Act (1984)

This law makes it illegal for employers to discriminate between candidates on the grounds of gender, sexual orientation or marital status. Direct discrimination has become very rare and is quickly challenged. However, indirect discrimination remains common in that rules are written which unintentionally disadvantage one group. Employers have a duty to recognise the implications of their actions in this regard and make correction in order to give the organisation greatest recruitment advantage as well as to meet statutory requirements.

Positive discrimination, favouring one underrepresented gender or group is illegal under the act, but positive action to remove barriers is legal and desirable. The law occasionally allows some posts to be for one gender only where there is clear evidence that the other gender would be unable to perform the duties involved.

Race Relations Act (1976)

The law makes it illegal for employers to discriminate between candidates on the grounds of race, colour, nationality or ethnic background. As with sex discrimination direct discrimination has become very rare and is quickly challenged. However, also as with sex discrimination, indirect discrimination remains common in that rules are written which unintentionally disadvantage individual groups. Employers have a duty to recognise the implications of their actions in this regard and make correction in order to give the organisation greatest recruitment advantage and to meet statutory requirements.

Positive discrimination, favouring members of an ethnic minority group is illegal under the act, but positive action to remove barriers is legal and desirable. The law allows some posts to be for one group where there is evidence that another group would be unable to perform the duties involved. Religion is not protected by this legislation, except where a religion such as Judaism may also be deemed a race.

This legislation was developed by the **Race Relations (Amendment) Act in 2000**, but this has no great impact on NHS and Social Services employment.

Workforce Planning (Manpower Planning)

In a rapidly changing health service, there is rarely an occasion when a vacant post can be filled without consideration of alternative possibilities. This exercise of deciding the ideal team constitution should not simply be performed when a vacancy arises. The service manager should at all times know the ideal make up of his/her department, and be looking for opportunities to move towards this position. In this way, the manager is proactively planning the service, rather than simply reacting to vacancies as they arise. (Torrington, Hall, Taylor, Atkinson 2014)

Workforce planning is a term given to the projection of staffing needs over a number of years in order to identify the extent to which training of new professional staff must be commissioned. Managers are asked to project their employee needs up to an identified point in the future. This information, when aggregated, tells how many of each profession will be needed at that future time. Taking into account the known rates for wastage from each profession, it would be possible to know how many new members of each profession should be trained each year. The NHS is unusual in that it carries out this exercise internally and pays for the training of its own workforce. Most other professions, lawyers, accountants, teachers, etc, have their workforce trained at the expense of Local Education Authorities (LEAs), and the market forces of supply and demand ensure that broadly the right number of people elect to be trained. However, market forces lead to short term periods of famine and of plenty, and it is only when seen over a period of years that a balance is achieved by these mechanisms. Recognising the great investment made in health care professional training and the importance of steady availability, the NHS seeks to control work force education. However, this exercise is imperfect for two reasons:

Lead-time

Allowing that the shortest training time for health professionals is usually three years and that Universities need at least a year to change recruitment numbers, the minimum lead time needed to make changes to supply is four years and projecting workforce needs forward for at least four years is inherently difficult. The changing NHS environment periodically calls for an increase or decrease in new recruits to a particular staff group. However, considering the lead times involved it may take four or five years before a response can be achieved (Weightman, 2004) and in the case of medicine, ten years.

Wastage rates

Work force planning requires predictable rates of wastage from a profession. The service must train, for example, enough new nurses to replace all of those who are expected to cease to practice and also to satisfy the need for a growing service. The number of nurses leaving the profession will, however, vary according to external and internal conditions, many of which are out of the control of the service. In conditions of economic growth, nurses and therapists leave the NHS to take work in other industries, or take career breaks supported by successful life partners. In times of recession, however, these opportunities are fewer, and wastage is less (Bratton& Gold 2012)

If the actual wastage coefficient is different from that assumed in calculating the future need for new staff, then the output from the Universities will be either too few to meet need or too many so that some people will have been trained at great expense and not employed. The DoH managed this exercise for some professions, and

District Health Authorities (DHAs) for others, until the NHS and Community Care Act (1990). The act passed responsibility for making work force plans and commissioning training to consortia of the NHS Trusts and DHAs who are to be the main employers.

This manpower planning exercise may be measured by its results. For the larger professions, such as nursing, the supply has been close to demand, although generally slightly low, but for smaller groups such as physiotherapy and occupational therapy, there has been frequent shortfall of supply amounting to fifteen to twenty percent for many years but with volatile swings such that in the 3rd millennium there have been periods of oversupply.

Skill mix analysis

To ensure that the most efficient and effective service is provided with the resource available, a service should routinely assess the tasks that are to be performed, the type of operative needed to perform these tasks and, by aggregating this material, the number and type of individuals needed (Bratton& Gold 2012) Clearly, not all of the tasks that could be done should be done. An exercise of prioritisation is required. This is the same as the exercise described under "Time Management". The task of the manager is to make prioritisation decisions for all of the resources available to the department. This will include the uncomfortable duty of deciding to leave some tasks undone, because they do not deliver adequate value to the organisation and the patient to justify the cost. This method of identifying ideal staffing by task analysis can appear reductionist, missing some of the more complex behaviours of individuals. The work of a department may be more than the aggregate of the tasks identifiable. It is necessary, therefore, to check the validity of a task based department plan, by asking whether the derived "Necessary team" feels right to the members of the current team. If the answer is "No", then it is necessary to ask whether the concern arises from tribalism a protectionist approach to one's own profession, or whether something needs to be added in order for the model to be comprehensive in its consideration of the responsibilities of the service. The ability of experienced performers to intuitively know when an answer is correct is a valuable tool. However, this should only be used as a way of checking validity of some findings, and not as a reason to abandon the scientific approach to workforce planning.

a) Skill mix analysis will result in changes, not just of skill mix within professions, but also between professions. Progress from uni-professional to multi-professional management resulting from the Griffiths Report (1980) and the NHS & Community Care Act (1990) have made it progressively easier to effect inter-professional skill mix changes. This skill mix analysis will replace a member of staff from one profession with one from another or with one of a different grade. However, although most managers routinely review intra-professional skill mix far fewer routinely review inter-professional skill mix. The emergence of generic employees at assistant grades in clinical settings has been a clear result of this change, but this occurs only in small numbers reflecting this reluctance to move resources between professions.

Staff development

Employees, once in post, need to be enabled to perform at their most effective and effective level. This entails a sequence of management actions (Brent, & Dent, 2013).

Induction

On starting in a new position, an individual needs to be orientated to the organisation and made aware of policies and practices (Weightman, 2004). This is achieved through an induction programme. The induction should be phased in order to give information and insights at the time they are required and at a rate that they can be usefully internalised. Knowledge of safety procedures cannot be left until the second month, while being told the names of forty colleagues on day one is unhelpful. A comprehensive program should exist at each supervisory level. This may be adapted to suit the situation at each appointment. If a new program is devised for each appointee then a number of failings are likely to occur:

1. The program is at risk of missing a key item, because it did not occur to the manager.
2. Inconsistency renders the employer open to a charge of negligence towards an employer if he/she was not given information that was given to another employee. This would be particularly important in the incidence of industrial injury. It is difficult to define what must be told when, and such cases are difficult to prosecute. However, it is easy to demonstrate that an employer has not performed to its own standards as defined by behaviour towards another employee. To tell one employee and not another would be very difficult to defend.
3. It is time-consuming and inefficient to repeatedly "Re-invent the induction Wheel".
4. The unnecessary time demand may result in procrastination over this important task.

Objective Setting & the Personal Development Plan (PDP)

As performance begins, a process of Individual Performance Review (IPR) should be initiated. This will set out the objectives to be achieved by the appointee, in doing his/her job during the period selected. It will also look at the skills needed to achieve these objectives. Any shortfall in skills will become the basis of a Personal Development Plan (PDP). Agreed employee aspirations regarding future objectives or promotional opportunities will also be reflected in the PDP (Druker, 1973), (Griffiths,1994), (Bratton& Gold 2012).

b) The PDP will show the agreed learning for the individual and identify the means by which this learning will be achieved. Routes to learning will include attendance at courses, but of equal importance will be mentoring and coaching, job swaps project work visits to other workplaces, shadowing etc. If qualification is felt to be essential, a University Accreditation Procedure for Experiential Learning (APEL) scheme might register this learning exercise. This would give academic credit for learning that has both free-standing value and currency towards undergraduate/postgraduate qualification. Most Universities will have an APEL mechanism, often accessible through an independent study module at undergraduate or post graduate level, although in many cases there will be a charge for the service. PDPs may be based upon a Profile that describes the balance of abilities in an individual and a Portfolio that contains the evidence to substantiate that profile

Individual Performance Reviews (IPR)

In the first IPR meeting, objectives will be set for performance and learning When the employee returns for a second IPR interview, typically after six or twelve months, it is possible to appraise the extent to which they have achieved the objectives that were set. This enables the interviewee to gauge the value of his/her work and to explore routes to enhance his/her contribution. Following this appraisal, there will be another round of objective setting and a review of the PDP. If the employee is subject to a Performance Related Pay (PRP) agreement, then this interview will set the value of the bonus to be awarded.

Goal Alignment

The objectives set constitute an agreement between the individual and the manager about the contribution that he/she is to make to the organisation. It is the responsibility of the manager to ensure that the objectives of all of the individual employees aggregate to the objectives of the department (Brent & Dent, 2013). If the objectives of the individual are well aligned with those of the organisation, these collectively will meet the organisation's needs and there will be no conflict between the individual's personal aspirations and those of the organisation. Therefore, there is an important task for the IPR interviewer, generally the manager, to ensure that the organisation's objectives for the individual are compatible with his/her objectives for job satisfaction and advancement. If this is achieved, then the individual is intrinsically motivated to perform the duties required of him/her. This will minimise conflict and maximise productivity

Industrial relations

For an organisation to negotiate individually with many hundreds of employees is impractical. Therefore, employers frequently encourage the involvement of Trades Unions (TU). A responsible TU seeks to maximise the benefits of employment for members but, although distribution of benefit may be contentious, TUs recognise that a healthy organisation is better placed to benefit employees. There is much common interest between employers and employee representative organisations. The TU is likely to come into conflict with managers over the treatment of individual employees, but again it is in the interest of an organisation that procedures are rigorously applied and TU attention helps to supervise this process. For these reasons trades unions are well recognised throughout the NHS and Social Services Departments TU representation has traditionally been through Whitley Council groupings in which the membership of each committee is understood and remains constant across the country. This makes management of industrial relations simpler and has ensured consistency of pay and conditions, thereby preventing the salary 'leap frog' and consequent cost escalation.

Salaries and broad conditions were initially agreed nationally by Whitley Council groups and the Department of Health, informed by independent pay review bodies. This continued until 2004. Local Whitley Council committees agreed local conditions (not pay) with local managers. With the amalgamation of many specialised TUs, the constitution of Whitley Councils locally and nationally become less complex.

from 2000, NHS Trusts had the right to depart from Whitley rates in order to reflect local conditions, but almost never exploited the opportunity, seeing it as an unnecessary 'can-of-worms to open. Following 'The Agenda for Change effective in 2004 all professional pay grades were condensed onto 9 bands, which in 2014 allowed for salaries ranging from £14K to £98K.

To obtain statutory rights, a registered TU must be demonstrably independent of the employer, and formally recognised by the employer. Responsible employers such as NHS Trusts and LAs are generally open to recognising TUs for the reasons described above. However, where an organisation refuses to recognise an independent TU, legislation allows for a ballot, to be held and if 50% of the workforce vote in favour of recognition, then recognition is mandatory. A recognised TU has the right of consultation, representation, with reasonable time off, protection for stewards and the appointment of Health & Safety Officers in each workplace.

Absenteeism and staff availability

Departments need to accurately estimate the time that employees will commit to their work in order to accurately plan the size and makeup of the workforce (Bratton& Gold 2012)

Departments can appear to operate on the assumption that employees work fifty-two, five-day weeks in every year. Managers can appear not to know that employees take holidays, become ill, undergo training and bear children. Notices advising patients that services have been curtailed due to routine and predictable staff absence might well be taken to indicate incompetent management. Taking emergency action in response to predictable events, such as maternal confinement, is unsatisfactory. Therefore a department plan, showing the work to be performed and the team that will perform it must be based upon the person-days realistically available to the manager, and this should reflect the certainty of many types of staff absence.

Case example

> Sign actually posted in hospital waiting room:
> **Clinic cancelled due to maternity leave**
> This being a hospital, it is surprising that nobody guessed...
> Predictable absences should be subject to advance planning, not emergency action.

Reflection of absenteeism will take two forms. The aggregate volume of work to be achieved must be based on a maximum of a forty-five week year, not fifty-two. Plans must exist to ensure that priority work is performed during periods of staff absence, rather than reactive action being taken with ad-hoc cover arrangements made.

Casual absenteeism in the form of un-certificated sickness leave and absence-without-leave are seen as a *performance indicator* to the quality of management and general morale of a service. This is an important area for monitoring and high levels of absenteeism point to departments in need of improved management attention (Bratton& Gold 2012)

Terminating contracts

Employees may leave an organisation by one of a number of routes. How the manager handles this separation is extremely important to the individual, those remaining and potential recruits (Bratton&Gold 2012).

Progressing to another position

The NHS and Social Services Departments operate a general principle that for employees to develop their abilities and increase their contribution to the service overall is desirable. Thus, individual employers will, normally, assist employees to develop new skills in order to move to another NHS Trust or a Social Services employer in a more senior position. The NHS Trust to which an employee moves will, normally, assist with the cost of relocation such as house sale and purchase expenses. However, this assistance is generally only available where there is evidence that the move is to the benefit of the service as a whole. The usual test of benefit is that the individual is moving for a promotion I.e. he/she is to contribute in the new position at a higher level than in the former position. Where an individual is moving from one employer to a very similar function in another then there is no net benefit to the NHS as a whole, and relocation expenses are not normally paid.

Career breaks

Many employees in the Health & Care industries will consider one or more career breaks. Most commonly, these will be relating to caring for children and other dependants. However, they may also be for further study, travel, sabbatical, etc. Career breaks including those for child rearing, should be considered for male as well as female employees.

It is not uncommon for individuals to plan a short career break, but never return to the employer or even the service. This loss rate can be reduced if the organisation offers a managed career break scheme. A scheme might involve continuous communication & social meetings technical updating, training opportunities, periodic episodes of employment and guaranteed re-employment. The cost of this scheme looks very good value when compared with training a replacement from scratch.

Dismissal

Employees who fail to perform the duties allotted to them, or who behave in an unacceptable manner, may be dismissed. The duty upon the employer is to manage this process by careful adherence to the recognised Disciplinary Procedure Where an individual is unable to perform as required, it is usual for the employer to support retraining explore alternative positions or to assist the employee to contact services capable of finding future opportunities.

Where unacceptable behaviour is concerned, there are clear procedures for warning the individual and where appropriate, helping them to correct their behaviour. These are described below, and must be observed scrupulously, if the disciplinary action is to succeed.

Redundancy & re-deployment

A post may become redundant where the work involved is no longer required. Individuals cannot become redundant, although they are affected if their post becomes redundant. Only where an individual's skill is in a redundant area, will employment become impossible without retraining. Redundancy in Health or Social Care is unusual. Members of professions and experienced managers are normally re-deployed within the organisation, if their post becomes redundant. Standard procedures exist whereby post-holders in redundant positions as a part of a re-organisation are considered for all emerging vacancies before formal recruitment may be commenced. This process normally accounts for redundant personnel. A duty to offer retraining is also attached to the re-deployment imperative. If re-deployment involves increased journey distances or re-housing, then it is normal for the employer to meet the costs involved.

There is a general rule in health care that there will be no voluntary redundancy. That is, the NHS will not pay redundancy expenses to an individual, who could be useful elsewhere, even if they elect to go. Only where there is no employment possibility is redundancy payment allowed. This, then, becomes compulsory redundancy. In the rare event that an individual cannot be deployed anywhere else in the organisation he/she will be compensated according to pre-negotiated rates. He/she should also be assisted with finding other employment if appropriate.

Retirement

When employees are approaching retirement in the NHS or Social Services, it is usual for the employer to offer assistance with planning for retired life. Planning will be in a number of areas:

The service will offer financial guidance to enable employees to maximise the value of their retirement funds.

Assistance may be offered with time management encouraging plans for use of increased leisure time. Experience shows that many people over-extend themselves in an attempt to keep busy. Health and social service personnel are frequently prized in their community. They may become 'targets' for local committees and other valuable works, and often report that they are busier after retirement than before, and have difficulty in reducing their workload. This reflects a number of factors, and retirement preparation aims to help staff plan a balanced workload that will result in their fulfilling their aspirations.

Staff will be advised about the rules and prospects regarding casual or sessional re-employment. Such employees are a valuable resource, because of their experience and the flexibility with which they may be deployed.

Early retirement is unusual in health care, unless it is on the grounds of ill health. However, some professional groups, such as Nurses who are designated Mental Health Officers are enabled to retire at a fixed earlier age, and the NHS Superannuation scheme alters its calculations of pension entitlement in order to allow this without disadvantage to the individual.

Accountability

Clinicians are separately accountable for their actions to four 'courts' (Andrews, 1995) (Andrews & Wheeler 1996). These are:

To the patient, to the profession, to the employer and to the country

Event	Incident	Incident	Incident	Incident
Action	Enquiry	Enquiry	Enquiry	Enquiry
Accountability	*accountable to patient*	*accountable to employer*	*accountable to regulator*	*accountable to society*
Offence	Damages	Breach of contract	Infamous Conduct	Criminal offence
Action	Civil claim	Disciplinary action	Conduct hearing	Criminal prosecution
Remedy	Compensation	Terminate employment	Removal from register	Criminal conviction

The Patient/client

Patients/clients may resort to civil law. They may look for compensation for damages caused by a clinician who fails to take reasonable care over treatment. If a clinician has not acted as a reasonable clinician would have, then he/she is negligent. If this negligence can be shown to have caused damage then the case is likely to succeed. The award of damages seeks not to punish the clinician, but to make the wrongdoer restore the injured party to the financial position he/she would have enjoyed if he/she had not been wronged. A successful suit requires:

a) **negligence** by act or omission, as seen by comparison to a reasonable clinician,

b) **loss**, by the injured party, in terms of financial loss or loss of well-being in the form of pain or distress

and

c) **causality** i.e. the loss can be shown to have been caused by the negligence

The client may sue the clinician directly, or the employer by invoking "Vicarious Liability" in which the organisation is said to be liable for the acts or omissions of those working on its behalf. It should always be remembered that although the employer pays for acts of negligence, the employee suffers the blight on his/her record, with consequent career limitation. It is also the case that the employer is not responsible for actions of employees while they are not working in the employer's behalf. Thus, if the error occurred because of a speech and language therapist exceeding his/her employment brief, then the suit may fall back on the employee. If a nurse gives careless advice to a friend in an informal setting, he/she is not working on behalf of any employer, and could be personally sued by the friend. It is sometimes mistakenly believed that issues of what is 'covered' are governed by a NHS Trust's insurance cover. In fact, NHS Trusts are not expected to rely on insurance as protection from legal action. Rather, they are required to guard against negligence through good quality management. Any successful negligence claim will effectively be paid out at the expense of future health service provision, either directly from NHS Trusts, or indirectly through the clinical negligence scheme for trusts (CNST) (York NHS Trust 2013)

The Employer

An employer dissatisfied with employee actions has recourse is to its Disciplinary Procedure This will be on the basis that the clinician is in breach of the employment contract Various levels of penalty exist including alteration of grading, alteration to location & supervision and ultimately dismissal.

Defence in these cases, in addition to understanding and observing the contractual obligations, as will be discussed later, is possible on the grounds of failure of the employer to comply with the requirements of that Disciplinary Procedure. Therefore it is of paramount importance for managers to know and follow the procedure carefully, keeping detailed records of each stage.

If a patient/client is not seeking compensation but wishes action to be taken against a clinician, they may ask the employer to take action under the clinician's accountability to the employer, utilising the complaints procedure.

The Profession

The professional supervisory organisation, The United Kingdom Central Council for Nursing (UKCC) or the Council for Professions Supplementary to Medicine (CPSM) for Professions Allied to Medicine (PAMs), etc, may call the clinician to account. The examination is of possible "Infamous Conduct" Generally the questions put, amount to "In view of what has happened, is the person a safe and suitable practitioner?" and "has he/she maintained professional standards?" There are a range of sanctions, but the ultimate penalty is removal of the individual's name from The State Register of Clinicians, and therefore prevention of the right to practice as a State-Registered clinician., Employment in the NHS, for example, would be effectively precluded to a clinician barred from state-registration. This removal may be permanent or for a limited period. If a matter causing concern to the client or the employer is of professional misconduct then they may refer the case to the CPSM for examination.

Society

The clinician as a citizen is accountable to society at large for actions and omissions. This is tested through criminal prosecution. It is rare, but not unheard of, for a clinician to be prosecuted under criminal law for clinical actions and a number of high profile cases have been in the press over recent years.

The prosecution must be in the public interest and will allege that the clinician has failed society. If it is found that the clinician has fallen short of what is required then criminal penalty will follow.

No personal insurance company, employer or professional body can indemnify the clinician against criminal prosecution or penalty. They may pay for legal representation, but cannot pay fines on conviction and, clearly, prison sentences will be served by the clinician in person and alone!

Repeated trials

An individual can be "punished" more than once for the same offence. In the case of the misbehaving health professional, this is often the case. This is reasonable when it is considered that each body is conducting its "trial" for a different offence, albeit arising from one incident. The employer dismisses the individual for breach of contract. Professional misconduct is considered separately and action taken. Neither of these events affects the patient's need for compensation and if a crime has occurred then it must be addressed by a criminal court. Beverly Allitt, was convicted of a crime, removed from the nursing register, and dismissed, all for different aspects of her misconduct and in different trials. None of these events address the right of victims and their families were able to seek compensation.

Dynamic Tensions

Sometimes, as with nurse Beverly Allitt, the views of all parties are in alignment and misconduct is agreed by all of the evaluating bodies. In other situations, the interests of the four parties do not so easily meet and there is a potential for conflict. Accountability can pull the clinician in several directions at once. It is the clinician's responsibility to resolve these contradictions. Conflict of demands does not excuse failure to meet a requirement and no one authority can indemnify the clinician against another. No "orders" from a doctor or manager, can excuse a breach of duty to any of the four groups to whom clinicians are accountable.

Accountability In Conclusion

Lawyers cannot stop people from exercising their right to call clinicians to account. Clinicians have a position of trust and authority in the community and they must work without fear or favour, in the best interests of the client, acting on behalf of the employer, striving to uphold professional standards and maintaining the trust which society has placed in them. If the clinician has acted professionally and recorded those actions accordingly, then they are not at risk. However, it is their personal responsibility to meet the high demands of patient/client, employer, profession and society, and whoever promises to stand by them, they will be alone when the complaint arises.

The Professions

The NHS employs a bewildering number of different professions. Members of each profession express regret about the limited and stereotyped understanding of their group by the wider service. However, this does not inspire them to learn about and adopt a sympathetic understanding of their colleagues. Each profession thinks it is unique in being poorly understood.

Case example

> *Interviewee*: As a S&LT *(Substitute any profession!)* I find it very frustrating that the other professions do not understand the breadth and depth of our practice. They only have a simplistic stereotype
> Interviewer: Do you feel you could explain the role of a chiropodist?
> Interviewee: Of course I can. They trim toe-nails

Below, is a description of the core role of each of the professions involved in the health and care industry, as defined by senior members of each of the professions.

Art Therapists

http://www.baat.org/

Art Therapists use all of the arts as a medium for analysis and treatment of health disorders. Most, but not all, of art therapy takes place in mental health and learning disability settings, where art therapists have an analytical as well as therapeutic role.

Art therapists are generally trained to degree level, over three or four years, and are required to maintain their name on a state register in order to practice.

Mental Health NHS Trusts and other institutions may employ an Artist in Residence, who engages patients/clients in artistic endeavour for general therapeutic benefit. The artist in residence may not be a registered Art Therapist, and in consequence, this function is separate from true Art Therapy.

Clinical Psychologists

www.bps.org.uk/

Clinical Psychologists are involved in the formal assessment, diagnosis and treatment of patients in a mental health or learning disability setting. Clinical psychologists are becoming progressively more commonly involved in physical medicine contributing to pain control etc. Clinical Psychologists are not supplementary to medicine and can, therefore, hold an independent case-load.

Clinical Psychologists are psychology graduates who have undergone specialist education to MSc or PhD level in the clinical application of Psychology.

Dieticians

https://www.bda.uk.com/

Dieticians are employed in Acute and Community settings. They prescribe diets that will contribute to the recovery of patients with illness, or will prevent deterioration, etc. They also recommend easy but adequate diets for individuals for whom cooking and/or eating is difficult. Dieticians play a significant part in health promotion and disease prevention through public education as part of Health Promotion services or Public Health departments.

Dieticians are educated in university to honours degree level.

General Managers

www.**ihm**.org.uk

Since the Griffiths Report (1983) The NHS has employed General Managers at all levels of the organisation. They have authority and accountability that cannot be diluted by notions of consensus management. General Managers are employed on renewable fixed term contracts, subject to annual IPR, and remunerated by a process of Performance Related Pay (PRP). There are no formal qualification requirements, although possession of Master's Degree in Business Administration (MBA) is becoming the norm. General managers may be drawn from any of the professions or have progressed through a succession of NHS administrative positions. Occasionally, general managers are appointed to the NHS after a career in management in other industries or the armed forces.

General Medical Practitioners

www.BMA.Org.uk

General Medical Practitioners (GPs) are the primary contact for patients with any health need, and the 'gatekeeper to secondary services. The GP and his/her primary health care team provide about 80% of NHS treatments. If specialist treatment is required in the opinion of the GP, then he/she will refer to a consultant in a secondary care service. Ordinarily, patients have no direct route to secondary services, with the exception of emergency treatment, through an Accident & Emergency Department

GPs play the pivotal role in Primary Care Groups (PCG) and Primary Care Trusts (PCT) which either advise Health Authorities in their commissioning role or take direct responsibility for commissioning or providing secondary services for the patients in their catchment.

GPs undergo normal medical education in Universities and as House Officer, followed by a vocational training scheme involving NHS Trust positions as Senior House Officer, and in designated GP Training Practices.

Medical Laboratory Scientific Officers (MLSO)

www.acb.org.uk

MLSOs are responsible for provision and technical management of scientific equipment in hospitals. They are also involved in the wealth of technically sensitive screening procedures that are conducted by hospitals. Qualification for MLSO is through professional examination.

Particular functions may call for Graduate, Master's or Doctoral level education.

Midwives

https://www.rcm.org.uk/

Midwives work in hospitals and the community, preparing parents for the delivery of a baby, managing the delivery and caring for the new family for the first six weeks of the baby's life.

Midwife training is generally over three years resulting in an Honours Degree and State Registration

Nurses

www.**rcn**.org.uk/

Nursing is a profession focusing on caring for people, individually or in groups, covering the whole life-span. They work with individuals to identify needs and plan together to address them. The viewpoint of individuals is fundamental to nursing in meeting needs. Nurses behave holistically, addressing physiological, psychological, spiritual, cultural and social needs, using scientific fact and empirical data.

Nurses are described as having two main functions.

They perform for people those tasks that illness or disability makes it impossible or dangerous for them to perform for themselves;

They administer a very wide of treatments prescribed by medical and other practitioners. Nurses are adopting a rapidly growing range of pharmaceutical and other treatments that they can prescribe and administer themselves.

Nurses are, usually, trained at University to Degree level, or through Project 2000 Diploma and Advanced Diploma courses over three or four years. Both routes allow State Registration with the United Kingdom Central Council for Nursing, Midwifery and Health Visiting and offer equal career prospects. All nurses are required to maintain their name on a state register in order to practice and maintain a portfolio of evidence which demonstrates Continuing Professional development (CPD).

Occupational Therapists

www.**cot**.co.uk/

Occupational therapy (OT) is concerned with the occupation of people. This is addressed in two ways:

1. The OT facilitates the individual performing all of the occupations to which he/she realistically aspires. This facilitation involves: teaching the individual new ways of performing where the old way is no longer possible, and altering the environment so that occupational performance is made possible. Environmental alteration may be as simple as supplying a handrail or as complex as building a new bathroom onto the home or workplace.
2. The OT uses activity as a therapeutic medium. I.e. he/she prescribes activities that will contribute to the patient/client recovering from illness or holding back the progress of incurable disease. In addition to prescribing activity for in or out patient application, the OT will prescribe ways of carrying out normal life activities that are intrinsically therapeutic and developmental.

OTs are trained to honours degree level, over three or four years, and are required to maintain their name on a state register in order to practice.

Pharmacists

www.rpharms.com/

Pharmacists are licensed to purchase, store and retail controlled and uncontrolled pharmaceutical materials. They therefore meet the need for supply of these materials. Pharmacists also act as a source of expertise about the effects, side effects and interaction of drugs and other agents. Clinicians and the public consult pharmacists about drug issues. Pharmacists may operate as small businesses or be employed by larger retail outlets. General Medical Practitioners employs pharmacists in rural settings to operate from surgeries or Health Centres. Pharmacists in hospital supply medicines for in patient use and to cover the period immediately after discharge. Hospital Pharmacists offer a sophisticated advice service to clinicians and may contribute to ward round and case conference discussions.

Pharmacists are trained to Degree level, over three or four years, and are required to maintain their name on a state register in order to operate.

Physicians

https://www.rcplondon.ac.uk/

Physicians are Registered Medical Practitioners who have chosen a non-surgical speciality, working in secondary or tertiary health care. Physicians may remain generalists (General Physician) or specialise in care groups such as The Elderly, Rheumatology, etc. Physicians in secondary health care usually only accept a patient when referred by a General Practitioner.

Physicians study medicine at University followed by a year in a NHS Trust as House Officer. They then seek employment in a NHS Trust as Senior House Officer, before joining a specialist training scheme as Registrar/Senior Registrar in posts approved by the Royal College of Physicians. When this period of training is satisfactorily completed and the relevant two stage examinations demonstrate attainment of specialist understanding they become eligible to apply for a substantive post as a Consultant Physician.

Physiotherapists

www.csp.org.uk/

Physiotherapists help people affected by injury, illness or disability through movement and exercise, manual therapy, education and advice.

They maintain health for people of all ages, helping patients to manage pain and prevent disease.

The profession helps to encourage development and facilitate recovery, enabling people to stay in work while helping them to remain independent for as long as possible.

Public Health Physicians

www.fph.org.uk/

Note: Public Health Services increasingly commonly employ public health nurses and non-medical specialists, in addition to physicians.

Public Health Physicians have a number of functions:
- to monitor health status & assess health needs and advise upon the appropriate health care to be provided. This includes the application of Evidence Based Medicine
- to monitor and control communicable diseases,
- to provide public health advice to the Health Authority, PCGs, PCTs LAs etc,

The Director of Public Health is required to publish an annual report of the health of the catchment population and the health care provided.

To play a leading part in clinical governance within the catchment.

Public Health Physicians study medicine at University followed by a year in a NHS Trust as House Officer. They then seek employment in a

NHS Trust as Senior House Officer, before joining a specialist training scheme as Registrar/Senior Registrar in posts approved by the Faculty of Public Health. When this period of training is satisfactorily completed and the relevant two stage examinations demonstrate attainment of specialist understanding they become eligible to apply for a substantive post as a Consultant Public Health Physician.

The Director of Public Health is a former Executive Director of a District Health Authority, now relates to the Local Authority, which is a reversion to the function of The Medical Officer of Health.

Podiatrists (formerly Chiropodists)

www.scpod.org/

Podiatrists formerly Chiropodists, offer advice and treatment regarding the health and function of lower limbs. The aim of the treatment is to maintain normal foot function and therefore mobility. The service is primarily to the elderly and people with disabilities, but there is an important health promotion role with children, focusing on the impact of lifestyle on foot health.

Assistants are taking a growing role in treatment of toenails etc, although this is closely supervised by a qualified Podiatrist.

Podiatrists train for three years, leading to an Honours Degree and State Registration (SRCh). Podiatrists may elect to undergo a further five-year training to gain the title Podiatric Surgeon and practice surgery on the foot.

Speech & Language Therapists

www.rcslt.org/

Speech and language therapists (SLT), assess and train/retrain communication skills. They are involved with children in schools and at home. SLTs work in Acute Learning Disability and Community NHS

Trusts assisting with treatment of patients whose illness impairs their communication, speech or feeding & swallowing function.

SLTs are trained to honours degree level, over three or four years, and are required to maintain their name on a state register in order to practice.

Social Workers

www.tcsw.org.uk/

Social Workers provide a problem solving service for disadvantaged people in the community. This may include ensuring that benefit income is claimed, but also can involve any other area of problem solving, such as housing, care services, education and employment opportunities etc. Social workers play a major part in the discharge of people from hospital and their aftercare and may act as Care Managers assessing and facilitating total care packages for people with disabilities living in the community and. In mental health setting the discharge plan is a formal requirement under the Care Planning Approach regulations

Many social workers undergo additional training to act as counsellors for people with mental health disorders. Approved Social Workers are agents for arranging compulsory admission of people under the Mental Health Act.

Social workers are normally trained in University to honours degree level or hold Certificate of Qualification in Social Work (CQSW). They are required to maintain their name on a state register in order to practice.

Surgeons

https://www.rcseng.ac.uk/

Surgeons are medical practitioners who employ surgery as their primary therapeutic medium.

Surgeons may remain generalists (General Surgeon) or specialise in an anatomical region.

Surgeons study medicine at University followed by a year in a NHS Trust as House Officer. They then seek employment in a NHS Trust as Senior House Officer, before joining a specialist training scheme as Registrar/Senior Registrar in posts approved by the Royal College of Surgeons. When this period of training is satisfactorily completed and the relevant two stage examinations demonstrate attainment of specialist understanding they become eligible to apply for a substantive post as a Consultant Surgeon. When a surgeon completes his or her RCS membership requirements, he or she may cease to use the prefix Dr. and be addressed as Mr. or Miss.

Tribalism

A clinician is a member of his/her profession and his/her NHS Trust, simultaneously and this can result in conflict if their demands do not match. Service politics (Handy 1980) politics in healthcare management might present as an attempt to increase the power of and resources allotted to the profession without consider that the same resources deployed elsewhere could have a greater patient benefit.

Successive attempts (DoH,1990) have been made to persuade members of professions to see the profession as their background, and the patient focused team in which they work as the area to which they give their loyalty and for which they campaign.

This places individuals in a position of dynamic tension. It is important for them to seek the progress of their profession, improving standards and taking part in Continuing Professional Development etc, but they are encouraged not to hide behind professional protectionist barriers.

Matrix Management

For most employees, this means existing in a matrix that shows them to be part of a professional and a patient focused group simultaneously, and allowing neither to operate to the detriment of the other.

	Surgery	Paeds	Elderly Care	Etc
Nursing				
Medical				
Physiotherapy			Elderly care PT	
Occupational therapy				
Speech & Language Therapy				
Dietetics				
Etc				

This shows a matrix management system the physiotherapists employed to work for the Elderly Care Directorate are encouraged to fulfil their duty to physiotherapy and Elderly Care equally in such a way as to ensure that loyalty to one will disadvantage the other.

Role Blurring

There has been a long-running debate about the extent to which professions should allow overlapping and role blurring (Sims, Hewitt&Harris,2014). This has been taken to the extreme where a single generic therapist is proposed whose members can provide all of the services currently associated with a wide range of professions. The emerging consensus is that a significant level of role blurring should be allowed in order to avoid clients being unnecessarily involved with a wide range of professionals, and to allow a clinician to deliver the care needed by an individual without unhelpful demarcation practice. However, there is very little support for the creation of one generic profession. Small rationalisations have occurred in the form of the merger of physiotherapy and remedial gymnastics and further discussions were held between physiotherapy and occupational therapy, although that proposal was not adopted.

The Practice

or how you might go about it

Recruitment & Selection

Confirming the post

Rarely can a vacant post be filled without revisiting the functions to be performed and therefore the person to be sought. This is explained in "Workforce Planning above. Therefore when you have a position vacated by a colleague or subordinate you should initiate a discussion about the best use for the released resource in line with existing strategy. Each vacancy is an opportunity to alter skill-mix to move closer to your strategic target make-up. This will involve discussing what profession and what grade of employee must be recruited. Skill mix may be between professions (*Interprofessional skill mix*) or within a profession (*Intraprofessional skill mix*). managers tend to find the latter far easier to contemplate than the former. A decision will generally be made by the immediate manager and ratified by a more senior manager authorised to appoint staff.

The Job Description

When you have confirmed the position, you must devise a Job Description This covers a number of areas, as described below.

The Job Description once published, becomes a part of the contract of employment. When an employee is in post, the job description may only be altered by agreement between manager and post holder. If an alteration is necessitated by a re-organisation and the post holder does not agree, then he/she is notionally redundant and the agreed re-deployment procedures are employed.

Job Description

Title of Post:

A succinct, but accurate representation of the core function(s) to be performed.

Job purpose:

A single paragraph that explains comprehensively, but in broad brush terms, the purpose of the post. *(This is frequently the most important and most difficult section to write.)*

Term:

Substantive Temporary/Fixed-Term/Fixed-term, rolling. (*See Types of contract above.*)

Location

Specifies the permanent base for the appointee

Accountable to:

The name of the post, *(not the post holder)* to whom the appointee will report. In the case of health and care professionals, this may be divided into:

> Professional accountability
> To a senior member of the profession, and

> Managerial accountability
> To a General Manager in charge of the clinical area in which the appointee will practice.

Relationships:

This section will explain the other posts to which the appointee will relate.

Duties:

This will be a detailed, numbered list of the duties to be performed, covering the whole job and aggregating to the Job Purpose above. The duty list should be restricted to about ten items.

A catchall clause is generally included of the type, "Any other duties that the manager may require". It is an error, however to believe that this clause allows managers to add responsibilities at will. In fact, the clause is generally limited to duties that fit within the job purpose and are broadly in line with the list of specific duties.

The Person Specification

When the Job Description is agreed, then you can define the skills, knowledge and aptitudes required of a person performing the duties involved. This is usually described in terms of *essential* qualities and *desirable* qualities. It is not possible to appoint candidates who do not meet the essential qualities. Any candidate failing to demonstrate these should be rejected before the shortlisting stage. The desirable qualities may be used to differentiate between satisfactory candidates.

Qualities are usually described under five headings. Examples are given for illustration (Churchouse & Churchouse, 1998).

Person Specification

Post Title:	Moving and Handling	Trainer
	Essential Qualities	**Desirable Qualities**
Physical	Able to move & handle patients	Highly Presentable
Attainment	SRN, SROT or SRPT Knowledge of H&SAW Legislation Knowledge of ergonomics	Experience of teaching Teaching qualification
Intelligence	Registered health professional Able to adapt to new culture	M level qualification
Aptitude	Attention to detail	Interpretation of legislation
Interests	Health & Safety	Quality Assurance
Disposition	Able to relate well to all categories of employees	Excellent communicator
Circumstances	Able to work day, night and week-end shifts	Able to attend international conferences

Advertising

You must advertise the post, in order to attract a wide range of candidates, thereby assuring the best available calibre of appointee. It may be possible to attract a satisfactory response through internal notification and word of mouth, but this is rarely considered acceptable, because it may not ensure equal opportunities to all members of the community.

Regulations to be considered are routinely published by the Equal Opportunity Commission (EOC) and the Commission for racial Equality (CRE).

ACAS (2010) and CIPM (2014)a publish guidance that includes the need for:
1) The Person Specification as the basis for the Advertisement;
2) A realistic description of the organisation;
3) Job location and salary or salary scale;
4) Clear instructions for application;
5) No discrimination on the grounds of age, gender, disability or race, unless within the exemptions in the prevailing legislation.

Your advertisement must attract and also inform. This maximises the recruitment trawl and yet ensures that the candidate list is appropriate by allowing individuals to screen themselves out if they do not meet the essential requirements of the post.

Advertisements must be appropriate to the medium. Therefore in a scientific journal, the language will be different from a daily newspaper. People do not read journals or newspapers as they do a novel. Rather, they skip read and browse. Most readers read the headlines. If they are interested by the headline, they read the first paragraph. This may satisfy the need, or they may decide to read to the end. This also applies to advertisements and is demonstrated below culminating in the advertisement.

Your headline must tell the reader if this is for them; self-screening.

Advertisement

Manual Handling Instructor - Manchester.

This tells the candidate whether he/she needs to read the advertisement further.

A State registered Nurse, Physiotherapist or Occupational Therapist is sought to teach staff of all grades and professions in this busy NHS Trust.

This further information allows he candidate continue assessing his/her suitability for the position. For those still in the running the next section tell the essential and desirable qualities in some detail.

Applicants should have good knowledge of H&SAW Legislation and ergonomics assessment procedures. They should have a keen eye for detail and be available to teach night and weekend staff. A Master's degree and ability to interpret policy & legislation would be an advantage.

A penultimate section should describe (honestly!) the attractions of the employer and locality.

Manchester is a thriving and vibrant city convenient for a variety of attractions, and The Manchester State General NHS Trust is ....

The final section should advise the readership, which has now been reduced to serious candidates only, how to apply.

Application forms are available from the HR Department tel: (*****) *********.

For an informal visit tel: (*****) *******

> **Manual Handling Instructor - Manchester.**
>
> A State registered Nurse, Physiotherapist or Occupational Therapist is sought to teach staff of all grades and professions in a busy NHS Trust.
>
> Applicants should have good knowledge of H&SAW Legislation and ergonomics assessment procedures. They should have a keen eye for detail and be available to teach night and weekend staff. A Master's degree and ability to interpret policy & legislation would be an advantage.
>
> Manchester is a thriving and vibrant city convenient for a variety of attractions, and The Manchester State General NHS Trust is ….
>
> Application forms are available from the HR Department tel: (*****) *********.
>
> For an informal visit tel: (*****) *******
>
> LOGO

Short listing

The applicant list is screened against the Person Specification Candidates who can be shown to fall short of the essential qualities are rejected at this stage. If this still leaves a large applicant list, beyond the preferred six, then further rejection is possible based on the desirable qualities.

Psychometric testing

Some qualities may not be assessable by reference to paper submission. For these, you may find it helpful to employ psychometric testing. Psychometric tests assess abilities and aptitudes. They predict performance, because they have been standardised upon large populations about whom much information is known (CIPD, 2003).

A standardised test result may be reported with reference to people who are known to be successful in the chosen career. They tests are able to comment on how well the profile of an candidate matches that of individuals known to be successful in posts similar to the one to be filled. They are, also, able to indicate where a person lies in relation to the general population in terms of reasoning and problem solving skills leadership etc. This is valuable if the person specification indicates need for a particular ability, such as verbal reasoning.

Specialists in Occupational Psychology or HR Management usually administer psychometric tests. The interpretation of this data is sensitive, and it is generally held that scores provide objective information to be considered alongside other information obtained from CV and interview observation.

Equal Opportunities

In all industries, you must recruit a workforce that reflects the population. This will ensure that you have the best possible pool to select from and thereby you will obtain the best possible workforce. Additionally, if your workforce reflects the local population, then you will have a resource able to explain to one another the special requirements of each segment of the catchment population. This imperative is reinforced by the wealth of legislation listed and explained above.

Interviewing

The purpose of your interview is to assess the candidates against the essential and desirable qualities that you have pre-selected and published in your person specification. (ACAS,2010) (CIPD 2014). The interview, particularly, looks at those qualities that cannot be assessed from a paper application.

Where an interviewer is unsure what he/she is looking for, because he/she is not working from a clear person specification, the interview is likely to be unsuccessful in choosing the best candidate. Furthermore, any appointment made will be very difficult to defend if an unsuccessful candidate makes an appeal, as the interviewer has no strong grounds to support the decision. Those who say *"I'll know it when I see it"* are usually wrong and likely to make faulty appointments drawn in by the 'Halo-effect' from one good quality.

Interviews may be by an individual selector, by panel or by sequential individuals (candidate moves from one interviewer to another until all 'panel' members have assessed him/her).

The interview environment

Attention to the room layout is important. 180^0 face to face seating makes the experience very formal and emphasises interviewer control. This effect can be enhanced if the interviewer(s) place a table or desk between them and the candidate. 90^0 seating, without a table and in informal seats will have the reverse effect. There is no one correct layout for a room. You must make the decision according to the extent to which you want control or affiliation with the candidates. However, you should ensure consistency of approach to all candidates. This may require you to make a special effort where the interviews are to run over a number of days. Distractions are to be minimised unless they have a value in testing a candidate. Comfort of candidates needs to reflect their individual circumstances and rights under race, religion, disability age and gender legislation.

The Questions

Your interview questions need to be primarily open in nature, aiming to achieve a balance where your interviewee speaks for about 80% of the time.

The first question is normally predictable and serves the purpose of establishing rapport between interviewee and interviewer. You might ask a question about the interviewee's journey or comfort for this purpose. This also enables the interviewee to speak on an unchallenging topic and thereby release tension. (ACAS,2010) (CIPD 2014).

Your subsequent questions are then asked. These may be very varied in presentation, but essentially, there are only three possible motives for your questions. These are:

1) to ascertain the extent to which the interviewee matches the Person Specification
2) to establish the interviewee's motivation towards to position;
3) to establish that the interviewee understands the post, the employer and the implications of the move well enough to be making an informed choice.

You will examine these areas through a series of questions. Answers are sought in order to assess the match of the individual with the person specification

Your interview might take the form:

Welcome & Introductions
Rapport question
Biographical details,
Questions about the candidate's Education,
Motivation for application for the post,
Career to date, focusing on achievements,
Candidates' opinion about his/her match with person specifications with reference to personal profile and portfolio evidence, aspirations for the future,
Outside interests
It is normal to allow the interviewee to ask questions of the panel during an interview, and these are often seen as indicators of insight and interest on the part of the interviewee.

Alternatives to interviews

There have been many studies of interviews and their effectiveness in personnel selection and they are consistently found wanting (Lasco, 2013) (Dana, Dawes & Peterson 2013) (Zee,K Bakker & Bakker 2002). Alternatives exist which may be considered, including:

- work simulation commonly exampled as typing tests for administrative appointments;
- group problem-solving activities and role-plays: used to observe candidates' performance in tasks similar to those to be performed by the successful candidate when in post;
- assessment centres where a profile of strengths, weaknesses and aptitudes is established over a period of days;
- presentations often used in conjunction with interviews to involve a wider constituency;
- predictive psychometric assessment described above.

References

References are traditionally sought as part of a selection process. You may consider references at the screening (short-listing) stage, the interview stage or only for candidates to be offered the position. References are unreliable because the referee may be ill informed about the candidate, or may be biased in his/her commenting. At the worst, a reference may be the reverse of the truth because the referee as an employer does not want to lose a good employee or does want to lose an incompetent worker.

The reference is, however, a means of checking the truthfulness of information about job history, given by the candidate, and may be used to reinforce detailed impressions gained from interview and application form. References are usually take up after short-listing, but may occasionally be taken up only for candidates to be appointed, in order to verify the accuracy of information given by the candidate.

Appointing

Each organisation has a list of official appointing officers. Appointments must bear the signature of one of these. Following an appointment a member of staff is statutorily entitled to a written contract that sets out all of the conditions of the employment (ACAS,2010). The contract is binding upon the employer, but has limited control over the behaviour of the employee. Should he/she for example leave without notice, then there is very little sanction that can be applied. The contract sent to an employee will normally have a copy to be signed and returned. This is good practice, because it encourages the employee to read and own his/her contract. However, the signature, given or not given, has no great legal status. The employee is deemed to have accepted the contract by attending for work, and therefore the normal employment conditions apply regardless of his/her written response. You must send the contract with full terms and conditions in order to be able to demonstrate that the employee had the opportunity to learn his/her conditions of employment and can therefore be held to account for compliance.

Offers

Employment offers are made verbally and/or in writing. Both are legally binding upon the employer. If you make an employment offer at interview, or by telephone thereafter, your organisation is bound to honour it, whether or not you have followed it up in writing. For this reason, it is important that you make explicit any conditions to the offers you make, such as 'subject to health assessment'. You cannot add conditions at the letter stage. It is important to be aware that any undertaking you make or receive at interview, such as "You will support the appointees' need for training will also constitute a part of a contract

It is important to use terms such as 'normally' or "We would explore the possibility" at interview if you are not certain about your ability to follow through for the candidate who is appointed.

Probation

It may be possible for you to continue the selection process in the early months of an appointment by making the offer of employment probationary (ACAS,2010).. If your appointee proves unsatisfactory, then he/she may be dismissed at the end of the probationary period before the employment has continued long enough for him/her to have rights against dismissal. You must, however, make the probationary nature of the employment clear at all stages of the recruitment and selection process and in particular in the verbal and written offers. Where workable, this is a satisfactory arrangement. However, many candidates already in substantive posts will consider this an unacceptable risk to take, and the recruitment pool would therefore be smaller. Additionally, in the case of internal promotions there may be continuity of employment, resulting in employment protection rights, making dismissal at the end of a probationary period impossible.

Rejecting

The majority of your applicants will be rejected (CIPD,2014). Many will be local residents and some will already be employees. Therefore, how you handle applicant rejection is very important for the reputation and image of your organisation. Some organisations have a policy of no response to unsuccessful candidates, but this misses a valuable opportunity to promote the organisation, and under no circumstances should it apply to existing employees seeking promotion

Your unsuccessful applicants ought to receive a respectful and regretful notification of failure, and you might offer counselling about how to improve their profile and make themselves more suitable in case of future vacancies. This is to the benefit of applicant and employer, particularly in the case of health and care professionals where the national pool is limited and informal "Grape Vine" communication is rapid. Reputations of organisations may be built or demolished very quickly, and the impact of careless rejection practice on the quality of future recruitment pools can be important.

Staff Development & Performance Management

Once employees have been recruited, you have a continuing responsibility to develop them so that they give the most to the organisation and obtain the most personal benefit from employment (CIPM,2014).

Induction

On starting in a new position, employees need information in order to perform safely, efficiently and effectively (ACAS,2010). Some of this information is required on the first day but much of it is better introduced in a phased manner, as the employee becomes ready to receive it. Essential information can be, as below, categorised as first day, first week, first month and quarter year. In some cases, where it is necessary to be able to demonstrate that information was given a signature may be obtained for each component of the program.

	These to be verified by employee signature	These are for employee's benefit
Day 1	H&S Procedures Fire procedures Rules of conduct, such as gifts policy	Tour of department Introductions to key colleagues
Week 1	Employee responsibility to the organisation Organisation responsibility to the Employee Terms and conditions Procedures regarding: grievance, complaints, disputes & disciplinary action Responsibilities such as State Registration	Tour of Hospital (or equivalent) Introductions to regular contacts Work Schedules with explanatory policies Workload apportionment Involvement in social bonding activities
Month 1	Payroll information Staff development & advancement practice Appraisal IPR & PDP procedures	Services provided by the organisation & context Organisational structure Enlightenment towards organisation Involvement in social bonding activities
Quar'r 1	First objective setting meeting Continuous Professional development: initial plans.	Detailed analysis of the organisation's training offer.

Drawing up an induction programme is the responsibility of the immediate supervisor. However, if desired, it can be made the responsibility of the employee to ensure that all information has been sought out, requested and understood. Any failure would therefore be the responsibility of the employee as well as the employer. This will improve the likelihood of a successful training being achieved.

IPR & PDPs

Throughout the period of employment, each employee needs an explicit statement of what he/she is expected to achieve within the chosen period (Druker,1973) (CIPD,2014). This takes the form of a set of objectives agreed between the individual the supervisor. Since an experienced individual will know more about his/her job than anybody else, it is not unusual for him/her to draft the objectives in the first instance and then have them adjusted and ratified by the supervisor. The duty of the supervisor is to ensure that the workload is reasonable and that the objectives represent good prioritisation. The objectives of all subordinates should aggregate to the total objectives for the area under the supervisor's management. "If you all achieve your objectives, I'll have achieved mine."

Objectives need to be couched in language that allows for no ambiguity in order that the later evaluation presents no difficulty. A useful test for the robustness of an objective is that it is SMART. (Specific, Measurable, Achievable, Relevant and Time-bound.) (Lawler & Bilson, 2013).

Specific	It is very clear what is to be achieved.
Measurable	Something can be measured to give an unambiguous indication about whether the objective has been achieved.
Achievable	It is realistic to think that the objective can be achieved in the time available
Relevant	The objective is clearly relevant to the job and the needs of the organisation
Time bound	It is clear by when the objective will be achieved.

An objective sheet might look as set out below:

OBJECTIVE SHEET

Objective No 1:

Broad statement of Objective:
To manage devolved budget

Processes:
I will control spend on budget for Mental Health Nursing, in order to achieve a spend of between 98% and 100% of target, while delivering the service requirements as per contracts held.

Caveats: (Subject to)
Secondment to training day on "Revenue implications of capital spend".
Receipt of accurate monthly statements of department spend;
Realistic funding of pay award;
Availability of human resources.

Signed: ....(appraisee)
Signed: ....(appraiser)

Progress report 1

Modifications
Signed: ....(appraisee)
Signed: ....(appraiser)

Progress report 2

You should agree ten to fifteen objectives and they should encapsulate the whole of the job to be performed. Some objectives will be of a maintenance nature, as in the above example, and some will be of a developmental nature, showing how your appraisee will change his/her service in the light of a changing environment.

If the individual does not have the necessary skills to achieve an objective, as above with "the revenue implications of capital spending", then this will indicate the need for learning and will form a part of a Personal Development Plan (PDP). The appraisee should also use this interview to discuss aspirations for promotion or enhanced duties in the future and if these are in line with service needs, then they, also, will form part of the PDP. As part of an IPR or appraisal interview, therefore, the employee will agree a PDP that shows how he/she will develop during the planning period. The learning opportunities agreed will include a variety of opportunities as described above.

Industrial relations

All professionals and ancillary workers in the NHS and Social Services are entitled to be members of a Trade Union (ACAS,2014). Members of professions will be members of their professional body each of which is also a recognised and registered, independent trades union. Ancillary workers may join any registered trades union that has been recognised by the employer for which they hold relevant qualifications. The pattern of recognition varies between NHS Trusts and Local Authorities, etc, but the largest trades union, Unison *www.unison.org.uk*, is recognised universally and represents the greatest number of public sector employees of all professions and grades.

Recognised trades unions are entitled to be consulted about all organisational changes, and to collectively represent their membership in discussions about the general organisational behaviour. This is normally achieved through standing consultative committees (ACAS,2014)..

Trades union representatives have a statutory right to be involved in all actions between staff and management (ACAS,2014). These include:

Grievances, where an individual employee wishes to take action against a manager;

Disputes, where a group of individuals wish to take action against a manager;

Disciplinary action, where a manager wishes to take action against an individual employee.

For each of the above events, the organisation is required to have a formal procedure, which has been agreed by the consultative committee, above. The Arbitration & Conciliation Advisory Service (ACAS) publishes guidance to each of the above procedures and this guidance forms the basis of local agreement Whilst the Code is not, in itself, legally enforceable, employment tribunals will take its provisions into account when considering relevant cases (ACAS,2014). Each action is a staged process. Each stage allows the opportunity for resolution and a route for escalation, if resolution is not possible. The procedure requires that a trade union official, or other representative for non-TU members, is notified at each stage and that the individual is apprised of his/her right to representation before each stage is conducted.

The outcome of any of these processes is largely at the discretion of the panel hearing them. Where decisions are successfully challenged, eg through claims for unfair dismissal, it is nearly always on the grounds of failure to follow the procedure not the substantive complaint. So, while managers can make rational decisions and expect them to be successful, it is crucial that these are conducted precisely according to the procedure.

> ## Case example
>
> An employee fails to attend for work for a sustained period of time and her employment is terminated. She later reported that she was unwell and that made attendance at work ill advised.
>
> A tribunal is asked to consider whether this is fair.
>
> The substantive reason for dismissal is undisputed, but the employing officer was unable to show written evidence of first or final warnings.
>
> The correct procedure was therefore not correctly followed and the dismissal not upheld.

Procedures vary in detail, but the general pattern is as below:

Grievance Procedure

Stage 1: The individual makes the grievance known, in writing and by interview, to the immediate manager who has the opportunity to correct the situation. If resolution is agreed, then the action is recorded and discontinued.

Stage 2: The individual makes his grievance known, in writing and by interview, to the manager of the immediate manager who has the opportunity to correct the situation. If resolution is agreed, then the action is recorded and discontinues.

Stage 3: The individual makes his grievance known, in writing and then by interview, to a panel drawn from the management board, who will decide the case. Generally, this panel will not include the CEO or the Chair of the Board of Directors of the organisation, as these will be held in reserve in case of appeal.

Appeal: If the individual is dissatisfied with the outcome of the hearing, then there will, normally, be the right of appeal to a more senior panel.

If failure of an appeal makes continued employment impossible, then the employee may leave the organisation, considering him/herself to have suffered "Constructive Dismissal Constructive Dismissal may be taken to an industrial tribunal as a form of "Unfair Dismissal". However, this action is unlikely to succeed if the procedures have been clearly defined and scrupulously followed.

At each stage, the personnel department or their TU representative may assist the complainants. In some organisations, all cases are routed through the personnel department.

Disputes Procedure

A grievance held by a number of employees is known as a dispute.

Stage 1: The group of individuals makes the dispute known, in writing and by interview, to the immediate manager who has the opportunity to correct the situation. If resolution is agreed, then the action is recorded and discontinues.

Stage 2: The group makes the dispute known, in writing and then by interview, to the manager of the manager who has the opportunity to correct the situation. If resolution is agreed, then the action is recorded and discontinues.

Stage 3: The group makes the dispute known, in writing and then by interview, to a panel drawn from the management board, who will decide the case. Generally, this panel will not include the CEO or the Chair of the organisation, as these will be held in reserve in case of appeal.

Appeal: If the group is dissatisfied with the outcome of the hearing, then there will, normally, be the right of appeal to a more senior panel.

At each stage, the personnel department or their TU representative may assist the complainants. In some organisations, all cases are routed through the personnel department.

Disciplinary Procedure

Preliminary counselling before a formal disciplinary procedure is commenced, the manager interviews the individual, alerts him/her to the problems and discusses the ways in which they may be corrected. It is required that the individual is advised that this is a counselling interview prior to and as a part of a disciplinary action. If this resolves the problem, then disciplinary procedure is not deemed to have been evoked. This is a verbal interview, but must be followed up in writing.

Stage 1 (verbal warning): If counselling has not resolved the problem, then the manager makes the unsatisfactory performance explicit, in writing and by interview, to the individual who has the opportunity to correct the situation by agreeing a set of objectives with timescales. If these objectives are achieved, then the action is recorded and discontinued. The record should be deleted after a period of six months' satisfactory performance. This is often described as a verbal warning. However, this is a misnomer, because the warning is given verbally and confirmed in writing.

Stage 2 written warning: If the objectives are not achieved within the agreed timescales, then the manager reaffirms the unsatisfactory performance, in writing and by interview, to the individual who has further opportunity to correct the situation by agreeing a further set of objectives with timescales. If these objectives are achieved, then the action is recorded and discontinued. This is often described as a written warning. However, once again, this is a misnomer, because the warning is given verbally and flowed up in writing.

Stage 3: If the objectives are not achieved, then the manager will dismiss the employee or otherwise alter his/her employment terms.

Appeal: The individual will have the right of appeal about the outcome of any stage to a panel drawn from the Board of Directors of the organisation.

Gross misconduct. In prescribed cases, a manager may skip one or more of the stages in the procedure. In extreme cases, Gross Misconduct may result in instant dismissal.

Suspension. Where serious misconduct is alleged, but not yet decided, it may be necessary to suspend employment, with or without pay, while the allegations are investigated and decided. This is usually done where the allegations, if true, would suggest that the organisation or its clients are at risk from the employee, or the employee is placed at risk by continued practice without resolution of the allegations.

Industrial Tribunal If the individual and his/her representative consider the dismissal unfair, then they may ask that an industrial tribunal consider the case as a possible Unfair Dismissal This avenue is only available to employees with over two year's employment. A major indicator to the fairness of a dismissal, as assessed by a tribunal, is the care with which the manager has followed and documented the agreed procedures in arriving at a dismissal decision.

Burden of proof. In an industrial tribunal, as in all industrial relations panel decisions, the test of proof is the civil one that "*In the balance of probability*" the misconduct occurred. This test of proof is far less stringent than that in criminal courts in which conviction requires that "*Beyond all reasonable doubt*" the misconduct occurred.

If an industrial tribunal finds that a dismissal is unfair, it can order reinstatement. If this is not possible, or the employer refuses to comply with this order, then the tribunal will order compensation for loss of earnings and other distress.

It is important that any decision being appealed is examined against the evidence available to the manager at the time of the decision. If a dismissal is made and contested, the manager must show that the dismissal was fair with the information held at the time of the dismissal. Further evidence that became known after the dismissal that may vindicate the decision cannot be cited as justification of a dismissal.

Equally, evidence that emerges after the dismissal vindicating the employee would not render the dismissal unfair. However, in this case the manager might consider reinstatement a reasonable course of action.

Accountability

As has been described above a clinician may be called to account by:

the patient/client,

the employer,

the profession or

the community.

The response to this should not be defensive practice, because this inhibits good patient/client care, but good practice and good record keeping.

Professional Good Practice

To be defensible to any of the four stakeholders above, the individual has only to behave as an exemplary member of his/her profession. This is a very simple defence and liberates clinicians from defensive practice. If the clinician always practices properly, doing what a reasonable clinician or manager would do, and keeping good records, then he/she will have nothing to fear when called to account.

Paradoxically, if the clinician becomes too focused on the law and attempts to become an amateur lawyer, instead of a clinician, this will impinge on his/her ability to act properly within his/her profession and will weaken any defence. The nurse in charge during an armed raid reported the event as she imagined a lawyer would speak, "When the gunman entered the room all of the patients evacuated themselves" Although possible, it is doubtful that the meaning conveyed was the meaning intended. Attempting to use "Law Speak" had prevented her from communicating clearly as a nurse. (Andrews and Wheeler, 1997). "Don't get involved for fear of being sued" - common bar room legal advice - will only result in being sued for your omissions. Omissions are as important as positive actions in deciding negligence. The only defence is to do what a competent clinician of your profession would do, and keep records to demonstrate it.

Record Keeping

A complainant will remember the events occasioning the complaint very clearly, because it has been central to his/her life for a long time. You as a manager or a clinician, on the other hand, will struggle even to remember consultations of many years ago, far less to recall the precise words that you used and the actions that you took (Andrews and Wheeler, 1997). The Judge decides the case on the balance of probabilities. Who has produced the best evidence? Your faint or non-existent recollection versus the plaintiff's total recall makes for a one sided contest.

You can overcome this problem by the production of detailed records. With good, accurate and detailed notes, your answer can be compiled. Without these, however good your treatment practice may have been in actuality, it is very difficult for you to mount a defence.

Your records must show: what information you elicited by the various routes; what underlying theory explained your action proposed; what consents you obtained; what actions you took; and what consequences resulted. Sometimes Kipling's six serving men can help: "Who? What? Where? When? Why? & How? (Kipling 1950), but they must between them answer the points above.

Team-working

Your work with patients and clients is inevitably conducted in teams in order to bring to bear the breadth of expertise necessary. Teams go through a predictable life cycle in reaching a stage of maturity (Tuckman, 1965). The stages that you will observe may be categorised as: forming, storming, norming and performing. You as a team member can usefully identify the current stage of each of the teams to which you belong and make contributions calculated to move your team forward. Further approaches, building on Tuckman's ideas are to be found in the Collaboration chapter.

Forming

Team behaviour

Making introductions and attempting to understand the other members of the team. Forming collegiate relationships and establishing communications.

You as a team member can help by

- Facilitating communication
- Helping members to better understand each other as people as well as professionals,
- Encouraging interaction between members on neutral issues as well as work problems,
- Organising social events, etc.

Storming

Team behaviour

Establishing a pecking order, forming strategic alliances, gaining a comfortable position, agreeing leadership establishing responsibilities and demarcations.

You as a team member can help by

- Mediating conflict
- Drawing out the special contributions made by each individual,
- Avoiding cliques,
- Seeking win/win resolutions to power conflicts,
- Ensuring that decisions reached meet all parties' needs rather that allowing one party to "Win" at the expense of another,
- Continuing to progress the endeavour to help team members to know one another as people.

Norming

Team behaviour

Settling down into workable patterns, agreeing protocols and procedures, establishing relationships and responsibilities that are comfortable to all members

You as a team member can help by

- Testing processes devised against client/patient need,
- Ensuring that no members are disadvantaged or disenfranchised,
- Ensuring that all skills and expertise has been considered and exploited.

Performing

Team behaviour

Getting the job done, running in line with agreed protocols, beginning the process of transcending the rules and allowing role blurring and overlaps for efficient co-operation.

You as a team member can help by

- *Testing performance against objectives*
- *Avoiding complacency,*
- *Driving up quality standards,*
- *Testing the rules devised above to find those that can be gradually relaxed.*

One might add:

Declining

Typified by: overconfidence, powerful individuals exerting excessive control, assumptions of team competence rather than challenge, acceptance of practice rather than criticism, reduced mutual support.

You as a team member can help by

Advocating a periodic shakeup!

Team Roles

In any team, there are a number of roles that are performed, and each of us has a profile of strengths in these roles Belbin (1981) (Myers & Briggs, 2014). It is important to know your strengths and perform team roles as are appropriate to you. You may perform different roles in different teams because of the roles dictated by strengths and position, of your colleagues. Your contribution in each situation will reflect the range of abilities across each team when seen as a whole. Conflict in teams may arise where two individuals have similar profiles and are unconsciously seeking to take the same role. This conflict may be overcome by explicit recognition of profiles and aptitudes. Conflict may also arise between two team members whose profiles and roles, although necessary, and in conflict. Recognising why a colleague is performing differently to you can make your relationship easier. The Shaper may be in conflict with the Completer Finisher, because of the nature of the contributions each make. However, each needs the other for the team to work. If both can gain an explicit understanding of the relationship, then they can learn to value one another rather than simply be irritated by each other.

Inefficient team working may also arise where individual team roles are not being performed by those best suited to them. Again, to achieve an explicit understanding of the aptitude of each team member, and to allocate roles accordingly will enable the team to perform at its best level.

Belbin (1981) describes team functions as:

Company Worker

The company worker is described as: conservative, dutiful, loyal and predictable. He/she will have organising abilities, common sense and discipline, and will be hard working. He/she may be inflexible and chary of risk.

Chair

The chair is described as calm, self-confident and controlled. He/she will have a strong focus on objectives, and will be unprejudiced and unconditionally welcoming. He/she need be on no more than average intellect.

Shaper

The shaper is described as: highly-strung, outgoing and dynamic. He/she will have restless drive, and will be challenging towards inertia and complacency. He/she may be impatient and be easily provoked.

Plant

The plant is described as: individualistic, serious minded and unorthodox. He/she will have genius, intellect, imagination and knowledge. He/she may be impractical, and disrespecting towards protocols.

Resource Investigator

The Resource Investigator is described as: extravert, enthusiastic, curious and communicative. He/she will be good at contacting people, responsive to challenge and enthusiastic about exploring anything new. He/she may be able to sustain his/her interest in anything for only a short time, before pursuing something new.

Monitor Evaluator

The Monitor Evaluator is described as: sober, unemotional and prudent. He/she will have judgement, discretion and hard-headedness. He/she may lack inspiration or the ability to motivate others.

Team Worker

The team worker is described as: socially orientated, mild and sensitive. He/she respond to people and promote a team spirit. He/she may be indecisive.

Completer finisher

The Completer finisher is described as: painstaking, orderly, conscientious and anxious. He/she will have a capacity to follow a project through to the absolute conclusion and be a perfectionist. He/she may worry about small, unimportant considerations and be unable to let go.

Identifying your team function

You may be able to allocate team functions from the above descriptions. To get a more robust idea, you might make your own assessment of yourself and compare it with that of a close colleague. In order to gain a more considered assessment you might complete an inventory and derive a score that allocates you to a role. You may find that you are adept at more than one function and you can therefore make a varied contribution in various situations. For an inventory list, see "Additional Reading", below.

Negotiation

Negotiation divides into two types: affiliative and distributive (Malhotra & Bazerman, 2012). In affiliative negotiation both parties seek to achieve a "Win – Win outcome (Covey, 2004) and (2004a). As an affiliative negotiator, you will seek an outcome where each party is satisfied. This may result in a degree of compromise on both sides, with neither gaining everything they want. However, long term benefits will ensue, because of the beneficial relationship established for future negotiation.

In distributive negotiation the parties are seeking a "Win – Lose" outcome. Should you be obliged to act as a distributive negotiator, you will be seeking to achieve advantage at the expense of the other party. This may result in benefiting from the negotiation at the expense of the other. The immediate benefit of this (to the winner) is great but the other party will be seeking to redress the balance in future negotiations, or if this is not possible, they may elect not to do business with you again. Distributive negotiation is inappropriate in long-term supply relationships, but may be inescapable where no future relationship is likely or where the other party is evidently operating according to a distributive paradigm.

Negotiating teams

Negotiating is commonly conducted between teams and each member will have a specific role.

Negotiator

The negotiator takes the lead in discussions, described as "Making the running". You will discuss the positions set out by both sides, introduce information as appropriate and make piecemeal steps toward agreement. You will start from a position demanding maximum benefit and give way on a series of points in exchange for reciprocal concessions until a point of agreement has been achieved. Each negotiator will, however, have a point beyond he/she cannot go.

---

for negotiator 1
Best outcome =====================minimum position
for negotiator 2
                Minimum position =======================Best outcome

This shows the range of acceptable outcomes for negotiators 1 & 2. Here the scope for agreement is represented by the overlap of the two lines. Each negotiator is seeking to agree an overlap position as near to his/her start position as he/she can achieve. In distributive negotiation these positions are not revealed, and therefore the negotiation exercise is one of exploration and controlled disclosure. The distributive negotiator may, however, reveal a false minimum point as a negotiating ploy.

In affiliative negotiation the positions are both revealed at the outset of the negotiations and evidenced as appropriate, and a conclusion reached that allows equal benefit to both parties.

Co-negotiator

A team may employ a co-negotiator who works in tandem with the negotiator, by listening and chipping in throughout the discussions. The lead "Baton" may even be passed from one to the other throughout the negotiation.

Recorder

The recorder is an analyst who knows and clearly understands what has been agreed and can quickly make comment when discussion backslides from this position or compromises an agreed position. The recorder does not keep minutes, but can at all times give a precise statement of what has been agreed and what remains outstanding.

Technical expert

A number of experts within their field may be present to advise during a negotiation. These might include clinicians, accountants, lawyers, etc.

Arbitration

If negotiation is badly conducted, overly distributive, or there is no overlap in the positions then the parties may agree to arbitration (ACAS,2014).

Arbitration may be binding arbitration in which case parties agree in advance to enact the arbiter's decision, or advisory in which case the parties may still continue the discussion. Arbitration may be of a pendulum arbitration type where the arbiter is obliged to decide in favour of one party or the other, or may be to find a compromise in which case the arbiter seeks a solution to the satisfaction of both parties.

In the case of NHS, where agreement between purchaser and provider cannot be achieved, the law requires binding, pendulum arbitration to be conducted by the DoH Outpost

Managing Oneself

Every employee is responsible for managing him/herself to the very best advantage of the organisation. This represents consumption of a very significant resource.

Time

The management of your time is the most important aspect of life at work and elsewhere, and is discussed at length in its own chapter, which you should read in conjunction with the material in this chapter.

Stress

Every modern work environment is a stressing one, but employment in health care is made more than usually stressful by the nature of the work to be done (Walton,1984) . The management of stress is essential, both to the individual and to the organisation. Stress and burnout may be a result of a mismatch between the degree of challenge experienced and the amount of support received. As the demand in a job, increases so should the support. It is healthy for a job to have periods of high demand interspersed with periods of lower demand allowing space for recuperation, tying up loose ends and creative reflection. When a job is in a demanding phase, it is appropriate for the employee to seek appropriate support. This might come from a supervisor, mentor peer or counsellor. Stress may also arise from poor time management. Stress may increase insidiously, arising from indistinct or multiple sources and through difficulties taking on a greater than necessary importance.

We can address stressful situations in a problem solving model, *removing the problem,* or an emotional model, *not minding the problem*.

Similarly, the management of stress might be considered in causal or reactive terms and cerebral or physical terms.
This might appear as a grid.

	cerebral response	Physical response
Cause focused action	Observe fluctuating stress levels
Understand the causes of stress
Reflect: on whether the individual causes are very important.
Decide upon changes that can be made to reduce identified stressors.
Improve time management	Break into vicious cycle stress patterns.
Practice relaxation techniques in stressful settings.
Diminish environmental stressors such as poor seating, lighting, noise, etc.
Avoid long unbroken meetings etc.
Reaction focused action	Gain increased support
Set achievable goals
Recognise and express feelings
Maximise the benefit of social contacts for emotional release
Question perfectionism: consider "Good enough" outcomes.
Adopt empowering language and attitudes.	Ensure suitable diet.
Take exercise weekly and daily.
Ensure a balance of work, domestic duties and recreation.
Practice active relaxation at some point every day.
Ensure deep relaxation periodically with holidays, short breaks and occasional days of indulgence.

We can also address stress with a problem solving focus or an emotion focussed response (Lazarus & Folkman, 1984) (Lazarus,1991).

Problem solving focussed approach	Emotion focussed approach
Commonly adopted by younger ambitious people	Commonly adopted by older people
Identify the cause of your stress and remove that problem. Confront people who cause you stress Solve problems that cause stress	Analyse the problem and see if it is really worth stressing over. Decide not to mind. Use a CBT approach, to rationalise the stressor.

Personal & Professional Development through Portfolios and Profiles

In order to control and maximise your rate of professional progress, you need to have a clear picture of your present attributes This may be achieved by drawing up a profile supported by evidence contained in a portfolio (Wheeler&Grice,2000)..

A profile is a statement of strengths and abilities that encapsulates your present position and helps you to monitor and plan your progress from novice to state registered clinician or manager and throughout your career (Wheeler&Grice,2000). It enables you to analyse the current position and, by reference to aspirations, decide and plan for your learning needs. It is sensible that you record your progress in discussion with a tutor, mentor coach or line manager at least annually. In this you are seeking to change your pattern of abilities. See the chapter on change.

The process of profiling provides an opportunity to reflect upon your professional and personal qualities. This can be a primary vehicle for addressing Continuing Professional Development (CPD) needs, which will affect your progress on the career ladder.

It is good for you to discuss your progress with a colleague and agree a series of scores that best reflect your position. The insights gained will help you to maximise your rate of progress. It may be helpful to discuss your profile with course leaders, when joining a course of study in order for them to tailor the learning opportunity to your best advantage. The same can be done with a new line manager in order that he/she tailors experience to your maximise benefit.

In a highly competitive environment, an explicit profile will show to prospective employers what skills knowledge and understanding you have gained during your education and thereafter. This, alongside a curriculum vitae document (CV), enables you to describe yourself in the job market. It is acceptable at interview to say that you have been a sister on an elderly care ward. However, it is better to say that you have been a sister and that you have gained expertise in managing money, selecting, training and supervising staff, etc, etc. To describe skills, knowledge and understanding is more persuasive than to simply refer to time served.

Point!

To achieve the career that you want you will need the right profile. At interview, in a few years, you may find yourself having to bluff and make your profile seem as close to the one interviewers desire as you can. Far better is to identify the profile you'll need now and slowly give yourself the experiences that will mean you have the correct profile when the time comes.

Example Profile

1	H&S	=	=	=	=	=	=	=	=	=	=	
2	Self Mx	=	=	=	=							
3	Problem solving	=	=	=	=	=	=	=				
4	Professionalism	=	=	=	=	=	=	=	=	=	=	
5	Communications	=	=	=	=	=	=	=	=	=	=	
6	Reflection	=	=	=	=							
7	Teamwork	=	=	=	=	=	=	=	=	=	=	
8	Legal/ethical,	=	=	=	=	=	=	=	=	=		
9	EBP	=	=	=	=	=	=	=	=			
10	Clinical skills	=	=	=	=	=	=	=				

This shows a practitioner skilled in Health & Safety (H&S) matters, highly professional, with good communications and teamwork skills He/she describes lower ability in self-management and reflection This profile is designed for a novice practitioner, covering those things necessary for the first year of practice. A clinician aspiring to a management career would have skills such as marketing, HR Management, Financial Management etc on the profile. Each individual should decide how many sections to have in his/her profile and what they should be. This may be influenced by published requirements from a professional body registration authority, course outcomes and personal preference for models of practice.

Where a practitioner does not explicitly examine his/her profile, he/she will have a tendency to further study those areas at which he/she is already expert and overlook those areas where he/she is lacking. Examination of your profile should help you to decide which are your priorities for advancement.

Case example

A senior Occupational Therapist approaches his manager asking for time and money to attend a study event on Orthotics.

Manager, "But you are already the best person at splinting in the county"

Applicant, "Yes. Good isn't it? This course will be great!"

Manager, "But your patients are frightened to be in a room with you. Shouldn't you be looking for a course to help with that?"

Applicant, "Oh I see what you mean. Why didn't I think of that?"

Manager, "Because you have not examined your profile"

Portfolio

A portfolio is a collection of evidence that supports and justifies your profile (Wheeler&Grice,2000). From your portfolio you can draw evidence with which to decide your profile and persuade others that it is valid. In order to substantiate the profile clinicians collect material showing their ability from their professional and personal life. This may include testimonials, examples of work, course marks and comments, reflective diaries, etc, etc. and is called a portfolio. Your portfolio may take any of a number of forms. Perhaps the simplest is a concertina file with sections created to match the sections chosen for your profile. As pieces of evidence occur you can easily file them for future attention. Periodically, your portfolio should be closely examined and an assessment made of each section. You are advised to be continually alert to pieces of evidence of an ability or an attribute to add to your portfolio. Bodies managing Professional registers may demand to see a portfolio as evidence of CPD. The HPC may require upon request, presentation of a written profile (which must be your own work and supported by evidence) explaining how you have met the standards for CPD. http://www.hpc-uk.org/registrants/cpd/

Evidence

It is important to be flexible about what constitutes evidence for your portfolio. Some evidence will come in a conveniently fileable form, such as certificates from H&S courses, but much will need to be canvassed "Would you write a brief appraisal of my communication with the next patient?" Evidence might also be the result of personal reflection. Reflections on an achievement can make rich evidence if captured quickly after an event, and particularly if seen in conjunction with other tangible evidence such as a certificate or testimonial. The notion of what is appropriate might be answered by considering the uses for which you might use your portfolio. If it is to win you jobs, then consider what evidence a panel might want you to describe.

Evidence to support a workplace portfolio may originate from many non-work situations. For example qualification as a scuba diver may be taken as evidence of experience of a strict health & safety culture. Work as a Cub Scout leader may demonstrate experience with children to support a transfer into paediatric care.

Self-evaluation

This involves looking through your portfolio and improving your opinion about your attributes. This requires only that the evidence is honest and gives rich information from which a profile can be deduced. This calls for reports of experience, reflections, testimonials, colleague and client comments, etc. You will critically examine your portfolio in order to decide what your balance of attainments looks like, what you want it to look like in the future and what experiences you need to make it so.

Evidence for Job interviews

Evidence for Job interviews from this your portfolio must be persuasive and incisive. An interviewer is willing to hear about experiences, courses, achievements and accomplishments, where they clearly indicate a skill that helps them to match you up against a person specification. The portfolio is not normally physically present at an interview except in unusual cases. However, the interviewee is called upon, metaphorically, to delve into their portfolio and refer to or describe evidence that can persuade the panel of their match with the person specification and therefore suitability for a position. An interviewer has a profile in mind, even if he/she does not always explicitly know that. The interview is to see if your profile matches that desired profile.

Evidence for supervision and personal development planning interview.

The profile and portfolio form the basis of Independent Performance Review (IPR) and Personal Development Planning (PDP), above. Here, you are seeking to draw the interviewer's attention to evidence of which both may have prior knowledge. The interviewee may refer to individual cases and projects, citing the outcome as evidence of ability and achievement. Alternatively, the evidence may be offered to demonstrate an ability that is not yet satisfactory and indicate the need for further learning by any of a number of routes. There might be a discussion between interviewee and interviewer until a common view of the profile is achieved based upon the evidence in the virtual or physical portfolio. A similar process might occur in an interview to decide Performance Related Pay (PRP). Possession of a portfolio and explicit understanding of the profile enables the interviewee to be more in control of these interviews.

It is important that you have ownership of your portfolio. That way, you can ensure that it gives best benefit for the time that you commit. If your portfolio is compiled mechanistically, simply to meet the demands of your professional body, then the value will be limited. If you compile your portfolio for your own benefit and ensure that it, incidentally, meets the demands of your professional regulatory machinery, it will prove far more useful.

Your personal development plan emerges from a study of your profile and portfolio. It may also be used as a vehicle for your PDP. Having stated a learning need, based upon study of the portfolio, it is possible to describe the learning in terms of the changes anticipated in the portfolio. Thus the evidence to be obtained is known, and from this, the best type of the learning opportunity is evident. This may help you to be more creative in recognition of learning methods. It may be more valuable to join a project team and thereby gain experience, than to follow a course and gain knowledge. Commonly, however, it is the combination of theoretical input and experiential learning that proves to be most educational and persuasive.

Job hunting

It always seems that there are not enough jobs and there is a temptation to apply for them all and be pleased to get anything. However, if you spread your energy too far, you will make a poor job of each application and a poor job will not get you any job. Identify the few jobs that you would really enjoy and at which you would excel and then put every effort into winning it (Cunningham, 2013).

A fully worked through application takes more work than you might expect but puts you in a strong position.

The process of job hunting can mirror the processes described above for recruitment

Job Specification,

Attracting potential employers,

researching potential employers,

passing screening,

being selected.

Job Specification

The first task is to define the job sought. If your desired job is not explicitly defined, then the job hunter is vulnerable to eye catching advertisements and may be seduced by attractive positions that will not adequately meet his/her needs. Posts may appear to be hard to find, but it is better to put energy into getting the right job than the wrong one.

There are a number of parameters to consider in your Job Specification. These are shown in the chart, below. It may appear that the candidate is in a poor position to define the position because the range is limited by availability. In this case, the parameters may be set wide. However, it is necessary to be explicit about the parameters in order to focus attention onto a manageable number of ideal jobs, and make a high quality application for these.

Quality	Essential	Desirable
Locality	Greater London	Inner London
Salary	£20,000	£25,000
Training	General support in principle	Funding for MSc
Client group	Mental Health	Acute Adult Mental Health
Assistance	Travel allowance	Lease Car
Supervision	Weekly supervision meetings	Peer Support Group

Attracting Potential Employers

Making contact with potential employers may be by response to an advertisement, introduction by current employee, cold calling.

Responding to an advertisement has the advantage that the employer is anticipating applicants and has set aside time to respond to them. The disadvantage is that such candidates are reactive, and have to use other methods to prove their creativity. Introduction by employee is a good route, because the introduction carries some recommendation and there is some innovation demonstrated by not waiting for an advertisement. Cold calling shows the maximum initiative, but faces the maximum expectation of rejection. Cold calling is best by letter, allowing the recipient to respond in his/her own time. Cold calling by telephone is not recommended, because this is likely to inconvenience and annoy the recipient although meetings and conferences may offer an opportunity for networking and informal enquiries, and responding to published research may create an employment prospect. The serious job hunter should consider all of these routes. When candidates have been generated by personal contacts it remains likely that a formal advertisement will be placed to ensure equal opportunity. However, those candidates who showed initiative in their approach will have an advantage in a position where initiative is important.

Once a desired employer has been selected, it is important to research the organisation. This research has three purposes: to confirm choice of employer, to persuade the employer of your enthusiasm, and to find out about the candidate qualities sought.

Information will be gained from the job pack sent to candidates, publications such as annual reports, personal contacts in the organisation and the traditional informal visit. It is important to collect as much information, by paper research as possible before the informal visit. This will allow insightful questions to be asked and the maximum to be gained from the exercise. It is important to use the informal visit to collect information that will strengthen the application. Candidates should not spend this meeting talking about themselves, although the employer may be impressed by the knowledgeable and insightful nature of their questions.

CVs

The purpose of a CV is to ensure that you pass the screening exercise and obtain an interview. It may, at best, ensure you a high place on the candidate order, but cannot bring about an appointment. The CV should be written to demonstrate how well you match the person specification described above. It must be rewritten for each application. That is not to suggest that the CV is not entirely honest, in fact, it is important that it is scrupulous. However, a great deal can be said about a candidate and it is necessary to select that which interests this employer. For this reason, commercial pre-printed CVs are of limited value.

Your CV is an example of the quality of the work that you can deliver and for this reason it should be drawn up with great care, over a number of days and finished to a very high quality. It is advisable to submit a number of copies of a CV in order that all panellists receive a top copy, rather than a photocopied one.

The notion of an ideal CV is specific to each industry. For health and care industries, a comprehensive CV is the norm. A good format is as below.

Curriculum Vitae

Name Address DoB

> **Résumé or Personal Statement**, summarising strengths and aptitudes, with some reference to experience and other evidence that might persuade the reader that these qualities are genuine. Max ½ page.

Education History in reverse chronological order, stating institutions and qualifications obtained. Add a script to a piece, if there is a particular point to make that is relevant to the position.
e.g.

Oxford Brookes University: EdD   Thesis: Public Sector Change Management

Uni of Keele: MBA   Note: A specialist MBA for NHS Executives

Employment History in reverse chronological order giving a list of responsibilities achievements and skills learned in each. Allow greater space for recent posts diminishing, as the positions become older. Focus of giving information that demonstrates your match with the person Specification.

Other attributes, such as clean driving licence, first aid qualification..

Hobbies and interests. This is to show a good balanced existence, but may also show a desire to live in the locality and evidence some qualities claimed in the Résumé, such as deep knowledge of H&S.

Publications

List all: Books, Book Chapters, Research Papers, Conferences presentations, etc. This list can be creative. Do not just list journal papers, as these may be few, but also include other times when you made your knowledge public. I.e. conference presentations, lectures given, work based training offered, papers written for managers, etc.

Interviews

The purpose of an interview is to allow the selection panel to match the candidate's profile of strengths with the person specification (essentially another profile)

Panellists will want to know that you are making a thoughtful and well informed choice of job and will perform well. They will then want to know that you have all necessary abilities and aptitudes to perform well and they will test you in each of these areas. Consequently, you should expect one of three questions, in a wide variety of forms. These questions are:

1. *Why do you want this job? and what do you know of the job/organisation/industry/ locality?*
2. *Where do you want your career to go?*
3. *What qualities have you that make you a suitable candidate; what evidence can you offer for these qualities; what knowledge can you demonstrate? E.g. by case example;*

A long list of questions can be generated from this base, and you might practice answers to each in informal role-plays with friends and colleagues.

Possible interview questions

It is worth your while to become fluent in answering any of the commonly asked questions. Not to have thought about these areas might be interpreted as lacking drive and initiative.

With others, rehearse the example questions below. You will notice that they all amount to variants on the three questions above. You should do this until you are comfortable talking about yourself while under a spotlight. Give feedback to one another and ensure that your performance is as good as it is possible for it to be.

1 WHY DO YOU WANT THIS JOB?
2 WHAT ARE YOUR STRENGTHS?
3 HAVE YOU ANY WEAKNESSES?
4 WHAT JOB DO YOU WANT TO BE DOING IN 5 YEARS?
5 WHAT JOB DO YOU WANT TO BE DOING IN 10 YEARS?
6 WHAT ARE YOU MAJOR ACHIEVEMENTS?
7 WHAT DO YOU ENJOY DOING MOST?
8 WHAT EXPERIENCES DO YOU THINK MAKE YOU SUITABLE FOR THIS JOB?
9 WHAT ABILITIES DO YOU THINK MAKE YOU SUITABLE FOR THIS JOB?
10 WHAT DO YOU WANT FROM THIS JOB?
11 WHAT WOULD YOU WANT FROM YOUR MANAGER?
12 WHAT WOULD YOU OFFER TO THIS JOB?
13 WHAT DO YOU KNOW ABOUT THIS TRUST?
14 WHAT DO YOU KNOW ABOUT THIS AREA?
15 WHAT DO YOU THINK IS THE FUTURE FOR THE NHS?
16 IF OFFERED THE JOB WILL YOU TAKE IT?
17 HOW DO YOU THINK THAT (eg) OTs SHOULD WORK WITH PTs/Psych/Etc*?
18 WHAT IS THE DIFFERENCE BETWEEN STUDENT AND BASIC GRADE?
19 HAVE YOU ANY QUESTIONS FOR THE PANEL?
20 YOU COULD BE GIVEN CASE EXAMPLES AS PROBLEMS TO SOLVE

In answering questions, consider the three ways in which you are expressing yourself. Mehrabian, (1971and 1972), has suggested that audiences are persuaded by three factors in a communication. Least persuasive are the words spoken. More persuasive is the intonation and voice quality when presenting. Of greatest importance are the body communications given when speaking. Mehrabian observed the relative importance of these three factors in persuading an audience and, more critically, pointed out that maximum effect is achieved when all three devices are in harmony

Other interview advice

At the interview, your research carried out before application will allow you to offer a very sophisticated match to the person specification and reassure the panellists that you really understand the organisation that you wish to join.

General points to note are:

Dress smart, but no more formal than the organisational norm;

Actively relax at the start of the interview, and smile;

Practice a firm handshake;

Rehearse answers. Mehrabian (1971) suggests to us that the least influential component of your communication is what is said. Tone of voice is of medium importance, and general demeanour is of greatest importance. Therefore to convince an employer, the candidate must not simply practice the right answers, but learn to use convincing tone of voice and demeanour;

Know exactly where the interview will be held, arrive early, park, eyeball the door, and then find a restaurant to relax drink tea and freshen up.

Carry the name and telephone number in order to call if you are delayed. If you do arrive late, late ask time to freshen up and thus perform well. Do not be rushed into a poor performance;

Answer the question asked, not the one you hoped for. If unsure ask for clarification;

Ask questions when prompted that show insight and demonstrate other skills e.g. "Would there be an opportunity to use and further my IT skills?" Do not ask about salary or holidays at interview.

Do ask about training etc. at interview. The answer forms part of the contract

Immediately after an interview make a reflective record. What went well/badly? What lesson have you learned? What will you do differently next time? In this way, interview technique will rapidly improve.

It is important that employers and employees are as honest as possible in the selection process. However, a degree of "Spin" is to be expected and as candidate, you should be cautious about what is said. Your broad knowledge of the situation should not be overwhelmed by a slick presentation.

Case Example

One day, a woman hospital manager was suddenly killed. She arrived at the gates to Heaven, where St. Peter met her. (The reader will see the problem straight away; healthcare managers do to go to Heaven,) "*You are very welcome,*" he said, but after a pause, he continued, "*although, you do present us with a bit of a problem. As you might imagine, we've never had a hospital manager make it to Heaven before and we're not really sure what to do.*" "*Just let me in,*" said the woman. "*I'd like to*" Replied the Gatekeeper, "but *I have my orders. What we are going to do is let you have a day in Hell and a day in Heaven, and then you can choose.*" "*Obviously, I prefer to stay in Heaven,*" said the woman. "*Rules,*" said St. Peter, and he put her into an elevator to Hell. She was surprised. She found herself on a beautiful paradise island. In the distance was a country club, and standing there were all of her former colleagues (naturally!). They were all dressed gorgeously and cheering for her. They ran up and shook her hand and they talked about old times. They played every kind of sport, and that night went to the country club where she enjoyed an excellent steak dinner. She met the Devil, who was quite charming. She had a great time telling jokes and dancing and before she knew it, it was time to leave. Everybody shook her hand and waved goodbye as she got on the elevator.

The manager spent the next 24 hours on clouds and playing the harp and singing. She had a great time there too, and before she knew it, her 24 hours were up. St. Peter came: "*You have spent a day in Hell and in Heaven. Now you can choose,*" he said. The woman paused for a second, and then replied, "*I never thought I'd say this. Heaven has been really great, but I think I had a better time in Hell.*" Accordingly, St. Peter escorted her to the elevator and back to Hell. When the doors of the elevator opened, she found herself standing in a desolate wasteland covered in all manner of filth. She saw her friends dressed in rags picking up garbage and putting it in sacks. Proprietarily, The Devil put his arm around her. "*I don't understand*," said the woman. "*Yesterday and there was a country club and we ate steak and danced. I had a great time. Now all there is wasteland and garbage. All of my friends look miserable.* "The Devil looked at her and smiled. " *Yesterday we were recruiting; today you're staff.*"

Conclusion

Health and Social services are human resource intensive organisations. A very large portion of revenue is spent on people, far in excess of the proportion in most other sectors of industry. How well these resources are managed and how efficiently they employed determines the efficiency of the service. Reduced staff turnover, increased activity, optimised co-operation and goal achievement lead to more and better patient/client care, so to achieve HR efficiency is an ethical imperative. You have a personal duty to enable maximum, harmonious performance for the benefit of the end user. Additionally, you are a human resource, and have a duty to ensure that you are delivering the best value that you can.

References

ACAS (2010) Recruitment and induction. London: ACAS *www.acas.org.uk* Accessed 02 11 14

ACAS (2014) Recruitment and induction. London: ACAS *www.acas.org.uk* Accessed 02 11 14

Andrews, A.. and Wheeler, N. (1996). Accountability. *British Journal of Occupational Therapy* 59 (10), 483

Andrews, A., & Wheeler, N. (1997) Accountability and Occupational Therapy. *British journal of Occupational Therapy* 59 (10) 483

Andrews, A. (1995)The road to the courts. *Health visitor* 68 (1):26-7.

Atkinson, J. (1989) Four Stages of Adjustment to demographic downturn, *Journal of Personnel Management*

Belbin, R, M. (1993). Team roles at work. Oxford: Butterworth Heineman.

Belbin, R, M. (2010) *Management Teams* London: BH

Belbin, R.M. (1981) *Management Teams: Why they Succeed or Fail*. London: BH

Bratton, J., & Gold, J. (2012) *Human Resource Management - Theory and practice* London: Palgrave Macmillan

Brent, M.& Dent,F. (2013) *The leaders guide to managing people* Kindle.

Churchouse, C., and Churchouse, J. (1998) *Managing People* Aldershot: Gower

CIPD (2014) *http://www.cipd.co.uk/hr-resources/factsheets/role-line-managers-hr.aspx*

CIPD (2003) *How to make use of psychometrics*. London: CIPD *www.cipd.co.uk*

Clark, A., & Taxis, J. (2003) Legal and Ethical Dimensions of CNS Practice: Developing Ethical competence in nursing. 17(5) , 236 - 237

Covey, S. (2004) *The seven habits of highly successful people* Bath: Bath Press

Covey, S. (2004)a *The eighth habit* New York: Free Press

Cunningham, A. (2013) *The essential Job Hunting Book*, Amazon

Dana, J., Dawes, R. M., & Peterson, N. (2013). Belief in the unstructured interview: The persistence of an illusion. *Judgment and Decision Making, 8*, 512-520.

Drucker, P. (1973) *Management Tasks, Responsibilities, Practices,* New York:Harper & Row.

Frances, R. (2013) *The Mid Staffordshire NHS Foundation Trust – report of a Public Inquiry.* London: HMSO

Gov.UK (2013) *Dismissal- your rights.* London:HMSO

GOV.UK (2013) https://www.gov.uk/set-up-a-social-enterprise

Griffiths, R (1984) *NHS Management enquiry.* London HMSO

Handy, C. (1980) *Understanding Organisations* London: Penguin

Handy, C. (1996) *Beyond certainty: the changing worlds of organisations* London: Arrow

Handy, C, B. (1990) - *Inside organisations* London : BBC Books

Handy, C, B. (1993) *Understanding organisations* London : Penguin,

Hull, C., and Redfern, L. and Shuttleworth (2005) A *Profiles and Portfolios: A guide for health and social care* (2nd Ed). Hampshire: Palgrave Macmillan.

IPM (1990) *Recruitment Code of practice* London: IPM

Johnson, C. (2011) *The Complete Guide To Managing People: A manager's toolkit for inspiring, challenging and developing staff* [Kindle]

Lasco. S. (2013) Want the best person? Don't interview. *Boston Globe*

Lawler, J. & Bilson, A. (2013). *Social Work Management and Leadership : Managing Complexity with Creativity.* London: Routledge.

Lazarus, R. S. (1991). Progress on a cognitive-motivational-relational theory of emotion. *American psychologist*, 46(8), 819.

Lazarus, R. S., & Folkman, S. (1984). *Stress, appraisal, and coping.* New York: Springer Publishing Company.

Malhotra,D., & Bazerman, M. (2012) *Negotiation Genius: How to Overcome Obstacles...* Harvard Business School

Mehrabian, A. (1971). *Silent messages*, Wadsworth, California: Belmont

Mehrabian, A. (1972). *Nonverbal communication.* Illinois: Aldine-Atherton,

Myesr, I., & Briggs, K. (2014) *www.myersbriggs.org*

Sims, S., Hewitt, G., and Harris, R. (2014) Evidence of collaboration, pooling of resources, learning and role blurring in interprofessional healthcare teams: a realist synthesis. *J Interprof Care.* 2014 Jul 22:1-6.

Torrington, D., Hall, L., Taylor,S., and Atkinson, C. (2014) *Human Resource Management* London: Pearson.

Tuckman, B. (1965). "Developmental sequence in small groups". *Psychological Bulletin* 63 (6): 384–99.

Walton, M. (1984) *Management and Managing: Dynamic Approach* London: Lippencot

Weightman, J. (2004) *Managing People* London: CIPD

Wheeler, N., & Grice, D. (2000) *Management in healthcare* Cheltenham: Nelson Thornes

Wheeler, N. (1995) Whither the Professions? *British journal of Therapy and Rehabilitation*

York NHS Trust (2013) www.northyorksresearch.**nhs**.uk/document.php?o=627

Zee, K. Bakker, A., & Bakker, P. (2002) Why structured interviews are rarely used *Journal of applied Psychology* 87 (1) 176

Managing Quality

Introduction

Optimising quality is an essential component of management, but is also the responsibility of all employees, especially clinicians. Those who directly relate to patients and clients exert the greatest influence on service quality (Darzi 2008).

Standards can always be improved by the allocation of additional resources and there is a duty to make maximum resources available. However, the management of quality requires the maximisation of standards within available resources. Frequently, managers say *"if I had more resources, I could..."* With more resources, anybody could do more; that's easy! The challenge of management and what makes a good manager is to be able maximise quality and volume within available resources.

Many quality improvements require no additional resource. Quality improvement may be achieved simply by taking time to consider the services delivered and improve empathy with the recipients. Management of quality is frequently a *revenue saving* exercise when the cost of making-good errors is added into the equation. Lean thinking is specifically a quality improvement approach that reduces costs (Cleaner Workplaces, 2014) (Ward, 2006). Additionally, achieving the very best quality is progressively important in winning contracts, customers or clients and thereby remaining in operation.

Service quality in the health and care industries has always been sustained by the dedication of professionals involved, sometimes in spite of rather than because of management practices (Einthoven, 1985). However, attention to consumer wishes was for many years subjugated in a paternalist paradigm *The Dr knows best* and it was only with the NHS Management Enquiry Report (Griffiths, 1983) that consumerism began to be respected. This was reinforced by The NHS and Community Care Act (DoH,1990), The New NHS - Modern and Dependable (DoH, 1998) and High quality Care for All (Darzi, 2008).

The Theoretical Framework

Quality

The biggest challenge can be first defining quality (Dickens 1994). If we are not able to say what we mean by quality it is going to be difficult to measure and improve it.

At the end of the 20th Century, much thought was given to this and the literature of that time rewards the reader with a wealth of ideas. Quality is a 'chimera', meaning a creature made up of pieces drawn from many other creatures (Taylor 1999).

If we run with Taylor's definition then it may help if we identify the parts of that beast.

Donabedian (1980) had already suggested three components: the *Technical dimension, the Non-technical dimension and the Environmental factor.* He then offers us *Structure, Process and Outcome* as three distinct focusses for quality (Donabedian, 1980).

Maxwell (1984) offers us four Es and three As, in the form of *Efficiency, Economy, Effectiveness, Equity, Access, Appropriateness and (societal) Acceptability*

Dickens (1994) favours: *Tangible evidence* of care, *Reliability* of service, *Assurance, Responsiveness and Empathy*

Ovratveit (1992) focussing on health and social care preferred to categorise quality as perceived by the three constituencies: *Managerial quality, Clinician quality and Client quality*.

Garvin (1984) Compiling very comprehensive literature identified five competing ways of recognising quality:

Manufacturing based quality: Conformance to requirements. If it is very well made it must be good quality.

Product-based quality: Differences in quality amount to differences in the quantity of some desired attribute. If passenger safety is the most important thing, then the safest car is the best quality car.

Value-based quality: Quality means best utility for the selling price. This can also be approached by picking a value in a product, such as safety in a motor car and calling the car with greatest safety the best quality car. This mirrors the notion of Virtue Ethics (Car & Steutel 1999), in which we decide what is 'good' and then we are ethical if we do as much of that as we can.

User-based quality: Quality is fitness for purpose. It should be aimed at the present and future needs of the consumer. If it is what the customer needs and wants it is good quality.

Transcendent quality: Beyond anything measurable, we just know what quality is.

Allied to Transcendent quality, Peters & Waterman (1982) point out that if we think it is good then in many ways it is good - *'Perception is all there is'*. We buy a motor car because we think it is good quality. Whether or not it is objectively good is no factor in the purchase decision, only whether we think it is.

The above components are diverse and Dickens' chimera is a complex beast but they may be aggregated into groups.

Non-technical dimension Environmental factor. Outcome Equity Access Appropriateness Acceptability Responsiveness Empathy Clinician quality Client quality Product-based quality User-based quality Transcendent quality Perception is all	... . Addressing the Patient & Clinician perception of need
Technical dimension Structure Process Effectiveness Tangible evidence of care Assurance Manufacturing based Reliability of service	. . . Addressing Reliability 'Right first time- Every time'
Efficiency Economy Managerial quality Value-based quality	. Addressing VfM. Must be the lowest possible price, or we are wasting money.

A service is of acceptable quality if it satisfies a number of criteria (Wheeler & Grice,2000). These are:

1) **It must do what the customer's wants and needs it to do (as agreed with clinician).**
2) **It must be entirely reliable.**
3) **It must represent good value for money.**

Meeting the Customer's agreed wishes

In health care, the issue of meeting "customers' wishes has taken a progressively prominence (Griffiths,1984) finding greatest prominence in the government's promise to patients in the NHS Constitution (DoH,2012). However, there remains a responsibility for the clinician to interpose his/her expertise thus modifying patient/client demands and reaching an intervention decision acceptable to both. This may be an informal negotiated contract if only one intervention is involved, but where the therapeutic relationship is a long-term one, the process becomes iterative. The patient/client makes a request of the clinician. The clinician responds adding his/her clinical expertise and there in a service provision. This service better informs the patient/client. There is a new situation and the patient request is informed by the previous iteration. Each party is modified by the other and by the outcome of former interventions. If this cycle is handled well, the requests and provision become ever more harmoniously aligned. In the final analysis, however well-meaning is the clinician, if service provision is not what the patient or client wants for his/her life, subject to resource limits, then it is not good quality. However, the "Customer" cannot be "King", as a market place requires, because of the gradient of expertise. Progressive alignment of clinician and consumer as in begins to overcome this conflict.

Patient request==Clinician Expert knowledge==agreement about care==informs next request

This is frequently an iterative process, where repeated cycles result in a steady convergence.

This progressive harmonisation of clinician and consumer is essential from the Next Stage Review (Darzi 2008).

Emphasis on 'customers' wishes is set out in The NHS Constitution (DoH, 2012). This is best studied in conjunction with the Handbook to the NHS Constitution (DoH, 2012)a. Both are available as free downloads from the DoH. They give some useful indicators, but are peppered with imprecise terms, leaving quality decisions subject to the discretion of clinicians.

Entirely reliable

Many providers of goods and services maintain a reputation for quality based upon an unquestioning willingness to replace faulty products. Therefore, in the final analysis, the customer always gets a good product or service (National Quality Board 2011). This is not possible in health or care, where the consequences of unreliable service are generally irreparable and always unacceptable (Wheeler& Grice, 2000). *"We regret that the operation was performed badly, but come back in a week and we will do it again completely free of charge"*. *"I am so sorry that the stair-rail came off the wall when you rested on it, but never fear, we will be back in the morning to put it right"*. Health and care providers must get the provision right first time or the consequences can be very serious. Again, in many industries there is an acceptable fail rate: "98% is pretty good". In health and care, no level of quality failure can be acceptable. *"We usually perform this operation properly"* will not do. Nor will, *"We usually place our frail elderly clients in a suitable residential home"*. Therefore, services must be right first time and every time.

Costing no more that it must

Quality must include the notion of value for money. Darzi (2008) defines quality as Safe, effective and with good patient experience. This is taken up by the National Quality Board (2011). However, Services and products in all price brackets may achieve high quality. Anybody can deliver a high standard if money is no object. So, an additional factor, absent in Darzi's initial definition (2008) in quality must be that the standard is very good considering the cost (Erlendsson 2002) (Harvey & Green 1993). Conversely, if the standard is fixed, then quality may require the notion that the cost is no more than it needs to be. If a product is unnecessarily expensive for what the customer is getting, then the quality is poor. A quality product is therefore provided at the lowest possible price for a pre-defined standard.

If we allow a service to cost more that the absolute minimum possible, even if it carries charming extras, then that extra resource will not be available for other treatments. This is not good quality health or social care when seen in aggregate, because resources are wasted and therefore not available for other care events.

Therefore, a quality service in health and social; care may be defined as one that meets the client/clinician agreed need, first time every time, at the lowest possible price (Wheeler & Grice, 2000)

Quality Control

In industry, an acceptable standard is defined with reference to customer demands and any product not reaching that standard is scrapped before the sales stage. That is why every radio purchased has a label attached indicating where, when and by whom it was checked before dispatch. The quality control approach is acceptable in many industries because the cost of a failing percentage is lower than the cost of ensuring 100% success. In health care, such a quality control approach is not considered sufficient because the cost of any unnecessary failure is unacceptable (National Quality Board, 2011)

Quality Assurance

Quality assurance (QA) is a multi-stage, iterative process that sets, monitors, assures and continually improves standards (Swage, 2004). The stages in the process based on the meaning and definition of quality established above, become:

1) Ensure that the service really does address the agreed need of patient/client;
2) Define the standards to be achieved, according to Specific, Measurable, Achievable, Relevant and Timely (SMART) criteria;
3) Audit these standards and take measures to assure that they are always attained;
4) Improve the standards;
5) Evaluate the process.
4) As this is an iterative process, there is no requirement that it be initiated at 1), above. In fact, it may be initiated at any stage, and it is when the cycle has passed through a number of iterations that it is really effective.

The NHS and Social Care organisations are given a wide range of standards and quality targets and these are used as a measure of the success of the organisation.

In the true spirit of Quality Assurance, these would be intelligently used to rapidly improve performance rather than simply evaluate services. A particularly valuable example of this is the **CECOPS Code of Practice** (Donnelly, 2011) which identifies standards relating to disability equipment, wheelchairs and seating, procurement and provision. CECOPS standards are widely used by clinicians and service managers to examine and improve their provision of these crucial services. Adoption of the code allows accreditation of individuals, departments and organisations through which they are able to reassure themselves, their regulators and commissioners that they strive towards the highest possible standards. http://www.cecops.org.uk/

Total Quality Management

TQM is 'a management approach, based on the participation of all its members and aiming at long-term success through customer satisfaction, and benefits to all members of the organisation and to society CQI (2012).

Total Quality Management (TQM) is a development of QA, attempting to reinforce the responsibility of the individual for a satisfactory outcome. The QA process, above, is retained, but every individual is encouraged to have the outcome of the intervention paramount at all times (Swage 2004). It may be that simply meeting agreed standards is not sufficient and that the need for exceeding or adapting standards is evident from observation of the results. In TQM, employees are expected to follow the spirit of the standard, going beyond the letter of the standard where necessary and ensure the best affordable outcome. This is to correct the possibility that a focus upon adherence to standards and policies moves the focus away from idiosyncratic needs of patients. TQM prevents complacency where standards are attained but the service is self-evidently poor.

Case example: TQM

A family goes on holiday leaving the neighbour to water the prized plant. The standard is 1.5 Litres of water at 6.00pm every day. However, there is a heat-wave and the soil dries out more quickly than predicted. The QA focused standard is observed at 1.5 Litres per day and the plant dies of dehydration. A TQM approach would have explained the degree of moisture required in the soil or the general health of the plant and the neighbour could have adapted the watering volume to maintain moisture levels and plant health, thereby protecting the plant. In a TQM approach the neighbour is enabled to relate to the end-result, plant health, and understands the requirements for this. He/she can therefore adjust the process standard to assure this quality outcome.

Audit

Audit was learned from the accountancy discipline - checking that agreed financial procedures have been adhered to, that no impropriety has occurred and that resources are well used.

Although an impressive version of clinical audit was employed by Florence Nightingale, the discipline was first formally adopted clinically in the NHS by the medical profession in 1989. The white paper "Working for Patients" required "the systematic critical analysis of the quality of medical care including the procedures used for diagnosis and treatment, the use of resources and the resulting outcome and quality of life for the patient." (DoH,1998)

Almost immediately thereafter this was expanded to include all health and care professions. It involves examination of processes employed in health care to ensure that procedures are followed, standards achieved, no impropriety occurs, stakeholders are optimally treated and best value is obtained from the resources consumed. The auditing process may be self, peer or supervisory colleague, internal or external, informal or formal and formative or judgmental in its nature.

Audit procedures are iterative It is essential to close the loop by ensuring that lessons learned from an audit inform and directly influence future practice. That means that there must be a system to ensure that the findings of any quality audit are systematically fed back into a forum that can change practice in response to what is found.

The Audit Cycle

= Service provision = audit = results = improvement plan = service provision=
Benjamin, (2008) adds focus on criterion and measurement, offering:
=preparing for audit=selecting criteria=measuring performance level= making improvements; =sustaining improvement=preparing for audit=

Further detail and explanation are offered by the Dartford and Gravesham NHS Trust in a free download *www.dvh.nhs.uk/EasySiteWeb/GatewayLink.aspx?alId=107264*.

It is also possible to conduct a non-criterion, qualitative audit, without measuring standards, but asking questions in a semi structured interviews or focus groups with service providers and/or users. These may be deployed in an attempt to elicit unpredicted information. Findings may be evaluated at a later stage through a more quantitative criterion audit in order to assess generalizability.

Clinical Governance

Clinical Governance is a sharpening of the focus of quality management introduced as part of "The New NHS - Modern and Dependable" (DoH, 1998). This is further developed by the NHS's National Quality Board (2011). The development formalises, and makes statutory, quality management in a number of areas. These are:

More formalised clinical audit responsibilities. These are placed on NHS Trusts and Primary Care Trusts, who will have to initiate continuous quality improvement, recognition of all national standards, procedures for reporting concern about practice, etc. This is the personal responsibility of the Chief Executive Officer (CEO) of all NHS Trusts. Quality reports to the board of directors are required to be treated with the same rigor as financial reports.

Establishment of guidance to clinical best practice based upon sound evidence emerging from the Evidence Based Medicine (EBM) movement. The National Institute for Clinical Excellence (NICE) publishes this information and fosters research where the evidence is inadequate. Further guidance is promulgated in the form of a National Service Framework (NSF) for each area of NHS endeavour.

Establishment of more rigid protocols for the supervision of individuals by each profession. This is to give substance to the self-regulation of health and social care professions

The Practice

Quality Assurance & Total Quality Management

The best choice of provision

Identifying the choice of provision for patients/clients and other stakeholders is a multi-faceted exercise for a provider NHS Trust or one of its departments. The parties they must consult may be broadly divided into consumers (who use services) and customers (who pay for services). A service is meeting customer and consumer wishes when the wishes of all such as those listed below have been addressed. Consumers and customers might be categorised as below.

Customers	Consumers
Purchasing SHAs and PCGs	Patients/clients/service users
The employing NHS Trust or SS dep't.	Carers
Private sector purchasers e.g. BUPA	Family
Fee paying patients/clients	Referring clinicians
Other service providers.	Society
Society in general.	

Ascertaining wishes is uncomplicated where customers know how to explain themselves to service providers. Then, it is only necessary to make it clear to stakeholders that their views will be well received, explain where and when they can be conveyed. At an individual patient/client level, specifically asking each what they want to achieve from their intervention.

To redefine a service provided, as required by QA, pt/client expressions of demand have only to be aggregated, modified to reflect resource availability and professional expertise and the services can be delivered accordingly. It is possible to devise complex mechanisms to learn what patients/clients want, but initially ask articulate people what they would like.

Some interested parties listed above may not find it easy to articulate their demands. There are a number of devices to access stakeholder views. It is usual to employ a range of mechanisms in order to obtain a rich spectrum of information (triangulation). Some deliver a better response rate than others; some deliver richer information than others. A high response rate is preferred to ensure representativeness of respondents. If a low response rate is achieved, then there is a risk that those moved to respond have more extreme views than others. This is known as a self-selected sample, and is potentially. To base service decisions on this sample may be undesirable. For the opinions collected to be valid, the department needs to employ a variety of collection devices and maximise the response rate achieved by each.

Suggestion boxes

Strategically placed boxes will allow service users to make comments and suggestions as they occur. It is essential that everything is available for the suggestion to be made spontaneously, as good intentions to make a comment are lost very quickly. A pad of paper and a pen must always be near a suggestion box. Boxes must be placed cautiously so that while they attract attention they also allow respondent anonymity. Therefore, a box must be sited so that it is eye catching but allows contributions to be made without direct observation from staff. Emptying must be routine, not in response to a specific comment. Good siting and resourcing of a suggestion box will make a significant difference to the response rate. Notices calling for suggestions and comments are valuable, but have a very poor response rate because once the respondent has accessed writing materials, spontaneous good intentions to may have been lost. The best response rate is achieved if respondents have the wherewithal to comment when issues are fresh and time is on their hands, e.g. in waiting rooms. The respondent using a suggestion box is a self-selected sample but the consequent bias is diminished if the box is very easy to use and the response rate is maximised. The measures described above to improve response rate will therefore also improve the representative nature of the comments made.

Suggestion boxes are the focus of hoax and "humorous" comment and this is often cited as a reason not to provide them. However, these comments take little time to deal with and the serious information gained has the great advantage of immediacy. As soon as an idea arises whereby the service might be improved, the respondent has the opportunity to report it. Any delay will risk their forgetting or losing resolve.

Questionnaires

Before, during and after intervention questionnaires offer the patient, client, carer, etc the opportunity to say exactly what service would be/have been preferable. The questionnaire may be closed, having questions needing yes/no answers or answers chosen from a pre-set choice of answers, or open, allowing the respondent to express their opinion in their own words. Closed questions in a questionnaire give quantitative information that is easy to collate and from which it is possible to draw conclusions that may be cautiously generalised to the whole population. Open questions give qualitative data that may be more informative and allow scope for unexpected responses. However, the conclusion drawn from closed questions cannot easily be so easily generalised to the whole population. Service quality questionnaires, therefore, need to be a mixture of open and closed style. A combination of open and closed questionnaires gives a range of information. The two types may be combined in one of two ways. Open -> Closed: Open questions are asked of a small population in order to establish the agenda, followed by closed questions to a larger sample to ascertain how many people share the views expressed. Closed -> Open: Closed questions establish the frequent areas of concern to respondents and open questions are then asked of a small number of respondents to better understand those issues identified as important. For detailed guidance on constructing a questionnaire, see "The management of Information"

Interviews

Patients, clients and other interested parties may be interviewed before during or after treatment. Interviews have the advantage of a very high response rate, few people refuse, and are therefore a more representative sample is achieved. Even if the sample number is low, as long as selection is randomised or purposive, the results will be valid if the rate of co-operation by approached respondents is high. In order to assure validity, however, it is necessary to ensure that a high proportion of those approached do agree to the process. If the interviewer simply keeps approaching respondents until a target, number is achieved, but the refusal rate is high, then the results will be potentially skewed. That is because those who responded are a self-selected group and may be willing to answer because they have extreme views.

Interviews may be to collect quantitative data, based upon closed questions, or quantitative, based upon open questions. It is usual practice to include closed questions followed by open questions, in order to satisfy the need for a range of data types, and to ease the frustration felt by respondents if faced with a string of closed questions. Interviewing is an expensive exercise and will therefore be used sparingly as a part of a broad strategy. For detailed guidance on constructing a interviews, see "The management of Information"

Focus groups

Respondents may offer richer information, if allowed to discuss the chosen issues in a small group. The patient who tells the interviewer, "Nurse was wonderful. They are all so kind" might be more willing to identify areas that could be improved if sat in a small group, with tea, to generally talk about the care given in the presence of an interviewer. Some focus groups involve the researcher simply making notes of the conversation as an observer or a participant observer, or they may go further and ask the group to form a consensus statement about possible improvements to the service. Conclusions of a focus group might usefully be checked out through a questionnaire to the whole population or, at the least, a representative sample. For detailed guidance on conducting focus group investigations.

Consultation meetings

Some interested parties, such as referring clinicians are difficult to consult. However, it is dangerous to assume that their collective view is understood, or that the views of a vociferous minority are representative of the majority. Such parties might usefully be canvassed in meetings for that purpose. These may, or may not take the form of a focus group. It is important to know your audience. In each locality and for each profession, there will be a different method recommended for gaining co-operation in this endeavour. You are advised to approach senior members of your target group and discover the best way to canvas their views about the service that you provide. There can be a temptation to entice an audience with gifts and meals etc. However, although hospitality may be in order, you want your audience to recognise that this is an opportunity to influence your service to their advantage. This should be the motive for co-operation and a free meal should not be allowed to obscure that point.

Writing standards

Having established the service most favoured by your stakeholders and moderated this with your knowledge of your service's capabilities, you must set the standards that are acceptable and affordable. This exercise is a team exercise. Standards should be owned by all stakeholders. This will include service deliveries from all professions and non-professions, users, commissioners, etc. These must be explicit and precise. Your standards have to be written in a language that allows for no ambiguity in their auditing. This is a four-stage process: Aim, Measure, Criterion and Quality standard (Wheeler& Grice, 2000).

1) State the overall aim of the standard. This is a clear statement of what is to be achieved. Example Aim "To ensure good note keeping"

2) Chose the measure to be employed. What scale is to be employed? Example of scale: "Frequency of entry on patient records"

3) Set the criterion. What score is required? Example criterion: "After every treatment"

4) Write the Quality Standard: "There will be an entry made in the case notes after every treatment session."

The standard is reached through a four-stage sequential process. Although it might be possible, in this example to write the standard without the stages 1 – 3, the process makes the standard more comprehensible. In areas that are more complex, the process may be essential to ensure that a representative standard is achieved.

The standard is Specific, Measurable, Achievable, Relevant and Time bound (SMART) (Druker, 1954). It is helpful to apply this SMART test to any standard in order to ensure that it addressed the right area and is subject to unambiguous audit.

Specific

A specific standard specifies precisely to what it references. Exactly what will be achieved?

Eg *improve timekeeping* is not specific. *Arrive at all meetings at least of 5-mins before the start* is Specific.

Measurable

A measurable standard is one that you feel you will have no difficulty in scoring, and to which any observer would award the same score. It is important to avoid words, such as "appropriate", that are subjective in their interpretation. If the standard was to require that content be appropriate the notion might be sensible, but the evaluation would be entirely subjective. As such, it could not be measured and earn a score upon which all would agree.

Achievable

A standard must be achievable. However, when setting a standard it is important that it stretches the service provider to achieve best quality possible. An excessively high standard will soon be abandoned as a lost cause and a low standard will be achieved without effort. Writing a standard, therefore, involves a balancing act so that the standard drives performance as high as possible, but is achievable.

Relevant

Standards must be demonstrably relevant to the service involved and, further, must be the most important area possible, allowing that not all areas can be addressed at on time. Ideally the standards set will map against the service objectives.

Time bound

It is essential to know by when an achievement will be made. If the time allowed for achievement is not stated, then there can be no audit point at which compliance or failure may be evaluated.

Detail

The above standard was:

> "There will be an entry made in the case notes after every treatment session."

This would ensure that you as a clinician write up records at what you consider the appropriate times. It might appear that this does not ensure that the record made is a satisfactory one. The clinician could perhaps write gibberish and yet meet the standard. You might consider a second standard defining the content of the record. However, it is unlikely that you as a qualified health or care professional will write rubbish in the case record. What is possible and even probable is that time pressure might lead you to put off writing notes until later, and in reality never get around to it. The standard suggested above would suffice if it were accepted that when clinicians are sat down in front of the case notes they will write appropriately. The risk that you will fail to write at all is addressed by the standard, and the risk of poor writing is too small to require policing. If nothing is left to trust, then the quality standard list will be very long and a very big rule book will be devised that is very unlikely to be read and followed. This is an example of TQM, where the spirit is clear and some discretion is permitted, rather than QA or QC where everything is defined and the intellect of the individual is not exploited.

By writing a small number of key standards *(performance indicators)*, a great deal can be achieved at an acceptable cost. There is a cost to writing, achieving and auditing quality standards. The resource put into this exercise must be justified by results in terms of improved quality of services. A number of key standards may be seen to be cost effective, but there will come a point where your exercise becomes bureaucratic and costs more than it delivers. Thus, you may feel that a standard ensuring note writing is justified where a string of standards dictating content is unproductive for a qualified health or care professional.

Example Quality Statements:

Aim (To ensure…)	Measure	Criterion	Quality Standard
good note keeping	Frequency of entry on patient records	After every treatment	There will be an entry made in the case notes after every treatment session
prompt handling of telephone enquiries	Number of rings	Four	The telephone will be answered during the first four rings
patients are interviewed promptly	Time from admission to interview	One day (working)	All newly admitted patients will be interviewed within one working day of admission
client/patient privacy	Availability of private place	Available & offered	A private place is available for all initial interviews and this is offered to all patients

In some areas, 100% achievement of the target score may be impossible. In these cases, a standard might be expressed in terms of a target score and secondarily, a target for the % of patients for whom this target will be achieved.

Patient satisfaction	Scale of 0 - 10	8	90% of patients score 8/10 on a self-rating satisfaction scale.

Auditing standards

You audit your standards in order to evaluate the success with which they are being achieved and to inform your planning for future services. There are a number of approaches to audit.

Schedule

Audit may be:

a) Continuous, in which case all standards are audited continually,
b) Random, in which case standards are selected randomly and then audited,
c) Focused, in which case an area is selected for special attention for a particular period of time, and audited in detail.
d) Retrospective audit, involving examination of records and other evidence of quality.

Continuous audit is expensive but guarantees compliance with standards. It may be adopted in areas where the consequences of any failure are unacceptable. The "Care Plan Approach" required by government as part of discharge from a mental health hospital, might be subject to continuous audit as may the procedures in an operating theatre.

A random audit is less expensive and yet all practitioners are aware that any of their standards might be scrutinised at the next audit cycle. This will inevitably focus the mind on high level achievement. The results may be generalised, resulting in a statement about quality that could be taken as an indicator of achievement throughout the organisation. The validity of any generalisation will depend on the number of standards audited and their representativeness within the organisation. Random audit may be conducted at any interval. It is common for a service to randomly select an area for audit every month.

Focused audit is used in an attempt to improve performance in a chosen, critical area. Repeated, detailed attention through several audit cycles rapidly improves the achievement of standards. When the area has achieved a performance plateau, then the focus is moved onto another area. This has the advantage of focusing the energy and resources of audit onto one area that is considered most in need of development. This may be a most efficient use of resources. However, the results are not generalizable, because the audited individuals were aware of the area of interest and would have paid particular attention to it.

A retrospective audit may be random or focused and can involve examination of evidence from a variety of quantitative and qualitative sources.

The Auditor

Audit is a great gift. There is little you want at work more than to do a very good job. An auditor looks at your work and suggests ways for you to be better. This is exactly what you want and a generous gift of the auditor's time. However, rarely is this the feeling that audit evokes. In some part, this is because the wrong auditor is used for the situation.

Your audit may be carried out by all of the following:

a) **Self**. You should monitor achievement of standards and ensure maximum performance at all times. This is intrinsically beneficial and ensures no surprises in the event of an external audit.

b) **Peer**. You can ask non-supervisory colleagues to check your standard compliance. This has the advantage of offering a critical audit without fear of penalty for failure thus enabling free and open scrutiny.

c) **Supervisor**. Your line manager might examine achievement of standards as a part of the supervisory process. This would, ideally, be conducted in an attempt to assist you to achieve the very best cost effective standards of service. If it is seen as a disciplinary scrutiny, then you will be less open to improvement through this route.

d) **Internal auditors**. Your organisation might employ auditors who have access to all work areas who periodically produce reports of achievement for the benefit of departmental managers, customers and senior management. Again, this will be a more productive exercise if it is conducted as a means to help individuals to continually improve rather than as a policing exercise.

e) **External auditors**. The NHS Purchaser, the Social Services Inspectorate and the DoH, etc employ auditors who can examine any aspect of care and report on the standards achieved.

f) **The Audit Commission**. The Audit Commission is a national body with the remit of auditing all aspects of public sector activity. Much of their audit focuses on the proper use of money, but they also report on value for money spent and can comment on quality standards.

You are recommended to employ all of these auditors in a mixed strategy. Your standards are of paramount importance to you, above all others. Consistent good practice is your ticket to success, promotion, etc, and you should take every opportunity to gain feedback and ideas for improvement about your practice. Every comment is an opportunity to improve, and every improvement is to your advantage. Therefore audit of your work is in your interest. Others will wish to audit you as well, but although this might appear threatening you should recognise that you also want these results and support the process as far as possible. External audit is an opportunity to improve your service, and thereby remain in employment/business.

Non-criterion audit. It is also useful to obtain free-wheeling feedback and observation about your service. This will not relate to any set standard, but offer general observations about how the service might better serve the client.

Case Example

> A patient satisfaction interview asks a long list of questions, such as 'Did the staff call you by your preferred name?
> At the end of the interview answers can be aggregated and an impressive report written.
> However, the interview never discovers that the patient is dehydrated being repeatedly given tea on a side of the bed which she cannot reach.
> Non-criteria audit would discover this very quickly.

Improving Standards

Whatever the type, frequency or means of audit it is essential that the results are used to effect change in future performance. Therefore it is essential that a systematic, iterative loop feeds audit findings into the provision and management of services. An ideal audit mechanism has this feedback as an automatic process. For example, the Performance Related Payment (PRP) for a manager might be directly linked to audit results. This will ensure that all managers closely monitor results and make improvements immediately a poor result is known. These mechanisms should feed results into any forum that can effect improvement. The primary focus in this is the individual clinician who is delivering the service. Feeding results back to this individual allow him/her to act for continuous improvement. Some service improvements require management action and consequently the audit results should appear at relevant management meetings. It is important that action plans are always made in response to audit reports and that the usual protocols of "Matters Arising from the Previous Meeting" are employed to ensure that planed action is carried out. It is not enough for an audit report to be made to the Board of Directors if it is to be welcomed and commended, but not acted upon.

A broader audit may, also, be carried out to collect information about the service going beyond simple compliance with standards. Such an audit might consult staff, customers and consumers about services in general or may ask questions about value achieved for money. Auditors may seek to make comparisons with other service providers making general enquiries or applying national standards resulting in a benchmark that shows how an organisation lies on a nation-wide spectrum ranging from poor to excellent.

Evaluate the process

Audit of the service may itself be audited. An analysis might be made of the appropriateness of the standards adopted and the extent to which they are owned by employees and valued by patients/clients. Examination should be made of the representativeness and rigour of the audit mechanism. Special attention will be made of the extent to which the findings from each audit exercise are used to improve performance. This is known as closing the audit loop. Assessment of the process would involve following an audit trail. This would involve assurance that the conclusion from an audit was thoroughly examined. There should be clear plans made for improvement, perhaps at a management meeting, and there should be clear evidence of the implementation of the plans with evaluation of the effectiveness of this implementation. This examination of the audit process should result in continuous improvement.

Some external auditors will be adequately reassured by the presence of a valid and robust internal audit system, with clear audit trails, thus negating the need for external audit. For example, it is common for DHAs to audit the audit procedures of NHS Trusts rather than the quality standards themselves. If the audit procedures are believed to be robust, audit loops are closed, then Trusts' audit results might satisfy purchaser enquiries into the quality of the services provided.

Quality Circles

A number of people with a shared interest in an aspect of quality but with different skills, may come together to consider possibilities for quality improvement. These groups may be called quality circles quality improvement teams etc. They may be set up for long or short-term operation. The performance of a Quality Circle is similar to a focus group It is important that they take a creative approach to the area under discussion and build upon the ideas expressed by one-another until an optimum proposition is arrived at. This may be achieved in a small number of meetings or in a standing committee may exploit the creative ideas occurring to participants on long journeys, on holiday, in the bath, etc. The group may conduct a brainstorm exercise in which ideas of tangential relevance to the subject are shared and participants build upon peer suggestions until a creative way forward is achieved.

It is important for quality circles to employ a creative, divergent thinking phase in their deliberations before converging onto a "Solution". There is often benefit in examining quite impractical solutions in order to draw out useful lessons for application.

Quality Circle Case example

A group of hospital staff formed a short duration quality circle to consider their very poor waiting facilities. Initially, convergent, problem-solving techniques said that they should improve the décor, the seating, the quality of reading material, etc. Although valuable, all of these solutions would be expensive to implement, and would have only limited benefit. A divergent thinking phase was introduced. What was the best experience they could quote of good waiting facilities? They quickly agreed that one such was the airport lounge, where passengers wait for, on average, two hours and rarely express distress. Hospital patients express dissatisfaction if kept waiting for ½ hour. Initially, team members felt reservations about the lessons that could be learned from that source. The hospital could not replicate the happiness of anticipated holidays, or the excitement of an atmosphere filled with Jumbo Jets. Therefore they thought that could learn little from considering an airport lounge. However, there were many factors at work in the airport lounge.

Customers in an airport do not sit and wait in one place for several hours. They spend a short time in one lounge and are then called to check-in after which they can move to another lounge. They spend time here and then they are called to a departure lounge. From here, they move to another lounge where they embark on the aeroplane. This process of movement gives the customer the feeling of progress. Sitting in a hospital waiting room denies any feeling of progress, which causes unnecessary distress.

Customers in an airport are given clear information about the time, for which they will wait, and they adjust accordingly. They engage in other activities commensurate with the time that they know they have to spend. Even when the delay time alters, appropriate information is given to customers and they adjust their expectations again. Hospital patients are simply asked to sit, and often have no information about whether they will be ten minutes or several hours. When they ask receptionists, "How much longer?" the receptionist is rarely in a position to answer, and may be too overburdened to find out. This can cause more irritation in the waiting room.

Customers in an airport have the opportunity to browse shops and spend money. This is possible because the facilities exist, and they know how long they have to wait. In hospital, little is available near the waiting rooms and patients will not visit the shops that do exist for fear of missing the call when it comes.

This conversation lasted for less than two hours and lead to three improvements that with minimal financial outlay improved the patient experience dramatically. The waiting rooms were made sequential. Patients on reception were directed to the first waiting room area. The nurse weighed them and they returned to a different part of the waiting room, they underwent a clerking process and returned to another part of the waiting area, from where they were called by the Consultant. Throughout this experience they knew how long they had to wait because they had a fixed appointment time and although clinics generally ran late, the delay was known and shown on a blackboard. Thus, patients could calculate the time when they would be seen. I.e.: 10.20 appointment; clinic running 45 minutes late; patient expects to be seen at 11.05. It was preferred that patients did not wonder off to shops, so vendors were given shelf space in the waiting areas, and self-funding diversion was thus provided.

Interestingly, these devices benefiting the airport were not a result of airport staff ingenuity. Rather they were essential actions making management of travellers possible. It was largely fortuitous that they improved customer satisfaction. However, when transferred to a hospital setting, they were exclusively for the achievement of customer comfort. This exercise was highly successful. Dissatisfaction because of waiting facilities reduced significantly and there were almost no cost implications.

Conclusion

Quality in Health and Social Care is dictated by those who deliver services. The appointment of a Director of Quality or a quality minded manager may assist in this process, but good or bad service is the responsibility of the clinician. It is essential for you to set the highest standards commensurate with patient/client numbers, have a robust means of assuring those standards and seek to constantly improve what is done. Always look for creative changes that will improve standards in your black-spots and ensure that quality audit is transparent and directly linked to your planning processes. Be open to feedback and audit wherever you can get it. That will enable you to continually improve. The excellence you will achieve is the best possible route to recognition, promotion and job security.

References

Appleby, J. (1995) *Acting on the evidence: a review of clinical effectiveness : sources of information.* Birmingham: NAHAT.

Baker,R., Lakhani, M., Fraser, R., & Cheater, F.(1999) A model for clinical governance in primary care groups *BMJ* 318: 779-783.

Benjamin, A. (2008) Audit: how to do it. *BMJ* 336:1241

Car, D., & Steutel, J. (1999) *Virtue Ethics* London: Routledge

Care Quality Commission Available at: *http://www.cqc.org.uk/national-standards* [Accessed on 05/04/14]

Cleaner workplaces (2014) 7 lean principles *www.kcprofessional.co.uk/lean-e-book (Free to download)*

College of Occupational Therapists (2010) *Code of Ethics and Professional Conduct.* London: COT

College of Occupational Therapists (2011) *The Professional Standards for Occupational Therapy Practice.* London: COT

CQI (2010) *The Chartered Quality Initiative.* http://www.thecqi.org/

Crawford, P. & Brown, B. (2008) Mental health communication between service users and professionals: disseminating practice-congruent research. *Mental Health Review Journal,* 14 (3), 31-39

Dartford and Gravesham NHS Trust (2010) www.dvh.nhs.uk/EasySiteWeb/GatewayLink.aspx?alId=107264.

Darzi (2008) *High quality care for all: NHS Next Stage Review final report.* London: HMSO

Dewar, S. (1999). - Clinical governance under construction: problems of design and difficulties. *http://guekufanb.ru/xugejib.pdf*

Dickens, P. (1994) *Quality and excellence in human services.* Chichester: Wiley

DoH (2004) *The NHS Knowledge and Skills Framework and the Development Review Process. Final Version.* London: DoH

DoH (2008) *High quality care for all: NHS Next Stage Review final report.* DoH. London.

DoH (2008) *Refocusing the Care Programme Approach: Policy and positive practice guidance.* Available at: www.dh.gov.uk/publications (Accessed on 13/04/14).

DoH (2010) *Preceptorship framework for newly registered nurse, midwives and allied health professionals.* London: DoH

DoH (2012 a) *The NHS Constitution* London: HMSO

DoH (2012b). *Compassion in Practice, Nursing, Midwifery and Care Staff Our Vision and Strategy.* Available at: http://www.england.nhs.uk/wp-content/uploads/2012/12/compassion-in-practice.pdf [Accessed 05/04/14]

DoH (2012c) *The handbook to the NHS Constitution* London: HMSO

DoH (2013) *Quality in the new health system: maintaining and improving quality* London: DoH

DoH: Commissioning Board Chief Nursing Officer and DH Chief Nursing Adviser (2012) *Compassion in Practice.* Available at: *http://www.england.nhs.uk/wp-content/uploads/2012/12/compassion-in-practice.pdf* (Accessed on 24/04/14).

Donabedian, A. (1980) *The definition of quality: A conceptual exploration.* Michigan: Health Administration Press

Donabedian, A. (2003) *An Introduction to Quality Assurance in Health Care.* Oxford: Oxford University Press.

Donabedian, A. (2005). "Evaluating the quality of medical care. 1966.". *The Milbank quarterly* 83 (4): 691–729.

Donnelly,.B. *Code of Practice for Community Equipment* Buckinghamshire: CES, Ltd.

Drucker, P. (2011) *The Practice of Management,* New York:Harper & Row.

Drucker, P. (1973) *Management Tasks, Responsibilities, Practices,* New York:Harper & Row.

Einthoven, A. C. (1985) *Reflections on the management of the NHS* London: Nuffield Provincial Hospitals Trust

Ellis, J. (2006). All-inclusive benchmarking. *Journal of Nursing Management*; 14(5) pp.377-83.

Ellis, R. (Ed) (1989) *Professional competence and quality assurance in the caring professions* London : Croom Helm. (This edited text contains very enlightening case studies from various health professions. Although the debate has moved forward since 1988, with the advent of Clinical Governance, the principles of quality assurance and their place in professional practice remain relevant and the cases are instructional.)

Erlendsson, J. (2002), Value For Money Studies in Higher Education *http://www.hi.is/~joner/eaps/wh_vfmhe.htm,*

Francis, R. (2013). *Report of the Mid Staffordshire NHS Foundation Trust Public Inquiry.* London: HMSO

Fryer, K., Antony, J. and Douglas, P. (2007) Critical success factors of continuous improvement in the public sector. *The TQM Journal,* 19(5), 497-517

Garvin, D.A. (2012) "Competing on the eight dimensions of quality". Harvard Business review. 1987.

Garvin, D. D. (1988) *Managing quality: The strategic and competitive edge.* New York: Free Press

Garvin, D. A. (1984) What Does 'Product Quality' Really Mean? *MIT Sloan Management Review* 26, (1) 23-29

Gotttwald, M., and Lansdown, G. E. (2014) *Clinical Governance: Improving the quality of healthcare for patients and service users.* Berkshire: OUP

Griffiths, R. (1984) *NHS Management enquiry.* London HMS

Handy, C. (1993) Understanding Organizations. London: Penguin Books

Harvey, L. and Green, D., 1993, 'Defining quality', *Assessment and Evaluation in Higher Education*, 18(1). 9–34

Health and Care Professions Council (2013) *Standards of Proficiency: Occupational Therapists.* Available at: *www.hpc-uk.org/assets/documents/*

10000512Standards_of_Proficiency_ Occupational_Therapists.pdf (accessed 29/7/14)

Iles, V. (2006) *Really Managing Health Care.* 2nd Ed. Berkshire: OUP

Leggat, S. (2007) Effective Healthcare Teams Require Effective Team Members: Defining Teamwork Competencies. *BMC Health Services Research.* 7 (17).London : King's Fund.

Lugon, M., & Secker-Walker, J.(1999) (Eds) *Clinical Governance: Making it Happen* Royal Society of Medicine Press.

Maxwell, R. J. (1984). Quality assessment in health. *British Medical Journal,* 288: 1470-1472

McSherry, R. & Pearce, P. (2007) *Clinical governance: A guide to implementation for healthcare professionals.* 2nd ed. Oxford: Blackwell Publishing

McSherry, R. and Pearce, P. (2011) *Clinical Governance.* Wiley-Blackwell (Location?)

Mickan, S., Rodger, S. (2005). Effective health care teams: a model of six characteristics developed from shared perceptions. *Journal of Interprofessional Care*, 19(4):358-70

National Institute for Health and Clinical Excellence (2006) *Violence: The short-term management of disturbed/violent behaviour in in-patient psychiatric settings and emergency departments.* London: Royal College of Nursing

National Quality Board (2011) *Quality Governance in the NHS - A guide for provider boards* London: HMSO

NMC (2008) *The Code: Standards of Conduct, Performance and Ethics for Nurses and Midwives.* London: Nursing and Midwifery Council.

NPSA (2004) *Seven Steps to Patient Safety - Your Guide to Safer Patient Care.* The National Patient Safety Agency. London.

O' Hagan, K. (2001) *Cultural Competence in the caring professions.* Jessica Kingsley, London.

Øvertveit, J. (1992) *Health service quality:An introduction to quality methods for health services*. Oxford: Blackwell Scientific Publications

Papadopoulos, I. (2003) The Papadopoulos, Tilki and Taylor model for the development of cultural competence in nursing. *Journal of Health, Social and Environmental Issues* 4 (1), 5-7

Parsley ,K., & Corrigan, P. (1994) *Quality improvement in nursing and healthcare : a practical approach* London : Chapman & Hall.

Parsley, K., & Corrigan, P. (1998). - *Quality improvement in healthcare: putting evidence into practice* Cheltenham : Stanley Thornes.

Peters, T. J., & Waterman, R. H. (1982) *In search of excellence: Lessons from America's best-run companies.* London: Harper Row

Peters, T. J. (1985) *A passion for excellence: the leadership difference* London: Collins,

QAA (2001). *Benchmark statement: Health care programmes*. The Quality Assurance Agency for Higher Education. Gloucester

Quality Assurance Agency for Higher Education (2001) *Benchmark statement: Health Care Programmes - Occupational Therapists.*

Quality Assurance Agency for Higher Education (QAA) (2001) *Subject Benchmark Statements: Healthcare Programmes.* Gloucester: The Quality Assurance Agency for Higher Education.

RCN (1987) *Nursing quality measurement: quality assurance methods for peer review* Chichester : Wiley.

RCN (1998) *Guidance for nurses on clinical governance* RCN London. This makes a good introduction to the mechanics of CG, intended for Nurses and Midwives, but proving very valuable for all health professionals.

Reile, R. (1987) *Evaluation of therapeutic recreation through quality assurance* London: Venture Publishing,

Sainsbury Centre for Mental Health (2000) *Taking your Partners: Using opportunities for inter-agency partnership in mental health.* London: Sainsbury Centre for Mental Health

Shaw, C. D. (1986) *Introducing quality assurance.* London: King's Fund

Simmons, P., Hawley, C., Gale, T., and Sivakumaran, A. (2010) Service user, patient, client, user or survivor: describing recipients of mental health services. *The Psychiatrist.* 34, 20-23.

Sinha, M. N., and Willborn, W. W. O. (1985). *The management of quality assurance* New York; Chichester: Wiley,

Swage, T. (2004) *Clinical Governance in Health Care Practice.* 2nd Ed. Edinburgh: Butterworth-Heinemann

The Quality Assurance Agency (QAA) (2006) *Benchmark Statement: Healthcare Programmes*

Timmins, F. (2007) Communication skills: revisiting the fundamentals. *Nurse Prescribing*, 5: 395–9

Walshe, K., and Ham, C. (1997). *Acting on the evidence: progress in the NHS:* HSMC, University of Birmingham

Ward, S. (2006) *Lean thinking* Health services Review.14(6) p12

Wells, M. I. (2000) beyond cultural competence: a model for individual and institutional cultural development, *Journal for Community Health Nursing,* 17, 287-296

Wheeler, N., and Grice, D. (2000) *Management in Health Care.* Cheltenham: Stanley Thornes

WHO (1982) *Quality assurance in diagnostic radiology* Geneva: World Health Organisation,

WHO (2007). *Communication During Patient Hand-Overs.* Geneva: World Health Organization.

Zoucha, R. (2000) Critical care extra: the keys to culturally sensitive care, *American Journal of Nursing,* 100(2) 24GG-24II

Managing Change

Introduction

The UK NHS has changed steadily since its inception in 1947 (Nuffield Trust, 2014). Successful management in this arena requires the successful management of change (Parkin, 2009). For that reason, the management of change is given close attention in this text. The chapter analyses and collates published comment and research and draws conclusions. This understanding will enable the reader to become an effective manager of change. Insight into the processes of change are generally considered to be necessary for a change agent as a formulaic approach is not always sufficient. However, the reader wishing to simply refer to "what to do" will find ample instruction in "The Practice".

This is a critical review of the literature collating material and identifying and evaluating emergent themes that may prove helpful to the clinician or health care manager and the management of human resources in change.

Inertia in enormous organisations such as the NHS is well described by writers from March and Simon (1958) to Pettigrew (2003) and effecting change takes a strong, active management action. There many sources of guidance to the management of change and these, although divergent, have a number of common features. These commonalties are examined and discussed in this thematic, critical review of the literature.

Many writers on change seek to describe a model which enables those involved to: predict the future, control the present and make sense of what is occurring. (Hogan 1997)

The discipline of Organisational Development (OD) suggests formulaic actions that may aid in change. OD may be described as being based in rationalism, pragmatism or existentialism. Rationalism and pragmatism based approaches allow for a degree of formulaic recipe exercised within an organisation to aid change (Freidlander 1976) (Dalin, 2004). Existentialism suggests a great reliance on individuality, context and environment, with the consequence that managing change is a far more intricate and difficult process. A post-modern approach to management theory might say that formulaic change paths seen in isolation could offer little of value. Pettigrew (2009), without abandoning the notion that good management practice is important in change, argues that change in organisations is a consequence of contextual pressures more than internal action and in many cases occurs with a significant fortuitous component.

There emerges, a diverse spread of views about the ability of managers and management consultants to control change. Buchanan (1997) studying change in Business Process Reengineering (BPR) in the hospital arena concluded that BPR might not be as context sensitive as has been recently claimed so that local drives can be very effective in changing an organisation. At the other extreme end of an emergent "formula - no formula" continuum, White and Jacques (1995) suggest that application of post-modern theories of organisational behaviour to a post-industrial community must cast doubt, almost by definition, on the validity of any business organisational theory. Taking a middle-way, Mabey and Mayon-White (1993) write that an approach to change management based upon a recipe of necessary and sufficient ingredients will fail because it can never take adequate account of the individuality of people, organisations and their external environment. However, they comment, certain process elements can be identified as necessary ingredients for successful management of change. This chapter identifies and explores those *necessary but not sufficient* elements that are relevant to health and care management.

In considering this subject, it is necessary to recognise that the UK NHS, and to a lesser extend social services departments, are not typical of UK industry for a number of reasons. Two particular idiosyncrasies are the absence of a profit motive, and the indistinct line relationships between managers and senior clinicians (Ham, 2009). The notions of clinical freedom and hegemonic control enjoyed by the medical profession described by Crozier (1976) (Ham, 2009) illuminate the limitations of line managerial control over medical and other health and care practitioners. For these reasons, it may be the case that approaches to change management devised for traditional industries need to be modified in order to be effective in this setting.

The Nature of Change

The nature, as well as the rate, of change has radically altered in the past two to three decades.

Thirty years ago, the company saw the future as predictable...more of the same only better . (Handy 1995 p5).

The altered nature of contemporary change is arguably more significant than the increased rate of change.

Incremental change suddenly becomes discontinuous change (Handy 1995 p7).

It is *discontinuous* change that is at work in modern industry in order to lift organisations out of their old tramlines and onto wholly new paths. Certainly, it is discontinuous change has been evident in the United Kingdom (UK) National Health Service (NHS), particularly exampled in the NHS and Community Care Act (DoH 1990). Subsequence reforms such as The NHS, Modern and Dependable (DoH, 1997), The H&S

Care act, 2001), Equity and Excellence (DoH, 2010) enhanced and redirected the structure created in 1990, claiming further discontinuous changes, although there is arguably as much reshaping as discontinuous remodelling.

Burnes (2009) describes the replacement of planned change, first defined by Lewin in 1958, by *emergent* change which is perpetual, open ended and not predictable and therefore not amenable to incremental planning as a continuous sequence. In agreement with Handy (1995), Burnes is describing emergent change as taking the organisation away from the route that continuous change would have devised.

A string of incremental, planned changes were made to the NHS since its origins in the NHS Act of 1947 (DoH 1947). These include the NHS (Amendment) Act 1949 (DoH 1949), the NHS Act 1951 (DoH 1951), the NHS Act 1952 (DoH 1952), the NHS Reorganisation Act 1973 (DoH 1973) and the NHS Reorganisation 1982 (DoH 1982). All of these changes sought to provide more and better patient treatment, through streamlining and decentralising responsibility, while reinforcing central accountability. These changes did not, however, alter the fundamental way in which health care was managed.

The NHS & Community Care Act in (1990) may be seen as the first emergent or discontinuous change, since it saw a total revision in the administration and management of health care. This was moving the service away from its forty-four-year-old *line management* tramlines onto the completely new ground of management by *market place economic forces*. This is a good example of the process described by Johnson

> *Typically, organisations go through long periods where strategies appear to be developed incrementally. There occur infrequently*

more fundamental shifts in strategy as major readjustment of the strategic direction of the firm takes place. (Johnson 1993 p60)

The movement between steady progression and periodic radical change is explained by Johnson (1993) as a consequence of strategic drift. Strategy exists as part of a cultural history and the inevitable drift leads to a periodic major strategic redirection that needs a dramatic unfreezing in order to occur. This redirection becomes a far more frequent experience in the context of current fast developing environment.

Pettigrew, Ferlie and McKee (1992) in their study of the effect on the pace of change of general management following the NHS Reorganisation (1982) found that there was substantial acceleration of pace of change in the NHS by the late 1980s. They also report that institutions may be intentionally transformed through the process of radical shock. The Thatcher experiment, they comment, may be considered an example of radical shock. In this they are suggesting that in addition to a radical redirection of strategy and management, there may have been a deliberate intent to shock the organisation throughout in order to facilitate unfreezing, described below (Lewin 1951), rethinking and redirection. This notion is supported by the literature and promotional media appearances in which both the Prime Minister and Secretary of State for Health repeatedly described the reforms as:

"Effecting root and branch changes to the NHS" (DoH 1989a).

Thus, rather than reassuring employees, there was an intent to maximise the perceived affect on individuals and thereby, perhaps, to prepare them to radically change working practices.

A New NHS - Modern and Dependable (DoH, 1997), the NHS reorganisation: the Health and Social Care (Community Health and Standards) Act (DoH, 2003) and then The White Paper, Equity and excellence: Liberating the NHS (2010) leading to Health and Social Care Bill (2012) have all endeavoured to present as further discontinuous change. This is in line with the needs of any new government. However each might equally be interpreted as progressing and refining the 1990 Act. Claims to abolish the marketplace are difficult to support as long as a commissioner/provider separation remains. Changes have been made to nomenclature, as PCTs become CCGs and SHAs become regional and local offices of the NHS England, but the functions although refined and improved retain many of the same functions.

The NHS will inevitable change and the rate of change will not slow, so that managers and clinicians need the ability to ride the whirlwind (Benton, 1990) and thrive on chaos (Peters, 1991) in an age of unreason (Handy, 2002). Players must not expect it to settle down, but must work effectively in a world of change. The following insights may help.

The Theoretical framework

The process of effectively bringing about change in the behaviour of people has been contemplated and researched for a very long period, with a great volume of important published work. This study considers publications from 1951, which saw the publication of Kurt Lewin's "Field Theory". Change management theory generally requires that a number of components be in place. Each is well described by commentators and to varying degrees tested by empirical examination. Empirical research in this field is predominantly of a case study nature, since there is limited opportunity or demand for controlled experiment in changing large organisations. Even the Hawthorn Studies which could be described loosely as a longitudinal: A-B-A-B design emerged as a fortuitous case study and one having limited participant numbers with questionable methodology (Gale, 2004).

Studies reported tend to be either cross sectional or longitudinal. Cross sectional studies compare different management units, inferring relationships between inputs and outcomes, which may or may not be causal (Bell, 2010). Further, it is impossible to eliminate the effect of individual idiosyncrasies and external factors. Any relationships demonstrated cannot be assigned certain causality (Easterby-Smith, Thorpe and Lowe 1991). Longitudinal studies, focusing on small samples over a long period, seek to use time series data to unearth the complex patterns that explain organisational behaviour. This process does not compare the wide range of possible relationships achieved by cross sectional study, but delivers a more robust model, particularly if the whole environmental and political context is taken into account. (Pettigrew,1985).

- Authors do not often claim generalizability and all studies are unrepeatable because they relate to events that occur once only in conditions that cannot, by definition, be caused to re-occur. None-the-less, the lessons drawn can be applied to future situations if active adaptation is continually made to bring about best fit.
- Thematic analysis of this descriptive theory and empirical literature sees the emergence of a number of clear areas for consideration as are discussed below.

Conditioning and Gestalt

Pavlov (1927), in *classical conditioning theory* described a system for changing behaviours through linking external stimuli in order to modify subjects' reflexes. A reaction normally produced reflexively in response to one stimulus might be progressively induced in reaction to another stimulus if those two stimuli are consistently experienced together by the subject. This discipline transfers from animal to human subjects, and is used to explain phenomenon such as motion sickness when it occurs as a response to the vehicle before motion commences. However, little success has been achieved in using classical conditioning to alter more than the most basic of human behaviours.

Skinner (1974), in *operant conditioning theory* describes systematic rewards for desired behaviours and ignoral of undesirable behaviours modifying future behaviour in animals. This discipline, as behaviour therapy, has been demonstrated to be very effective when used with human subjects, with some very complex behaviour being altered in this way.

However, in *gestalt field theory* the manipulation of external stimuli described in conditioning theories are considered insufficient. The notion of gestalt is that the whole organism or system is more than simply the sum of its component parts. This leads some observers to consider that the reductionist approach used in behaviour therapy, which reduces complex behaviour to simple components that may be modified, is insufficient to alter a complex being. A lasting change in behaviour requires a change of the subjects' understanding of themselves and the context in which they exist as well as simply a change to stimulus/response through rewards. The effect of a change of stimuli through reward and ignoral as described by Skinner is considered important in gestalt. However, there must also be attention to cognitive functions, and the place of the individual in a community, before change can be effective at more than a cosmetic level. (Smith, Beck, Cooper, Cox, Ottoway, and Talbot 1982).

The need to consider change in terms beyond reward for desired behaviour is developed by many theorists on the change process. Nadler (1993), echoing Smith et al, points out that the forces of equilibrium tend to work against any localised change. Only when the change considers the stimuli on individuals, the conceptualisations of individuals and the manner in which individuals make up an organisation wide system will changes become permanent.

In all, there are many approaches recorded to managing stimuli in order to bring about alterations to individuals' understanding in order to effect a change in behaviour. These have formed a part of change management and organisation development theory.

Theories of the management of change

In the study of general, and NHS specific, change management theory there is considerable divergence in approach to be found, however, there are also a number of constant themes and large areas of agreement. These may be presented as *necessary-but-not-sufficient* conditions. Each must be addressed for the project to have the possibility of success but adherence will not guarantee it.

Involvement of employees

Employee ownership of the unsatisfactory nature of the present and desirability of the proposed future is generally reported to be critical in gaining enthusiasm and co-operation. This was described by Beckhard and Harris (1987) in

The Change Equation: $(D+V+S)>R.$

Where D is a dissatisfaction with the present, V is a vision of a better future, S is step one and R is the resistance to change expressed by employees. This is an important part of change management theory. It suggests that where change is not progressing at the desired rate, then the situation may be improved by increasing D, V or S rather than simply attempting to eliminate resistance R, which is commonly the first line of approach. This model complements the force-field analysis described by Lewin (1951).

Forcefield analysis

Positive forces driving the change	Negative forces resisting the change
Opportunity to save revenue→	← general fear of change
Client benefit→	← concern about skills
Staff benefit→	← concern about redundancy
Community benefit→	← concern for social network
	← concern for patient care

The purpose of the analysis is to make explicit the forces at work affecting worker enthusiasm, and then - crucially - to devise a plan to enhance the positive forces and reduce the negative forces, thereby driving the change forward. Involvement in the planning of change gives employees confidence and enables them to understand what is being done (Lippitt, Langseth & Mossop 1985). It exploits the insights of those intimately involved with the processes concerned and consequently results in improved planning. Also, they comment, managers making it possible for subordinates to own and solve problems and then supplying the new conditions that subordinates have prescribed for themselves is more effective than offering a *fait accompli* change. This, they consider, results in employees effecting change because they wish to and believe that it is right rather than under instruction.

Vail (1982) also pointed to this notion, commenting that the whole system must be the object of change. All employees must be involved, in order that the entire system has been taken into account in change design and also in order that the whole system is actively changed. Change of a single facet, involving only a small part of the work force carries the risk that the remaining unchanged 'rump' will undo the change effected in the minority

There is a need for the level of involvement of the individual to be proportionate to the extent that he/she will be effected (Burnes 2009). *[handwritten: → Support proportionate to needs NSG]*

Mabey and Mayon-White (1993) describe the emphasis on participative change management as the most important change to change thinking over the past few years. In the same year, Nadler said that one of his most consistent findings in the research on change is that participation reduces resistance, builds ownership of solutions and motivates people to make changes work (Nadler 1993).

Van de Ven (1980) and Quin (1980) both describe involvement of employees as essential to assist them to see issues in a wider context and enable a natural process to occur which leads to institutionalisation of new management ideas and a natural move over to new working practice. This supports the notion of change as a complex, contextually based occurrence and yet offers simple practical means of manipulation. At a simple level, employees are able to see the reason for change, and co-operate. At another level, the individual is exposed to the, difficult to conceptualise, context based rationale for change and by sophisticated behaviours will steer the change through an environment too complex for a single manager to manipulate.

Michael Walton, a clinical psychologist and Organisational Development (OD) consultant in the NHS, considers in that setting that a significant determinant of the outcome of a change exercise is the agreement among staff that the changes are needed. He also expresses the view that it is essential that they have been involved in that decision to change as well as the choice of path to be followed. (Walton 1997)

The first action step has to be to identify and surface dissatisfaction with the current state as perceived by the workforce (Nadler 1993). Upton and Brookes (1995) report on the need bring to the surface dissatisfaction with the present and also with the planned changes, if any exist. In a case study of a NHS community resettlement scheme for patients, they found that passive resistance to change was more difficult to deal with than active resistance. Where a workforce is involved with the process and will voice concerns and state reasons for preferring not to alter practices, then these can be the subjects of negotiated settlement. Where resistance is not expressed but simply results in failure to co-operate, then it is far more difficult to find acceptable avenues of compromise. A common reason given for the recognition of trade unions is the desire to bring concerns into the public arena and thereby to begin the process of reconciliation. The NHS, through its Whitley Council Committees for staff recognition has strong machinery to ensure this dialogue.

Burns (1996) reported finding infrequent exceptions to the need for comprehensive communication. In fact, he occasionally found that changes are adopted very rapidly without careful management preparation. Burnes and James (1995) also note this phenomenon and suggest that Cognitive Dissonance might explain this phenomenon. In cognitive dissonance theory, individuals will alter their perceptions of the world in order to resolve paradoxes and contradiction between the various models or ever the total paradigm with which they explain their beliefs and behaviours (Festinger 1957; Jones 1990). Burnes and James (1995) suggest that, on occasion, detailed involvement of staff is not required to effect change, because if staff perceives a dissonance between their underlying beliefs and their behaviours then they experience discomfort and intrinsically are motivated to change either their behaviour or their beliefs. This intrinsic motivation replaces the extrinsic motivation achieved by high level involvement and explains occasional co-operation with profound change in the absence of adequate involvement

However, in a cautionary note, Vrakking (1997) points out that consultation is time consuming and this time lag may reduce the success of the change drive. Studying change in the Netherlands taking account of the health service reforms based upon The Dekker Report (Dekker 1987), Vrakking considered that there was an inverse relationship between the time taken to implement a change and the extent of change ultimately achieved.

> *Preparations must be made during the innovation phase to ensure that the target level can be achieved as soon as possible. This requires well-planned and irreversible actions, which are implemented in big steps (Vrakking 1997 p37)*

Therefore, although involvement and ownership are universally valued, time is a qualifier. These conditions are not of necessity contradictory, but the time concern might temper the enthusiasm for endless consultation.

Participative leadership is tested empirically by research conducted by a variety of studies. Peter Langseth was management consultant to the World Bank leading its major restructuring and redirection concluding in 1982. His longitudinal, case study is reported extensively in Lippitt, Langseth and Mossop (1985). In this study, Langseth et al describe the importance of employee participation as a major learning that was derived from the exercise. Participation, he found, identified needs, created trust, generated ideas, and offered expertise specific to the industrial area concerned. However the tendency to raise unrealistic expectations was noted and a need for guarded realism advocated. This is the informed report of a commissioned project. Findings are the considered conclusions of expert deliberation. However, the project cannot be described as a formal experiment, control of outside factors would not be appropriate and the study is not replaceable. It is not claimed that the population studied (bank employees) is representative of wider populations and in particular is not very similar to health care.

Participation requires reciprocal communication regarding the need to change, the consequent proposed changes and progress towards the chosen condition. Many analysts describe the importance of this communication.

Communication and feedback

There is a crucial need for change managers to continually reiterate the superiority of the vision of the future and the way in which the change process will bring the organisation to the desired state.

> One of the first and most critical steps for managing change is to develop and then communicate a clear image of the future ... resistance and confusion frequently develop during organisational change because people are unclear about what the future might be like. (Nadler 1993)

Nadler describes the importance of multi-channel communication, repetition and variety in this communication. This, he observed, might include small group meetings, large group briefings, newsletters, videotape presentations, etc. Lippitt echoes this observation commenting that it is crucial to inform individuals about the change effort before it commences and to ensure that they understand the intended result and the mechanism by which this change will bring it about. In addition, there is a need for managers to hear responses in order to modify the process as appropriate and to permit expression of concerns and catharsis. These concerns might otherwise lead to resistance. In catharsis, employees feeling aroused and distressed by proposed changes, release this energy constructively, in this case through dialogue. Even when dialogue is heated, it may perform a constructive part by enabling release of strongly felt emotions.

Changes may be usefully modified to become more acceptable to employees who have legitimate concerns. Interactive communication elicits concerns not otherwise evident to change managers. Lippitt, Langseth & Mossop, (1985) propose a situation where reasonable change might be resisted, merely because it moves an influential individual away from a window thereby reducing his/her enjoyment of the working environment It, therefore, may be critical to successful change management that such issues are surfaced and resolved.

The importance of developing feedback mechanisms specifically targeted on the effectiveness of change initiatives in train is clear. participants in change need constant and timely information about the path of the event (Nadler 1993). Steady state feedback mechanisms often break down under the turbulence of change, particularly in response to the increased influence of the grapevine.

Michael Walton (1997) observed that change leadership is effective only if it addresses a number of communication components. The need for change must be made clear and evident to all; the practical scope for change must be made clear and evident to all; the resources must be identified and transparently allocated to the process; an explicit commitment to change must be obtained from all affected.

The communication process will expose conflict. Failure to acknowledge this conflict and to allow its expression will prevent individuals from resolving tensions and restructuring their personal models and paradigms. This exercise requires an allocation of time in which employees make the journey which has already been made by the change agent in arriving at the need to change. The exercise also shows up the need for internal communication opportunities among subjects of change as well as hierarchical communications between change agents and subjects of change. (Marris,1993).

Empirically, the part played by complex communication in effecting change is comprehensively explored. In the World Bank Study, Lippitt, Langseth & Mossop, (1985) report the importance of communication before and during change. It was found necessary to establish new mechanisms, and even language for communication under the new conditions, with reference sources for individual access, and constant feedback about achievements.

Price and Murphy (1987), in a longitudinal case study, reported the effect of their work on OD in British Telecom: Western London District. The study was with a broad skill-mix of employees, in a technically demanding field, working in a multi-million pound organisation with 6,000 plus workforce. As such the subject group have some commonality with a larger NHS Trust. The report is, as described by Mabey and Mayon-White (1993),

Anecdotal and unsystematic...but realistic (p153)

The study found that that there was a need to simplify and publicise information. This, they observed, needed to be comprehensive and multi-channelled. A simple information cascade used in isolation, they found, could not give adequate coverage or clarity. They observed that meetings for idea formulation and information needed to be visible within normal working circumstances. They found it to be damaging when decisions happened mysteriously, e.g. out of hours, through an away-day in a hotel, etc.

The importance of recognising the inevitability of conflict was found by Burnes (2009) when in a cross sectional case study he examined the merger of five colleges of Nursing and/or Midwifery into one large college of Midwifery and Nursing. This 1993 study was of a longitudinal, descriptive and analytical nature and involved academic members of the health service. As such, Burnes considers the lessons relevant to the NHS and other public sector industries in the UK. The five colleges were drawn together under one management and in partially new premises. There was conflict described between the two professions and between the various management teams. This conflict was inevitable, and it was necessary to recognise this and make it explicit in order for it to be addressed. This explicit attention to conflict made resolution possible. Failure to recognise and address conflict lead to continuing resistance at various formal and informal arenas in the organisation and an increase of inertia and resistance. The critical importance of addressing conflicts through sophisticated and robust communication is reported as the main lesson from the study.

The importance of devising and communicating a clear strategy was found by Burnes (2009) in his case study of GK Printers Ltd, as they made radical changes throughout their organisation to deliver dramatically improved quality and flexibility in their product. The longitudinal study tests a variety of inputs over a number of change phases, with some clear conclusions. Significant among the conclusions is the importance of success through attention to the customer and the critical contribution of communicating a well-constructed strategy.

> The company had a strategy for the future, and therefore was able to take an overview in all areas of its business in relation to future objectives. Because the company was strategy driven it was able to establish not only where problems lay, but also whether the problems were high, medium or low priority. (Burnes1996 p258)

Tom Peters (1989), from a detailed study of a very broad spectrum of USA organisations, observed the same point commenting that:

> *Communicating a strategic mind-set, focused on skill building, is more important than ever. (Peters, 1989 p394)*

Buchanan (1997) studied BPR in hospitals using a case study design. He found that where there was not an adequately precise definition of focus and methodology, politically driven actors manipulate the exercise to subvert the outcomes. This, he found, was compounded by the absence of a clear and well-understood strategic direction for the organisation.

The issue appears to reduce to a requirement for reciprocal and open communication over a sustained period of time to allow employees to adjust their models adopt a new strategy and contribute into a proposal to such an extent that they can own the change effort. Many organisations use formal and informal education opportunities in part, as a vehicle for this time and communication based personal development to occur.

Education

Change agents will have assimilated changes and reformulated their models so that the proposed system makes sense to them. This may have occurred over a long period. Subjects of change need to hear this new vision clearly and, crucially, be given the opportunity to actively reform their own constructs before they can work positively towards a changed model. Many observers and managers recognise the value of educational opportunities in facilitating this developmental process.

Walton (1997), in examining NHS change, observed that understanding the emotionality of change is critical to outcome. Staff need the time to reassure themselves that change is worthwhile and that it leads to a future in which they are needed and in which they are able to be influential. This process requires time and may be enhanced by the opportunity for detached education.

There is reference in the literature to the importance of time out and an opportunity for contemplation to help employees to move through the threshold represented by major change.

Handy (1995) observes that there has been an explosion in MBA degrees, as part of a rush by organisations to link their development plans to some form of qualification.

Plant (1987) argues that the learning process is the key to the self and organisational change. Handy (1995) and Marris (1993) describe time for reflection and development, associated with educational opportunities. The impact of educational opportunity on the ability to change is more than anecdotally demonstrated. In the World Bank project report Lippitt et al.(1985) report the importance of direct education in change management, observation and various technical specific areas.

Goodstien and Burke (1991) in the British Airways (BA) study found that many training programmes were required to enable staff to generally improve their understanding of the industry. This was an example of the benefit of more general educational opportunities, not simply to inculcate skills but to change insights and attitudes to work. In the movement phase of the exercise, a very heavy emphasis was placed on manager training in management and leadership. As part of their re-freezing exercise, the organisation has adopted executive "Academies" leading to MBA awards.

Graham Benjamin (Benjamin, and Mabey 1990) reporting his work as consultant to Billton International Metals in The Hague during their major reorganisation drew a number of conclusions around the nature of time needed to change attitudes. A major reorganisation will require individuals to question their vision. This, he found, required time for individual values, attitudes, beliefs and behaviours to be worked on participatively, alongside business and organisational imperatives. Leaders needed to change their behaviour in a visible form in order to model required behaviour.

Burnes (1996) in his study of The Rover Group between 1989 and 1994 found success firmly based in a belief in education of the workforce. Through the creation of the Rover Learning Business (RLB) as an independent organisation within The Rover Group, the situation was achieved where at one time over 50% of the workforce are engaged in learning activities. Burnes found that the RLB to be a dynamic and very effective device for bringing about change. The introduction of the Land Rover Discovery range was managed by the RLB and described as,

> the smoothest and quickest change project ... ever (Burnes 1996 p248)

Chair of British Aerospace during the period building up to their purchase of Rover, Sir Austin Pearce, had already expressed his recognition of the essential part of education in industry by accepting the position of Pro-chancellor of the University of Surrey and chair of the Science Museum. (Ezra & Oats 1989)

Lawler and Hearn (1997) in a cross sectional case study examined the rise of managerialism in Local Authority Social Services Departments, found manager training to be a major predictor of successful change. They did not, however, encounter the organisation wide learning culture described by Burnes (1993) in his study of The Rover Group.

Leadership and Trust

The critical nature of the communication, involvement and education process leads to examination of the nature of the leadership involved.

Nadler observes the importance of using leader behaviour to generate energy in support of change. Change needs to consider formal leaders deriving power from their position and informal leaders whose power derives from one of many other sources. Concert of leaders is essential.

Sets of leaders working in co-ordination can have a tremendously powerful impact on the informal organisation. (Nadler 1993 p96).

The importance of symbols and energising language to support leadership is reported by Peters (1978) and this, he observes, may be an essential adjunct to the energising behaviour of leaders.

It is not possible to ensure that the reasons for every component of a change are explicitly understood by all parties affected. Therefore, successful leadership requires that some management actions can be taken 'on trust'. Equally, leaders will benefit if they can be seen to trust employees to make decisions and act in the best interest of the organisation without the need for tireless supervision.

Lippitt, Langseth & Mossop, (1985) express the importance of trust and observe that mistrust arises when information given is incomplete or misleading and that trust might be earned by open and candid communication.

Burnes (2009), based on a longitudinal case study, looked at Process Control Inc. which employs 395 staff of various skill levels in management, technical and support roles as they restructured in response to business expansion. Strong conclusions are drawn in relationship to the leadership role. The study concluded that strong and directive leadership was essential to the change achieved and that this leadership needed to display consistency and continuity. Managerial changes were found counterproductive. Commitment from the team was found essential in promulgating the leadership message, and emergent/iterative strategy development was found unhelpful. Therefore direction, which does not preclude participation, from managers was found essential. Burnes found that no new ingredients were required to effect change. Rather a fortuitous coincidence of factors can spontaneously lead to desirable outcomes. This reflects the comments of Pettigrew (1985, 1989) when he observes that chance and opportunism play major parts in effecting change. These findings must be tempered by the limited similarity of the midlands based organisation to the UK NHS

Attention to the impact of change on individuals

Change to the processes, outputs and outcomes consequent upon an organisation's new endeavour will have profound effect on the lives of those concerned with it. Careful attention to the effect of change on what, how, where, when people work with whom and to what personal benefit, are described as critical to the success of a change effort.

Lippitt et al (1985) point to the need to consider disruption to congenial working groups and the consequent impact on issues such as vacation possibilities, dining groups, etc. Fear of alteration to base, commuting arrangements, car pool deals etc. can result in resistance that is hard to bring to the surface and therefore hard to address. Upton and Brookes (1995) point out that staff will be concerned about the possibility of their becoming a part of a different group. They might be concerned about their status and influence in the new setting. They may also have concern about the acceptability of the change agents in relationship to the current informal hierarchy.

Changing to a new model of operating requires abandoning an old model, and may amount to letting go of a former way of life. For many individuals, this constitutes a distressing loss. An experience similar to bereavement is often described. The feelings experienced in times of dramatic change are often categorised into the stages of: shock, denial, bargaining, acceptance and performance. These are the same stages described by people experiencing other forms of bereavement and some commentators propose similar support mechanisms. Nadler (1993) observes that change frequently creates a feeling of loss that is "not unlike death". He suggests that people need to mourn for that change. Plans might usefully allow the time for mourning to occur and the various stages of bereavement to be recognised. In a transition stage, bereavement can obstruct progress and there may be benefit from permitting it to follow its natural course to resolution before expecting active change.

In health and social services, the scope for loss of power and status for leaders of individual professions or other groups that will be fragmented by change is considerable. This potential for the feeling of loss may be of great importance. Marris goes further, suggesting that bereavement is the paramount consideration:

> We need to recognise the element of bereavement, above all, in the process of a major reconstruction (Marris 1993 p218).

Major effects on the individual may be anticipated or experienced early in the process and successful change management requires the careful management of this experience.

Recognition of the importance of the impact of change on individuals and groups is supported empirically by Iles and Auluck (1990) who in a longitudinal study of a health and social care teams, concluded that team building exercises considering the meaning of proposed changes for individuals contribute to diagnosis and problem solving in OD. It is essential, they observed, that the team achieves personal commitment and consensus on mission and vision with consequent commitment to objectives. The study involved small teams of between ten and fifty people, and a full range of health and care staff. Although the numbers

208

are small and the case reports anecdotal, the study is particularly valuable because it is specific to the Health & Care industries.

The early experience of benefit

In many settings, the early experience might be one of benefit if management effort was exerted to ensure this end. As change begins to deliver results, it may become possible to ensure reward for those who have been affected. Alternatively, the change process can last for a considerable time, and the promised end benefits can appear to be a long time away. Many writers advise change managers to ensure that some small benefits and successes are achieved in the early stages of a change process (Lippitt, Langseth & Mossop,1985), (Wheeler & Grice, 2000), (Burns, 2009).

Clearly, early experience of benefit fits well with Skinner's notion that reward encourages the repetition of desirable behaviours. In this case desired behaviours are change-supporting behaviours and these might be amply rewarded. Lippitt, Langseth & Mossop, (1985) echo Skinner, when they describe the importance of rewards for desired behaviour in the early transition stage of a change process. They observe that reward systems devised during relatively static phases of an organisation's existence may be ineffective or even obstructive in the enactment of change.

> *(rewards) ... need to be carefully examined during major reorganizational changes and restructured to support the direction of the transition. (Nadler 1993 p93)*

Lippitt, Langseth & Mossop, (1985) say that managers should facilitate early implementation of a tangible component of the change and reward those who contributed. This is an example of extrinsic reward, in that the reward is applied externally to recognise contributors. An intrinsic reward, i.e. one that is a direct benefit of the change can be shown to have an even greater value. Thus, if the change is manipulated to be to the direct benefit of change subjects, then this will better ensure future co-operation than a reward applied by a manager. However, if an intrinsic reward is not possible, then an extrinsic reward should be applied as a very good second best.

Unmodified reward systems can contribute to the cultural factors that hold individuals' loyalty to the present system of practice and thereby hold back change. The change of reward systems is therefore a factor in freeing up a structure in order to allow it to change. This should include consideration of official formal rewards such as bonus schemes and informal rewards such as peer recognition. All rewards should be considered for their possible effects in locking up the present or motivating a change to a future state. New reward systems are needed, to confirm and establish a new way of working. The notion of manipulated reward appeared in a number of change models particularly in Lewin's Field Theory.

Models of change management

There have been a number of models of the managed change process, which although different, have much in common. Many models derive from Lewin's Field Theory. Lewin (1951) describes the need to unfreeze, change and refreeze the organisation. Lewin, in force field analysis, also described the notion of examining the forces at work and manipulating any or all to achieve movement. In particular, force field analysis shows how change can be aided by reducing resistive forces as effectively as progressively increasing driving forces.

Johnson (1993) describes unfreezing the paradigm by making explicit the constructs within the paradigm. He points out that people who are not part of the system to be changed more easily do this. This supports the need for employment of formal change consultants from outside of the organisation. Once a new process has been established, Johnson observes, it is necessary to refreeze by adjusting infrastructure and systems to ensure that it is easy to continue with the new system, and to prevent backsliding. In addition, he considers it necessary to extend any new process to other parts of the organisation rapidly and thereby maximise the benefit achieved while minimising the risk of reversion to the old.

The re-freezing component is described by Lippitt et al as critical and prone to being overlooked:

> *Perhaps the most critically overlooked and vital part of change is that of timely assembly of a human support system dedicated to maintaining the new.* (Lippitt, Langseth & Mossop, 1985 p.101)

The implementation of new systems will not always receive the support of the workforce. Hogan (1997) observes that, in the NHS, poor usage of a revised or new system can often be seen. This has the effect of preventing stabilisation and a failure to re-freeze the system. This rejection of the new, or regression to the old, radically reduces the efficiency of the organisation and may be taken as a failure of the implementation process.

The steady state model for before and after the change may or may not be the same, but it is inevitably unsuitable for the change period. Consequently, special structures to manage the change need to be developed. Further different structures may be needed for employment after the change, to institutionalise the new structure. (Nadler & Tushman 1979)

Pettigrew (1985) reflects the unfreezing process, expressing of the need to de-legitimise the ideas associated with inertia. The old model will have had legitimacy in the past and this legitimacy must be removed rather than simply countered. This supports the model of force field analysis where removing a force supporting inertia is as important as adding as force for change and demonstrates unfreezing in action.

As is made clear by gestalt theory (Smith, et al 1982), the management of change cannot be conducted at singe points in the organisation. Nadler (1993) says that multiple and consistent leverage, recognising the interdependence of the components of the organisation bring about successful alterations. Therefore, he considers, the unfreezing and refreezing process needs to be considered throughout the organisation.

Walton (1997) describes a process in NHS change that mirrors field theory while recognising the medical model of intervention. Change, he observes, requires diagnosis, building a basis for collective change action, enabling change and maintaining changed systems.

Systematic manipulation of the paradigm employing models such as force field analysis is identified in field research by Goodstein and Burke (1991) who used it as a model to evaluate the restructuring of British Airways between 1982 and 1987. The study is of a very large organisation having 60,000 employees. The organisation was in the service sector, had a skill-mix similar to the NHS and like the NHS was experiencing the change from bureaucratic state control to market control.

The study was able to match occurrences in the reorganisation closely to the Lewin force-field model, with unfreezing involving a 37% workforce reduction and change of CEO and Chairmen. A broad range of educational opportunities were introduced to allow staff to develop a better understanding of the industry facilitated in addition unfreezing.

The movement phase of the Lewin model again involved education, this time for senior and middle managers in the area of management and leadership. This phase was characterised by the use of diagonal-slice task forces and extensive team building activity. Support for individuals at all levels was reported and involvement of the new CEO in formal and informal contact was found critical. This echoes the comments made by Peters in1989 and 1994 when he observed the importance of *Managing by Wandering About in* his studies of the USA's most successful organisations. Re-freezing was achieved by human resource management changes, including the promotion of those who exemplified new practices into higher management levels. Re-freezing was further achieved by the instigation of new performance appraisal mechanisms based on behaviour and results in line with new practices. This clearly demonstrates the value of introduction of new human resource practices to re-freeze the system as described by Lippitt et al.

Goodstein and Burke express a strong belief, following the lessons from the BA reorganisation, that an understanding of the social psychology of change through models, such as those of Lewin, assists in achieving the desired outcome.

Price and Murphy in their BT study (1987) noted the critical nature of the re-freezing after change, establishing processes and systems capable of institutionalising an entire new paradigm. They observe that a steering group was an effective venue for spotting the time for re-freezing thereby identifying a comprehensive yet efficient means of fixing the new.

Burnes in his study of the Midshires College of Midwifery and Nursing, pointed to the importance of considering the stage at which the process is, because

> *A style of management suited to a stable state may, as in this instance, be totally unsuited to a more dynamic situation. (Burnes 1996 p228).*

Thus, different behaviours need to be consciously adopted during the unfreezing, moving and refreezing phases of a change.

Upton and Brookes in a case study of an NHS community resettlement scheme found the destabilising exercise to be crucial, even where the acceptance of change was suggested by superficial observation,

> *While change may be agreed on the surface, it will not happen unless there is some real dissatisfaction felt within the staff team (Upton and Brookes, 1995 p44).*

Since Lewin, theories have evolved in a number of directions. A distinction exists between the more internally and systematically focused pragmatic and rational schools of OD with a choice of rational, linear, longitudinal analyses and the, far richer but less manageable, expanded focus model as described by Pettigrew (1985). Pettigrew considered that change is not simply a prescribed management action but a natural process resulting from external and internal elements acting in, often fortuitous, combinations. Changes may not be a system-wide planned exercise but the result of the action of a small subset of people in the organisation responding to perceived mismatch between environmental demands and organisational performance. Some attempt to reconcile these views exists in open systems thinking in work by Spurgeon and Barwell (1991). They consider that, whatever the personal belief preferred, successful management requires the existence of a personal model of the organisation which is dynamic enough to explain current performance and the continuous changes which it is undergoing. The degree of simplicity or holism of this model may depend on the individual and the situation. Schwenk (1988) describes models as "schemata" being devised personally and applied diagnostically to situations. Schwenk points to the tendency to adapt old models to new problems, using metaphor and analogy. This practice is natural, but may result in faulty diagnosis. It is helpful to be explicit when a proven model is adapted to an untried situation and thus to exercise caution and guard against false assumption.

Change, as a process consumes energy over and above routine management of the organisation, which is frequently continuing alongside the change process. Nadler (1993) finds that resources such as financial, human, training, consultative input, etc. must be provided for the transitional stage in order for change to occur. However, it is not assumed that these are entirely new resources. Resources may be redirected for this purpose and short periods of exceptional managerial productivity are frequently harnessed for the change process.

Nadler points to the stark need for new resources to be applied to the change process since it constitutes activity over and above the routine of operational management. Johnson (1993) considers that the extra resource should take the form of a change agent from outwith the organisation that can therefore recognise a separate role as well as a new function and new manpower. The effectiveness of change agents has been richly examined, although the rigour of the evidence offered is limited.

In the World Bank project, Lippitt showed that a separate change management project group was essential to effect a reorganisation, but this group, they found, needed to be closely linked to operations management This was found necessary to support operations managers a well as in order that operations managers may operationalise new systems to refreeze after changes.

> *The use of internal and external consultants is helpful, but these must be controlled and integrated. (Lippitt et al.1985 p153)*

Price and Murphy (1987) in their BT study reinforced this concern finding that too much reliance on change consultants worked against sustainability in changes achieved. Where they are not working in close concert with operational managers, the effects of the change cannot be sustained in the absence of the consultant. Additionally they report the importance of early recognition of the time requirement and the need for injection of resource for this period.

Vrakking (1997) went a stage further in quantifying this resource with his X 2X formula. This formula said that whatever the cost of planning and designing the change, the cost of implementation would amount to double that figure. This conclusion was drawn from studies of a number of organisations in the Netherlands, including some health service changes.

In the NHS, however, although the planning resource is frequently provided as an extra to operational costs, the resource for enacting the change is commonly achieved by redirection of normal revenue.

Subsidiarity and Levels of Interference: breadth and depth of intervention

Many writers discuss limiting the scope of change to that which is necessary. Destabilising an organisation is essential to enable change. However, the relationship between reduced stability and increased ability to effect change extends only to a limited point. Just as the Stress Curve relates stress positively to learning performance but recognises a critical point where performance falls away (Walton 1997), so stress can be related to change performance, with a critical stress level at which the ability to change is adversely affected. Nadler (1993) recognises that the increased anxiety associated with destabilisation, while initially beneficial, may reach a point where it has a detrimental effect. Therefore, Nadler points to the need for protected sources of stability through systems, which do not change. Walton in examining NHS change considers that it is crucial to limit disruption, confusion and consequent anxiety in order to secure positive commitment from staff involved. Thus the unfreezing phase involves destabilisation, but this needs to be tempered in order not to disable the workforce.

As Stress increases, so does learning. However, there comes a point s1 at which stress is too great and learning rapidly declines.
(Walton,1997, p90)

Change managers need to alter swathes of an organisation, but they are advised to consider that this is an invasion and only intervene where there is clear benefit anticipated, and in any event not to the extent that constructive co-operation is disabled.

Harrison (1970) suggested that managers should interfere at a level no deeper than that required to produce an enduring solution. In addition, he observed that it is pointless to interfere at a level where change energy is not available. To do so would not achieve results and may discredit the change process by setting about a task that was not to be completed.

Senior management within an organisation should not make change decisions for lower levels of the organisation which could have been made at that lower level. Subsidiarity suggests that no decisions should be made at a level of an organisation that could have been made at a lower level. Handy (1995) considers it an injustice for an organisation to arrogate to itself a decision that could be made efficiently by a lower body.

Pettigrew (1993) observes that intervention needs to take account of all internal and external levels in an organisation in order for changes to be effective. Smith et al (1982) re-enforce this point, observing that multi point leverage is needed to bring about directional change. Goodstien and Burke (1991) in the BA study concluded that multiple level management lead intervention was essential, with many leverage points and multifaceted support including maximum contact between the CEO and all levels of the organisation. However, Burnes (1996) identified the importance of allowing decisions to be managed at appropriately low levels in the GK Printers study. The company was moving to a state where change was the norm.

Without devolving responsibility to those affected, change either would not take place, or would not be successful

When the MD went back to taking decisions... the company failed to maintain behavioural changes (Burnes 1996 p266).

This suggests a need for comprehensive intervention, but with constraints around unnecessary interference. Although Handy and Harrison define conceptual cut off points little evidence exists to answer the question of how much and how deep? In addition to consideration of the above local intra-organisational cause and effect considerations, it is critical to address the context and the environment in which the individual department exists as part of an open system. Therefore, it may be argued that no change process can have enduring benefit unless it works at all internal levels. Pettigrew (1985, 1989) says that there is a tendency to attend to the content of changes and consequent outcomes at the expense of consideration of context and process. Context and environment affect the behaviour of all levels of the organisation. Formulaic change management must be insufficient if it fails to account for individuality, and much benefit is gained from chance and opportunism when individuals make inevitable responses to the wider environment in which they exist. It is evident that insight into the broad organisational context and attention to processes that occur at all levels in an organisation can have a substantial benefit.

Pettigrew (1987) makes it clear that although it is not practicable to integrate the operational context of change into a prescriptive formula it is essential to have a good understanding of context in order to effect lasting change. This is reinforced by a study of Oticon in which Burnes (1993) found that a deep understanding of the market place in which they operated was central to their effective reorganisation. The Oticon organisation is a small international organisation described by Peters in 1994 as having visionary leadership which enabled it to change the rules of their endeavour. The significance of context is powerfully expressed by Burnes. It is further emphasised that understanding and exploiting societal values has played a major part in the success of this reorganisation..

Burnes in his study of GK Printers during their radical change, found that the context in which the organisation operated was central to its successful transformation.

> ...understanding what the customers wanted and were willing to pay for. In speaking to customers, GK also identified what competitors were offering. (Burnes 1996 p264)

There is only limited similarity between these organisations and the UK NHS, and transferring this conclusion requires caution

Summary of the theory

The literature is complex in nature. It ranges from simple opinion, through anecdotal observation to soundly constructed case study analysis. It appears that the *necessary but not sufficient conditions* that consistently emerge are:

Reward

Ensuring that perticipants see rapid, personal benefit and are thereby rewarded for their co-operation is consistently advised. This recognises theories of learning through condidtioning and is demonstrated through recent and applicable case studies. The change manager could usefully engineer early opportunities for those affected to experience advantage. It may be advantageous if the benefit was focused upon those whose part in the change process was of a high profile nature. It is aslo important to ensure that participants are not adversely effected if it can be avoided. This will involve close examination of the situation to uncover and adress possible areas for personal inconvenience and disadvantage.

Communication systems

Much is said about the importance of communications. The machinary in place for steady state communications will need to be dramatically upgraded in order to meet the needs during a change event. Informal communications will immediately accelerate and it is necessary for the formal routes also to accelerate to keep pace. The machinary introduced needs to be varied in nature this could include all media and a full spectrum from highly formal to spontaneous and very informal.

The communications need to be reciprocal, so that concerns can be identified and addressed, and so that those involved may develop a perception of ownership of the decisions that emerge from the planning exercise. Ownership of the unsatisfactory present and the improved future sought among the workforce is essential. Change is rarely gratuitous, but unless the workforce is allowed to recognise the need for change, through this protracted communication exercises then they are unlikely to be intrinsically suportive of the development.

Time, and time out

Managers partake in "Away-days" and interminable executive meetings through which avenues they will have made the developmental journey that enables them to recognise the unsatisfactory components of the present and the need for the proposed developments. The other members of the workforce have not "enjoyed" this advantage. Therefore, all of the workforce will need time to digest and accept the development proposals if they are to give active co-operation. Thus, a period is needed to allow the ideas to germinate and develop to the point where the change manager can harvest the benefit. This will happen naturally, if the issues are held current in employees' thinking and patience is practised. However, the process can be accelerated if active opportunities are created for discussion and exploration. The literature refers to the adoption of educational exercises to facilitate this development. Exercises reported range from short study sessions in the workplace to facilitation of long courses such as university based degree study. A note of caution is introduced, however, since there may be a time when the "Iron is hot" and the benefits of action may decay if the initiative is not swiftly grasped.

Leadership and Trust

The importance of credible leadership is clearly demonstrated in the literature. Leaders need to earn the trust of employees if they are to co-operate without needing to know the reason behind every move. The literature suggests that trust is earned by consistent open communication and that it may be lost rapidly and permanently if a manager is found careless with the truth. A perception of fairness will also develop trust.

Subsidiarity

There is a paradox to consider when deciding the extent to which a change should permeate the whole organisation. It may be that a change effected in one part of the organisation will not take hold if the bulk of the organisation continues to operate unaltered. This suggests that the more wide ranging the change, the more likely is the success. However, there are repeated observations that it is unhelpful to alter portions of the organisation from above where that change was not directly needed or where that change could have been managed internally. To make gratuitous change is ethically questionable and results in a destabilisation that causes unnecessary stress to employees. This is ethically unsound and may result in stress levels sufficiently high to disable more-vulnerable individuals and detract from patient/client care.

Models

The Lewin model may be seen at the heart of more current change management protocols. This model is also identified at work in current research. There are examples cited where the force field model can be recognised in successful change exercises and others where the model was not respected in exercises that were not successful. Clearly, these are associations only and the evidence is not powerful enough to definitively demonstrate a causal relationship. The necessity to respect the stages of "Unfreezing" and "Refreezing" as well as "Changing" are repeatedly reported. Failure to unfreeze is given as a cause of failure to effect change and failure to refreeze is given as a reason for reversion to old ways of working when the change driver is removed.

Discussion

Is the literature advocating an outmoded "Country club" (Blake & Mouton 1964) approach to management in a sector where "Hard-nosed" management is essential in a ruthless environment? The health and care sectors are managerially driven and operate under ever more tight constraints. The responsibility of the manager is to use the system to achieve the best quality and value for patients and clients. NHS trusts and Social services departments are not sheltered employment schemes for the benefit of staff. Clearly, this is so, and management practices should be adopted only if they result in the maximum benefit for patients and clients as end users of the service. Applying this principle to the conclusions of the literature search results in discussion, but it can be argued that generally good behaviour from managers will result in optimum services to users.

Staff must feel benefit from changes. However, changes may not be to the benefit of staff and this must be recognised. Employees can always be coerced to co-operate with change by threat of grater disadvantage if they do not. This results in a coercion paradigm in which developments occur only where they cannot be avoided. This will minimise the amount of change that is achieved and demand a large amount of management effort at all stages. Alternatively, benefits can be identified and made evident to individuals thereby maximising their recognition. Disadvantage can be identified and actively negated wherever possible. Positive rewards can be engineered for those who actively drive change or the entire workforce where a point is to be made. Redundancies may be unavoidable in change, but if these are seen to be managed with scrupulous fairness and individuals are given all of the help possible, then the effects on residual and future personnel will be considerable. If perception is all there is, (Peters, 1985), then there is benefit for the change manager to be careful to be seen to be minimising disadvantage wherever possible, maximising benefit wherever possible and rewarding loyalty religiously. Then he/she will be seen as caring for the workforce and may expect more support. This costs very little in terms of management effort or other resources and might be rewarded by co-operation based on loyalty. The output in terms of achievement is maximised and the input in terms of management resource is minimised. Therefore, taking a ruthless economic approach, this approach is the most efficient.

Communication systems and time out, even sponsorship of courses are advocated in the literature as a means of gaining ownership of the change exercise among the workforce. Is this necessary, when employees would co-operate out of fear, or out of a wish to ingratiate themselves with their managers? The benefit of ownership appears to be that the workforce that owns the problem and the solution, and will actively cause it to happen rather than passively allowing it to happen. They will want the exercise to succeed and might be expected to find creative ways to enhance the project or solve problems rather than simply following received guidance.

Earning the trust of the workforce is advocated, which requires care and attention. The workforce can be caused to co-operate through fear of redundancy or discipline, and it is easy to find anecdotal examples of this style of management. However, this again an example of gaining co-operation through coercion and that paradigm has been shown inefficient as well as unethical. It is largely because of the inefficiency of this approach to management that so many organisations have published anti-bullying policies that refer as much to bullying managers as other grades. This prevention of bullying has an efficiency driver as much as an ethical one.

The Lewin model may be seen as arcane and overly fussy in the prevailing fast moving culture. However, there is strong evidence supporting its effectiveness in practice. The logic of removing the factors that wed us to the way things are done now is clear in freeing us to consider other ways of being. This often requires managers to undermine and discredit old ways of thinking in order to allow new ones to develop currency. This is an exercise in destabilising the system in order to allow it to move, because a stable system while very secure, is unable to change. The inherently unstable fighter aircraft has far more manoeuvrability than the very stable passenger airliner. The business of undermining an old paradigm risks causing damage to those individuals who hold them dear. However the discrediting can be seen in the context of current developments and not in terms of the environment when that paradigm was prevalent. It may also be important to ensure that it is the paradigm is undermined and not its proponents. Thus any conflict can be around issues and not around people. The refreezing argument is a mirror to the unfreezing argument. Just as it is necessary to release the ties in order to permit movement, it is equally essential to create new ties once the new model has been achieved in order to keep it at work. Thus, the gardener takes great care to release the roots of a plant before attempting to move it and then firmly to bed them in the new situation in order to hold it there. Any other approach will damage the plant.

Why is it that the pace of change accelerated so dramatically over the past decade? Virtually all commentators observe that the pace and nature of change has accelerated and altered dramatically over the past one or two decades. Little discussion satisfactorily explains this phenomenon. It may be that the pace of technological advancement has accelerated and organisations move ever faster to exploit this environmental change. Additionally, there is a move from an industrial age to an information age, and this may be causing a change similar in impact to the industrial revolution of the 19th century. Alternatively, it is the rapidly expanding population with explosively improving communications and mounting expectations are at the heart of this drive. One explanation, less frequently discussed, is to look at the individuals who are now running the major industries and services in the western world. In the 1960s and 1970s, there was the emergence of an unusually challenging cadre of post-war youth, perhaps facilitated by mass communication, who did not accept the ways of life of their forbears, questioning and changing the entire nature of adolescence. That generation is now in its fourth and fifth decade and there are many anecdotal examples of this very turbulent generation holding very influential national positions. In developmental terms, we do not leave behind earlier developmental stages, but transcend and integrate them. Therefore the adult still has the adolescent within. This explanation might be paraphrased "The Hippies and Punks are now running the world!" if that is true, and it is difficult to see how it cannot be so, then a turbulent period can be no surprise.

Limitations

No scrutiny of theory can be truly comprehensive and this one does not claim such. Case study and anecdotal evidence does not lend itself to meta-analysis as would quantitative data and therefore the aggregation of information must be imperfect. The greatest limitation of this chapter, however, may lie in the attempt, through reductionism, to identify a list of instructions for the successful management of change. This chapter therefore claims only to have discussed *necessary but not sufficient conditions* in change management, i.e. those that must be considered, but will not guarantee success. The intent is to highlight areas where insight and consideration would benefit the manager.

Conclusion

In conclusion, if there are recipe ingredients, a clear list emerges. These are: staff involvement, communication, education, leadership, attention to the impact of changes on individuals, the early experience of benefit, a system wide model, care about the breadth and depth of intervention and integrated consideration of the context in which the organisation operates. These might be condensed into Rewards, Communication, Time, and time out out, Leadership and Trust, Subsidiarity and the aplication of models .

Attention and thoughtful insight into each of these factors may be seen as a necessary condition for successful change, although they are not proposed as always sufficient. The additional factors in success are the open system in which the organisation exists, the unique individuality of the players and sheer chance. The extent to which formulaic practice alone will lead to a desired outcome, is questioned by the post-modern trend towards longitudinal, open systems attention to the widest possible contextual model. However, this uncertainty is not a licence for inactivity. Rather, there is an imperative to ensure that all components are in place and dynamically addressed and then to maintain constant vigil to understand and reflect the part played by the additional factors.

The Practice

or how you might go about it.

If you are going to bring about change in the area under your control you will need to do a number of practical things for and with the staff who are to be part of that change. These are "*Necessary, but not Sufficient*" conditions. That is to say that they are essential if your organisational change is to be effective, but they will not of themselves guarantee success. They cannot be treated as a recipe that will always gain a consistent outcome, but should be in place before you address the more idiosyncratic concerns of individuals and the way that they interpret the environment in which they operate. In addition to the issues below, there are contextual issues that will influence the open system that is your workplace. These will have a significant bearing on outcomes. There will be benefit to you in being well informed about the context in which you operate and taking such account, as you are able. This will allow you to better understand, when outcomes are not as you expected even though you have done everything "According to The Book"

Models of change management: Forcefield analysis

Good change management requires a sound internal logic. This gives credence to the process and

Allows you to understand when the process does not go as you have expected. The Lewin (1951) models have passed the test of time and retain considerable currency.

Force field theory suggests that you use a three-stage process: Unfreeze, Change and Refreeze. Two commonly found errors in change management are to attempt to change without unfreezing or to fail to refreeze the system and lock up the new situation afterwards, thereby allowing backsliding to the previous state.

Unfreezing

Unfreezing requires the change manager to remove those forces that hold the present practices and processes in place. Many possible forces encourage a workforce to remain with an existing mode of practice. These may include:

1) Administrative processes that ensure the present arrangements persist. I.e. because of the way the infrastructure of the organisation operates it is easiest to continue with existing practices. These processes must be removed, in order that they do not encourage inertia.

2) Reward systems will have been established to encourage operation in a particular way. If a new way of operating is to be established, then the old reward systems may be unhelpful and may need to be dismantled. This may include alteration of formal rewards such as bonus and overtime payments, or informal rewards such as deals regarding leave opportunities.

3) Satisfaction with current processes militates against change Therefore, it is necessary to establish an agreement that current working is not delivering the best possible results for patients and clients in order to enable the workforce to contemplate changing.

4) Loyalties to groups other than the employer may result in resistance to change if those groups are to be disrupted by the change. This is countered by asking employees to consider that they are a part of a different group alongside the existing one. It can be achieved in most cases, only with patient attention. A

number of phases of the various NHS reforms have involved breaking down tribal loyalties to professions and encouraging new loyalties to client related groups. This process has operated over a long time frame with some success, allowing professional clinicians to consider themselves a part of a group serving for example People with Learning Disabilities as much as a group of people who are Speech & Language Therapists.

Many other factors may be implicated in freezing the current situation and thereby preventing change. It is your responsibility as a change agent or as a professional involved in a changing service to identify and unfreeze these forces.

The Forcefield Analysis may be useful in identifying and describing some of these pressures.

You can use the force field analysis. to show the direction and strength of all of the forces freezing the paradigm. These can then be examined explicitly and removed, or undermined, wherever possible. The diagram also shows the forces supporting the change such as each of the benefits anticipated for patients or clients.

You will achieve change when the forces for change outweigh those for stasis from the perspective of all employees. However, it is a mistake to force change by simply building the change forces so that they overwhelm the forces for stasis. In such a model, as you will see, the forces may become massive and the organisation can be very volatile with unsatisfactory results for employees. Reducing the forces for stasis will allow change to be effected with only small change driving forces. This change will be more harmonious.

The Change Equation: **(D+V+S) >R** will also allow you to balance the positive and negative forces and decide when you are in a position to effect change. When the positive forces D, V & S in the change equation. exceed the resistive forces R then change is to be expected. However, reducing resistance will create a better change than simply escalating the forces for change.

Changing

Once freedom to change has been achieved through careful unfreezing of the existing paradigm you can bring about change. This requires a sequential plan that is well understood by all stakeholders. A sound and robust plan can be developed by a process of divergent and convergent thinking involving stakeholders. The divergent phase of the plan might involve exercises such as brainstorming where all possible angles and opportunities are expressed. A brainstorm may be conducted by inviting all participants to offer ideas, which are recorded on open display such as on a "flip chart". Participants should not judge the comments of peers, since it is often the quixotic suggestions that can point to the most creative developments. However, colleagues should be encouraged to build one upon another's comments and in this way help creative plans to emerge.

> *If for example, there is a need to change arrangements for notifying a plethora of community colleagues about frequent changes to responsibilities in the department, a quixotic suggestion might be "We could always try sky-writing". Nobody expects that to happen, but the build might be, "Of course we couldn't do that, but we could post it on a secure Intranet site, and put the address on all referral forms."*

Thus, a creative, but impractical suggestion has led to a creative and very practical solution. This ability to build on the suggestions of colleagues, rather than seeking to solve all problems individually can be a mark of an effective team.

The Plan

The change plan must cover all aspects of the change in order to proceed smoothly and not to involve frequent redirecting, thereby losing the confidence of the participants. Aspects to consider include:

Mission Statement

A reminder should be given of the purpose of the organisation, showing how the proposed change. will advance that mission

Strategic Direction

It should be made clear how this change. will advance the agreed strategic direction. of the organisation. This will reassure those concerned that the change is not a whim of the manager, but a logical. move in the already agreed direction.

Summary of Business

The plan should show what is achieved now with current systems, and what will be done after the change. demonstrating clear benefit.

Market Analysis

Where appropriate, the plan should show the evidence for a belief that the customers. purchasers. clients, patients, etc want these changes.

Assumptions and contingencies.

The plan will involve assumptions. If these are proven wrong by developments, then you do not want the workforce to see this as a mistake. If assumptions and contingencies. are made explicit at the planning stage, then when they are enacted as a result of environmental changes, it will be seen as good planning. rather than correcting an error.

Details of the changes planned

Each move must be described in careful detail. If it is possible to delegate these choices, then the objectives. and outcomes required might be detailed and the subordinate department allowed to devise careful plans that will achieve these targets.

The plan should be checked and challenged through wide consultation before publication in order that it is seen as robust. Responsiveness to comment at the design stage will be perceived as flexibility, but alterations after the launch will appear as incompetence.

Financial Implications

How changes will alter the financial position must be made explicit, and where any new resources will be accessed must be agreed before publication of a plan. New resources must include short-term resources to drive the change as well as new resources to run the organisation in its future state.

Human Resource Plan

The plan must consider and explain: negotiation, retraining, re-deployment and recruitment. of workers. Each of these actions will have different lead times. and the plan should show when they are to be initiated so that necessary workforce comes on line at exactly the time for the service needs. A hold-up in a plan, while staff are recruited, although common, must demonstrate incompetent planning.

Plant and equipment

The plan will show any changes needed to equipment and buildings. These developments must be initiated so that they are delivered at just the right time for service needs. This is simply a matter of advance planning.

and reduces the resistance from employees based upon absence of needed resources.

Critical Path Analysis and Plan

In order to visualise and communicate a plan a Critical Path Analysis (CPA) might be drawn up, showing the relationships between the various components of the plan and indicating when each task should be initiated. The critical path is the sequence of activities dependent one upon another, that decide the length of time needed for the change. Items on this path must occur exactly to schedule or the change will be delayed. Other activities will have some allowance for slippage. The CPA, below, shows when each activity is to occur. Working backward from project completion in Dec and allowing the known lead-time for each component will enable you to calculate start times for each aspect of the change.

Jan	Feb	Mar	April	May	June	July	Aug	Sept	Oct	Nov	Dec
Consult						Recruit					
	Audit	plan	Devise	Syste	ms m						Train
							Instal l	equi p	men t		

The critical path is: Consult, Audit. Plant, Devise Systems, Recruit and Train staff. Install equipment.

GANTT Chart

	Jan	Feb	Mar	April	June	August	Sept	Oct
Consult	====							
Audit plant		=====	====					
Devise Systems			====	====				
Install						====	====	

Equipment						▓▓		
Recruit					=====	====		
Training							====	====

Re-freezing

Once the new paradigm has been established, action must be taken to lock it into place, and thereby prevent backsliding to the old systems. Re-freezing requires consideration of a number of issues. These might include;

Administrative procedures. You may need to alter reporting arrangements, referral arrangements, etc if you are to prevent employees, colleagues and patients/clients reverting to the old arrangements, because they are accessing their old administrative contacts.

Rewards systems. Rewards such as grading structures may have been put into place to support the old paradigm. If salary depends upon how many subordinate staff you had, then moving to a system of collegiate working will disadvantage you and you will be at risk of rebuilding your empire. The grading structure would need revision to reward the new collegiate working.

Informal networks. If employees choose exclusively to interact socially with a former team. then the new team will not adequately gel. You may benefit from organising social events, such as informal sport meetings. BBQs, treasure hunts, etc in which new colleagues may form loyalties.

Make explicit the benefits enjoyed by all stakeholders. A newsletter might regularly focus on the benefits of the new paradigm. thereby creating an ownership of the new arrangements.

Tactics to enable Change

When applying a change process as described above, a number of broad conditions will help. The following considerations have been shown to help and may play an essential part in your planning.

Communication and feedback

The quality of communication within your service and between services needs to be even more effective during a period of change. than at other times. Change plans make the grapevine for communication become more than usually active and convincing. Incomplete information, promulgated by informal routes will create anxiety about the changes, leading to unnecessary stress and resistance. The counter to the grapevine is good accurate and timely communication. This must be readily available, multi-channel and comprehensively understood. Devices to consider include:

Team Briefing

Here you create a formal updating message, containing accurate and simple packages that are passed from the top to the bottom of the organisation thereby dispelling the most alarming of the rumours that abound. Team briefing should be short and swift. Information is cascaded through agreed channels very rapidly. The briefing exercise involves ensuring that everyone knows and understands the message, but it must not become a discussion forum, because that will make the exercise too time consuming to be effective, and the message may become distorted.

Newsletter

A special edition of an existing newsletter might be introduced to carry change information, or it might be necessary to create one for the purpose. A newsletter has the advantage of being the result of careful thought and attention to wording and it has permanence. If departments are encouraged to keep a file copy, then individuals can refer back as appropriate and can take some responsibility for dispelling incorrect information that is the subject of rumour.

Bulletin boards

Where a new project is established, it may be helpful to establish a short lived notice board through which information can be disseminated. For multi-site organisations, several will be needed. The Intranet for your organisation may be able to offer a virtual bulletin board for public display of information. You may even want to allow the board to carry staff questions as well as management answers. Such a process allows the entire workforce to see the dialogue that surrounds the change. and therefore better understand the decisions that emerge. This is particularly effective in the case of virtual bulletin boards on the Intranet. It is important, if you develop this system, that it is frequently serviced and questions do not go long unanswered.

Suggestion schemes

Offering your staff the opportunity to make suggestions and contribute to the exercise will make the process seem far less remote. You may be concerned about the less constructive contributions that such schemes attract. However these are easy to 'bin' and should not prevent your harnessing the good will that exists. It is important to attract a high response rate, perhaps by offering a prize, and to find suggestions to publicly adopt, demonstrating the value of the communication exercise.

Roadshows

As a leader in change you need to get among the people affected. This involves travelling to the involved sites, if more than one is involved, and setting aside time to explain the plan and hear reactions. You might also address the various constituencies involved. For instance, domestic staff may be unwilling to raise concerns at meetings where medical consultants lead the questions. They might be more forthcoming at meetings dedicated to ancillary employees. This communication exercise enables the workforce to feel valued and involved and may supply you with useful information and insights. Be willing to hear trivial as well as substantial comments because both can explain resistance to change. In a smaller department, this might involve no more than time in a staff meeting and in larger settings may become a vast semi-public meeting. Whatever the scale, the rule is that you must make yourself visibly available to explain and listen. You must be seen to be putting yourself out for staff benefit, and must couch your communications in terms relevant to the audience. You must also talk about benefits that are applicable to the staff group, not simply the organisation.

Management by wandering about (MBWA)

It will be helpful if you can make informal time to talk, and listen to affected staff. You might also encourage managers from higher in the organisation to accompany you on some tours. This partnership will show the workforce that they are respected and valued in the process, because managers at all levels take the trouble to visit. "Wandering About" with senior managers will reassure staff that you have access to more influential management tiers and that they hear you. This will encourage your staff to confide in you, because you are seen to be able to act on their behalf.

Ownership

For enthusiastic co-operation with change plans, employees need to know that they have been consulted about plans and have played a part in their development. Thus, they are implementing plans that they constructed. Gaining ownership will require involvement of staff at all stages of the process. As soon as change is anticipated, it may be appropriate to commence a dialogue, so that staff are able to work through the issues and accept the need for change, before the planning stage is reached (Unfreezing).

Once the need for change is accepted, the nature of the objectives can be discussed. Once the objectives are agreed, the means by which they can be achieved can be discussed. Clearly, these stages are sequential. It is a common error to be trying to gain acceptance on one stage, when the previous stage has not been agreed.

If you have authority to design your own solutions, you can work with interested staff to produce a solution. This change will be very easy to implement, because the workforce owns it. If you write your own solution and then try to sell it to the workforce, you can expect resistance, even if the solution is the one that the staff would have chosen had they been given the chance. If you are going to be required to implement a solution from another tier of the organisation, over which you have little influence, then the consultation process should be conducted as a fact finding exercise, with small groups. Thus, if an idea is offered that, although sensible, is not in line with "orders" then you must not be in the position of failing to honour what staff may perceive as an agreement.

Wherever possible, be seen to make or modify plans in line with staff suggestions and thereby maximise the impression that it is their solutions that are being implemented. Do this at the planning stage if possible. To do it at the implementation stage might appear indecisive.

Education

Education gives a perspective that cannot easily be achieved at the workplace. You are advised to increase the opportunities for key staff, and yourself to become involved in short or longer courses. This may appear to be diverting a resource, when there is extra work to be done, but the benefits in terms of improved perspective and insight, as well as ensuring that individuals feel valued. Elevated loyalty can improve the prospects of success, and justify the investment.

Leadership and Trust

You will need to show strong leadership in a time of change. The staff are to follow you into a situation that is unknown. Therefore you must be informed, confident and decisive in your actions. You will consult throughout the process, but this is out of courtesy and respect for their insights, and must not appear as indecision. Trust is achieved by open, comprehensive and candid communication. Some messages will be carefully planned in order to demonstrate decisiveness, and surety, but it is important that information is consistent and honest. Where a change in direction occurs, this should be admitted and explained, rather that shrouded in vagueness. Information that is incomplete, dishonest or inconsistent will lose trust in you, and develop a local grapevine that will convey harmful ideas.

Attention to the impact of change on individuals

Very few people are truly altruistic. They cannot easily accept a change that is for the greater good when it causes them considerable personal disadvantage. You will effect change more easily if you can recognise simple dis-benefits affecting individuals and counter them. This may be alteration of working relationships to protect successful teams or funding additional home-to-work transport. However there may be far more difficult issues to resolve such as redundancies. How these are handled will affect the remaining workforce as much as the redundant individual. All of the assistance described in The Management of People should be offered and the individual helped in every imaginable way.

Some disadvantages affecting individuals may not be immediately evident. Fears and inconveniences must be brought to the surface in order for you to help. Therefore you will need to create an environment where individuals can raise concerns, however trivial or foolish they may appear. If you fail to realise that a change is depriving a staff member of some small but cherished benefit, then you may encounter incomprehensible resistance that could have been avoided by better insight.

The early experience of benefit

Reward those who contribute to the change. Also, contrive to ensure that the early stages of the change bring benefit to all staff. Thus, they may gain enthusiasm for the process and help it to continue. Generally, the higher you rise in an organisation, the longer will be your time focus. Therefore, where you may be happy to know that there will be advantages in two years, staff lower in the organisation might need far swifter evidence of benefit.

There may be benefit that is missed by some staff. The newsletter or staff meetings should be used to ensure that all benefits receive maximum publicity. For instance, patients might be receiving better services because of the early stages of a change, but then this may not be obvious to those staff without patient contact. Ensure that this becomes well known and discussed, while, of course respecting the need for confidentiality.

Subsidiarity, and Levels of Interference: breadth and depth of intervention

Devolve responsibility for designing change and then implementing it as low in the organisation as possible. This will minimise resistance and respects the autonomy of staff members. A manager taking this approach will gain respect from staff and build a healthy organisation. It is essential that the objectives are agreed and that the plans drawn up will be acceptable to the wider organisation. However, there are frequently a number of ways to achieve one objective and if individuals can chose their own solutions, they will implement them with greater enthusiasm and strive to ensure that they work well.

Conclusion to tactical endeavours to enable change

Health and social care provision is in a state of permanent change. It may be tempting to look forward to the time when it all settles down, however, there is no reason to believe that it will and, therefore, good clinicians must perform in a constantly changing environment. Additionally, clinicians and managers must strive to make change as smooth, positive and patient/client friendly as possible. That requires a sound knowledge of the issues above, in order to contribute to an environment delivering the necessary although not sufficient conditions for smooth transition. This is the personal responsibility of the change manager, all other managers in the system and all professionals operating in that arena.

References

Beckhard, R. and Harris, R. (1987) *Organisational Transition* London: Addison Wesley.

Bell, J. (2010) *Doing Your Research Project* McGraw-Hill International

Buchanan, D. (1997) The limitations and opportunities of business process reengineering in a politicised Organisational Climate *Journal of Human Relations* 50 (1) pp 51

Burnes,B. (2009) *Managing Change* London: Pitman

Crozier,M. (1976) *The bureaucratic phenomenon* London: Tavistock Publishing.

Dalin, P. (2003) *School development theories and strategies* London: Continuum Studies.

Dekker,W.(1987) *Willingness to change* The Hague: DOP

DoH (1947) ; *NHS Act* London: HMSO

DoH (1949) ; *NHS (Amendments) Act* London: HMSO

DoH (1951) ; *NHS Act* HMSO London: HMSO

DoH (1952) ; *NHS Act* London: HMSO

DoH (1973) ; *NHS Reorganisation Act* London: HMSO

DoH (1979); *Patients First* London: HMSO

DoH (1982) ; *NHS Reorganisation* London: HMSO

DoH (1989a);*Working for Patients* London: HMSO

DoH (1989b); *Caring for People Community Care in the Next Decade and Beyond* London: HMSO

DoH (1990); *The NHS and Community Care Act* London: HMSO

DoH (1997); *A New NHS - Modern and Dependable* London: HMSO

DoH (2003) *NHS reorganisation: The Health and Social Care (Community Health and Standards)* Act London: HMSO

DoH (2012) The White Paper, *Equity and excellence: Liberating the NHS (2010) and Health and Social Care Bill* London: HMSO

Earl,M. Sampler,J. Short,J. (1997) Strategies for business process reengineering *Journal of management information systems* 12, 31 - 56.

Easterby-Smith,M. Thorpe,R. and Lowe,A. (1991) *Management Research* London: Sage

Ezra,D and Oates,D. (1989) *Advice from the Top* London: David and Charles:

Farachex,C. Amado,G. and Laurent,A.(1982) Organisational development and change *Annual review of Psychology* 343 - 370

Ferlie, E., Cairncross, L., and Pettigrew,A.M. (1993) *Perspectives on Strategic Change*, Dordrecht The Netherlands :Kluwer

Festinger,L. (1957) *The theory of cognitive dissonance* Stanford University Press: California: Stanford

Friedlander,C. (1976) OD Reaches adolescence *Journal of applied behavioural science* 12 (1) 43-47

Gale, E. (2004) The Hawthorne studies-a fable for our times? *Journal of QJM* 97 (7) [online]. accessed: 12 November 2007

Goodstein,L.D., And Burk,W.W.(1991)Creating successful organisational Change *Organisational Dynamics* Spring 151 - 164

Ham,C. (1991) *The New National Health Service: organisation and management* Oxford: Radcliffe Medical Press

Ham,C. (2009) *Health Policy in Britian* Radcliffe Medical Press: Oxford:Palgrave Mcmillan

Handy,C. (2002) *The age of unreason* London: Business Books Ltd.

Handy,C. (2009) *Gods of Management: The Changing Work of Organisations* London: Arrow Books

Harrison,R.(1970) Choosing the depth of organisational intervention *Journal of Applied Behavioural Science* 6 6 (2) 118 - 201

Hogan,K. (1997) *Change in the NHS* in Clark,J. and Copcutt L Management for nurses and health Oxford:OUP

Johnson,G. (1993) in Mabey,C. and Mayon-White,B. (Eds) (1993) *Managing Change* London: OU Press

Kent, R. (2001) *Installing Change:* An Executive Guide for Implementing and Maintaining Organisational Change. Winnipeg: Pragma Press

Lewin, K. (1951)*Field Theory in Social Science.* New York: Harper & Row

Lippitt,G. Langseth,P. Mossop,J. (1985) *Implementing Organisational Change* Jossey – London: Bass

Lippitt,G. Langseth,P. Mossop,J. (1985) *Implementing Organisational Change* Jossey – London: Bass

Mabey,C., and Mayon-White,B. (Eds) (1993) *Managing Change* London: OU Press

March,J.G., and Simon,H.A.(1958) *Organisations* New York: Wiley

Marris,P. (1993) *the management of change* in Mabey,C., and Mayon-White,B. (Eds) (1993) Managing Change OU Press: London

Mullins, L. (2005) *Management and Organisational Behaviour.* Harlow: Pearson Education Limited.

Nadler,D.(1993) *Organisation Development* in Mabey,C., and Mayon-White,B. (Eds) (1993) *Managing Change* OU Press: London

Nadler,D.and Tushman,L.(1979) Feedback and organisation development Using data based methods *Journal of human relations* 50 (1) 52 - 72.

National Institute for Health Clinical Excellence (2007) *How to Change Practice: Understand, identify and overcome barriers.* London: NICE

Nuffield Trust (2014) *http://nhstimeline.nuffieldtrust.org.uk/*

Parkin, P. (2009*) Managing Change in Healthcare: Using Action Research.* London: Sage

Pavlov,I.P. (1927) *Conditioned Reflexes* Oxford University Press: London

Peters,T. (1991) *Thriving on Chaos* New York: Harper Perennial

Pettigrew, A.M. (2003) *Strategy as Process, Power, and Change*, in Cummings, S., & Wilson, D, *Images of Strategy,* Blackwell Publishing, pp. 301-330

Pettigrew,A.M. (1985) *The awakening Giant: Continuity and change in ICI* Oxford: Blackwell

Pettigrew,A.M *change in ICI*. (1993)a in Luca,Z Zambon,S and Pettigrew,A.M. *Perspectives on Strategic Change* Kluwer London: Academic Press,

Pettigrew,A.M. (1993)b in Tilly, I. *Managing the Internal Market* Chapman London

Pettigrew,A.M. Ferlie,E. and McKee,L.(1992) The leadership role of the new health authorities *Public Money and Management* ,April 39 – 43

Plant,R. (1987) *Managing change and making it stick* London: Fontana

Price,C. and Murphy,M (1987) Organisational Development in British Telecom *Training and Development* July 45 - 48

Qiun,J.B. (1980) *Strategies for change* Homewood Illinois: Irwin

Skinner,G.,E. (1974) *About Behaviourism* Cape: London

Smith,M., Beck,J., Cooper,C.L., Cox,C., Ottoway, D., and Talbot,R. (1982) *Introducing Organisational Behaviour*. Macmillan: London

Spurgeon,P. and Barwell,F. (1991) *Implementing Change in the NHS* Chapman and Hall: London

Upton,T.& Brooks,B. (1995) *Managing Change in NHS* L'don: Kogan Page

Vaill,P. (19820The purposing of high-performing systems *Organisational Dynamics* 2 (2) 23 - 39

Van de Ven,A.H. (1980) Problem solving, planning and innovation *Human relations Journal* 33 Nov 10 - 11

Vrakking,W.(1997) The implementation Game *Journal of Organisational Change Management* 8 (3) 31-46

Walton,M. (1997) *Management and Managing: Leadership in the NHS* London: Stanley Thornes

Walton,M. (1997) *Management and Managing: Leadership in the NHS* London: Stanley Thornes

White,B. and Jaques, A. (1995) *Managing Change* London: OU Press

White,R. and Jacques,R. (1995) Operationalising the post modernity construct for efficient organisational change management. *Journal of change management.* 8 (2) 45 – 71

Wilson,T,A. (1994) *A Manual for Change* Aldershot: Pitman

Benton,P. (1990) *Riding the whirlwind* Oxford: Blackwell

Leadership

Introduction

Leadership is the crucial factor in effecting change and maintaining excellent service provision (Storey, 2013). Leadership is found throughout the organisation, not just at the top (Bolden, Gosling, Marturano & Dennison 2003). Therefore, it is essential that all clinicians as well as managers develop a strong leadership ability. It is not required that all players are leaders at all times but a distributed notion of leadership (Barr, & Dowding 2012) suggests that we all have to take a lead at some point and the ability to know when and how is critical to health and social care efficacy.

Leadership is defined in many places with differing results: Mullins (2007:363) considers that *'leadership is a relationship through which one person influences the behaviour or actions of other people'*. This cannot be disputed, but allows leadership to be influence, regardless of purpose. It may be possible to identify leaders who consider that as long as they are *'in control'* then they are good leaders. Of course to be in control is not necessarily desirable and if not used to the benefit of the organisation is worthless or worse. Leaders may be driven by a wish that team members are doing what they as leaders say, imagining that makes them good leaders. As we have seen in chapter 1, good management is that which gets the greatest value output, in terms of volume and quality for the resource available. This may or may not be achieved by being in control of people. In many cases relaxing control and allowing autonomy will result in greater and better output. Control without purpose and output is an abuse.

> **Case example**
>
> **Manager 1**: "I am a good leader because I am in absolute control of what *'My Staff'* do. You are a poor leader because you allow *'Your Staff'* to make their own decisions."
>
> **Manager 2**: "I am a good leader. These people are not *'My Staff'*. I do not own them; we both work for the firm. By agreeing ideal results and allowing autonomy, I get a very high level output from "*My Colleagues*". You are a poor leader, because although your bullying results in tight control of "*Your Colleagues'*" actions, the output is poor because they are not motivated. They do exactly what you demand, but are not driven by a desire to do the very best they can for you or for the firm."

Northouse, (2012:15) offers us *'Leadership is a process whereby an individual influences a group of individuals to achieve a common goal.'* This is useful because it allows that control is not essential and influence may be more effective and reminds us that it is only valuable where it is focussed on the common goal. In a situation of employment, a common goal will be the goal set by the organisation.

Gill (2011:9) develops the notion further by saying that 'Leadership is showing the way & helping or inducing others to follow it. This entails envisioning a desirable future, promoting a clear purpose or mission, supportive values and intelligent strategies and empowering an engaging all those who are concerned.' The leader may be seen as a servant, helping rather than controlling.

So, a notion emerges that Leadership is a communications exercise, clarifying the vision, aim and objectives and then causing the team members to actively pursue that goal. As will be clear, below, from discussions of Distributed Leadership, Transformational Leadership and high-level motivators an autonomous team member enabled by a leader can achieve exceptional results because he/she wants to; far higher than can a controlled person subject to over directive leadership and micro-management.

This chapter sets out to explore how a powerful leader achieves dramatic results by correctly electing to enthuse, enable, support, persuade and direct as required by the situation and even facilitate an autonomous team member driving him/herself far harder than any manager could do.

Bullying management and leadership can force the team member to do the minimum necessary to avoid discipline and dismissal, whereas with inspiring leadership and management there is no limit to the excellence that team members can seek to display.

Leadership thinking can be tracked from the beginning of the 20th Century. These might be taken as: Great Man Theories, Trait Theories, Behaviourist Theories,
Situational Leadership, Contingency Theories, Transactional Theories and Transformational Theories.

Great Man Theories

Closely based on the European and UK Class structure, the great man notion was that leaders are exceptional people, who were born with innate qualities and destined to lead.

People were thought to have the right strengths as a right of birth. It was assumed that only men could lead (with only a few very memorable exceptions) and that they were superior as a matter of breeding.

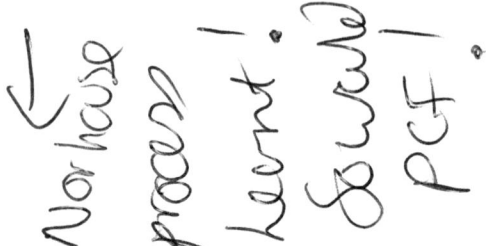

This applied very strongly in the military where social class dictated rank and industry where the same was true. Since wealth and ownership was also inherited, the system and belief was self-perpetuating

Trait Theories

Living with great man theories invites an attempt to identify the traits that were being transferred by this inheritance. Many lists of traits or qualities associated with leadership exist and continue to be generated. They draw on some positive and virtuous human attribute.

The military continue to assess for traits that predict leadership ability and this is still replicated in Assessment Centres frequently employed to select senior managers in health and care organisations.

However, research carried out to demonstrate an association between leadership success and specific traits has been largely inconclusive (Stogdill, 1974). The best that can be offered is a set of traits common to most schemata. Although they are rather predictable, they are at least available in all social classes and learnable.

Traits	Skills
- Adaptable	- intelligent
- Alert to social subtlety	- able to conceptualise and visualise
- Ambitious	- Creative
- Assertive	- Diplomatic and tactful
- Cooperative	- Fluent in language
- Decisive	- Knowledgeable about group task
- Dependable	- administrative ability
- Dominant	- Persuasive
- High activity level	- Socially skilled
- Persistent	
- Self-confident	
- Tolerant of stress	
- Tolerant of Paradox	
- Willing to assume responsibility	

As will be seen, later, these qualities fit well with the emerging notions around *Emotional Intelligence* as a predictor of leadership ability.

Psychological Behaviourist Theories

As traits studies have been inconclusive leadership and management analysts considered the way in which leaders behave rather than what they were like. This is commonly referred to as adopting different Leadership Styles.

Theory X and Theory Y

In 1960 McGregor reported observing two basic beliefs about a workforce each having its own consequent approach to leadership. These McGregor (1960) described as 'Theory X and Theory Y' managers.

Theory X managers and leaders were said to believe that workers have an inherent dislike of work and will avoid it if possible. Therefore, people must be coerced, controlled, directed, or threatened with punishment to get them to work hard.

The worker prefers to be directed, wishes to avoid responsibility, has relatively little ambition, and wants security above all else.

Theory Y managers and leaders were said to believe that hard work is natural as rest, and the worker, under proper conditions, learns not only to accept but to seek and enjoy responsibility. All workers will exercise self-direction and self-control to achieve objectives to which they are committed.

Workers have capacity to exercise a relatively high level of imagination, ingenuity, and creativity in the discharge of work and the intellectual potentialities of the average human being are only partially utilized under the conditions of modern industrial life.

The point of this theory, the irony and the joke, is that both of these leaders can be shown to be entirely correct. Leaders and managers who assume theory X will develop an unenthusiastic workforce that needs constant driving.

Managers who assume Theory Y will develop an enthusiastic workforce who need enabling, not driving.

Blake and Mouton's Managerial Grid

In the *Managerial Grid* Blake & Mouton (1964) focus on task and employee orientations of managers and plots five basic leadership styles. Blake & Mouton, observed that some managers and leaders considered that the task was the only point of the team and others believed that concern for the people was the key to success. They expressed the view that concentration on one to the detriment of the other would work against good performance and that success required close attention to both factors.

High people focus	*Country club Mx*		*Team Mx*
Medium people focus		*Organisational Mx*	
Low people focus	*Impoverished Mx*		*Authority/obedience*
	Low task focus	Medium task focus	High task focus

This was further developed by John Adair (1973) who added to the Blake & Mouton list suggesting three constituencies: task, people and additionally the team. Again, leaders must not focus on one to the detriment of the others. In Adair's Action-Centred Leadership Model a 3-circle Venn diagram based on mathematical 'sets theory' (Devlin, 1993) describes a 'sweet spot' in which managers and leaders are focussed all three constituencies and achieve the best in long-term as well as short-term results.

Situational and contingency Leadership

Lewin, Lippitt & White (1935) identified three types of manager:

1) **Autocratic Manager** who dictates and expects obedience, evidently associated with McGregor's theory X.
2) **Democratic Manager** who allows the team to contribute to decisions on the best way to achieve the organisation's aims. Evidently associated with McGregor's Theory Y.
3) **Laissez Faire manager** who offers minimal managerial intervention. (Why did he give that one a name in French?).

It can appear that one of these will bear fruit more rapidly than the others, especially after considering the later ideas of McGregor (1960), Adair (1973), and Blake & Mouton, (1964)., However, it rapidly becomes evident that each has its place in different settings:

If the building is on fire, or the patient has an arterial bleed, the leader is not expected to call a meeting and ask for suggestions; he/she takes immediate and strict control. Autocratic Leadership has a place.

This leads to the idea that different situations need different leadership and management. A number of 'contingency theories' or situationally based theories emerged.

The Hersey-Blanchard Situational Leadership Model

The Hersey-Blanchard Leadership Situational Leadership Model (Hersey & Blanchard, 1996) develops this thinking by suggesting that the developmental levels of team members play a role when deciding which leadership style is most appropriate.

The amount of direction (task behaviour) and support (relationship behaviour) a leader must provide depends on the "level of maturity" of the followers. These may be categorised as M1, M2, M3 and M4.

Enthusiastic Beginner M1:

>keen to learn = low competence

>has clear vision of what they want to do = high commitment

Directing Leader The team requires high level of direction from leader

Disillusioned Learner M2

>some skills = increasing competence

>frustration at all there is to learn = low commitment

Coaching Leader - The team requires high levels of direction and support from leader

Capable but Cautious Contributor M3

>mostly capable = moderate to high competence

>some clear successes and challenges = variable commitment

Supporting Leader - The team requires high level of support from leader

Self-reliant Achiever M4

      independently capable = high competence

      able to create success = high motivation

Delegating Leader - The team requires low level of support from leader

Leadership skills are therefore applied in response the team member's needs. They are:

Directing: The leader provides clear instructions and specific direction.

Coaching: The leader encourages two-way communication and helps build confidence and motivation on the part of the employee, although the leader still has responsibility and controls decision making.

Supporting: The leader and followers share decision making and no longer need or expect the relationship to be directive.

Delegating: The leader allows the competent and motivated team member to take full responsibility.

Feidler's Contingency Leadership Model

Feidler (1967) devised a model focussing not on the people being led but the leader and task, suggesting that there are three conditions to consider:

The *power* of the leader, the *relationship* between leader and led, the *structure* of the task. By scoring each of these as high or low an overall score can be derived. If that score is very high or very low, the leader can be directive in style. If the result is neither high nor low, then the style would be better as affiliative and collaborative.

So, if you have power, a good relationship and a very structured task, then you can be quite directive.

If you have none of the above, then you will also resort to directive leadership.

However, if there is a mixture of strong and weak in your analysis, as is commonly the case in healthcare, what Feidler describes as 'Moderately favourable' situation, then you are advised to adopt a relationship focussed approach.

Transactional and Transformational Leadership Theory

Burns (1978) and then Bass and Alvolio (1994) identified a divergence between two approaches to Leading people.

Transactional Leadership

In transactional Leadership, a 'transaction' occurs – a deal. A worker agrees to perform a duty and in exchange an organisation gives pay and other reward. These rewards are said to be 'contingent' upon performance.

This is a clear, explicit and fair approach to agreeing work. However it is in the nature of a transaction that the worker seeks to obtain as much reward for as little input as possible and the employer seeks to achieve the opposite. That is the strength of a market place. The result is that a negotiation occurs and each party is contented.

However, although this is OK for buying a pair of shoes, in an ideal employment relationship, an employee is committed to the work and does as much as he/she can rather than as little; the employer does the most possible for the employee, not the least. A transactional approach to leadership does not get the most it can from employees. Rewards given tend to be lower order motivators, as described by Maslow (1943), hygiene factors as described by Hertzberg (1987) and follows a McGregor (1960) Theory X management approach.

Transformational Leadership

Transformational leadership seeks to change or 'transform' the situation such that workers perform to the highest possible level, because they want to, based on high commitment to the firm and the client. Individual and organisational goals are in concert so that employees do well by causing the organisation to do well. Generally, it can be assumed that professional people entering health and social care industries want to serve clients to the maximum and therefore fit well within a Transformational Leadership model. However, it is not impossible by deploying a Theory X, Transactional model and to damage this situation and achieve Theory X workers. In a Transactional Leadership model, Hertzburg's Health motivators, from the apex of Maslow's pyramid are used.

Northouse (2012) considers that Transactions can deliver expected outcomes, but only a transformational approach can result in performance beyond expectations.

Motivation theories associated with Transactional and Transformational Leadership Theories

Two approaches to what motivates people, offered by Maslow (1943) and then Hertsberg (1987), exemplify the difference between Transactional and Transformational leadership.

Maslow's theory of motivation

It is easy to recall the notion of five general motivational factors, but rare to see leaders deploy the full concept.

Simply, there are five needs experienced by humans and these might be fulfilled, in part, by their employment. These are given as:

Self-actualisation needs

*************Esteem needs***************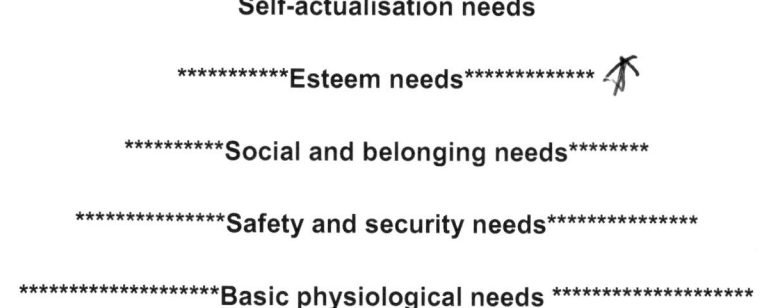

***********Social and belonging needs**********

****************Safety and security needs*****************

********************Basic physiological needs** ********************

Leaders can seek to fulfil these as part of rewarding employment. If the reward is made contingent upon particular performance then this is a Transactional approach. If they are offered in good faith then this is part of a Transformational approach and the result can be a dedication and drive far beyond that achieved by a negotiated transaction.

What makes Maslow's notion powerful is the dual notions that needs are *hierarchical* and *satiable*.

Hierarchical means that a higher level need is unlikely to motivate a worker if a lower level need is unfulfilled. It is hard to consider the pleasures of social contact when you are cold and hungry.

Satiability tells us that a need once satisfied ceases to be a motivator. There is little use telling a worker that this project might set you up for a promotion if he/she is already satisfied with her status (esteem need is satiated), but discussing how valuable the project is to customers would have motivated strongly.

> **Case example**
>
> A manager approaches a teacher and asks her to take on a major and time consuming project.
>
> "This is great experience. You will be able to apply for a promotion to a more senior job!"
>
> "Thanks, but that is not really what I want"
>
> The manager was shocked. The worker did not want what she (the manager) would have wanted in her place. The manager was offering what she would have wanted and assumed other people wanted that too. Had she asked herself 'What does this worker want?' she might have realised that she had already satisfied her drive for status and was driven by a need to self-actualise - to feel that she was doing something worthwhile with her life. Had the reward been phrased as, 'This will *really* help the students', then the worker would have made a different response.

So, being able to list out possible motivators offers little practical guidance to leaders. To consider which need an individual is currently working on and to find ways that their employment can contribute to that is very powerful indeed.

Each of us at any time has satisfied a number of our need groups and has others which we have not satisfied. We all, therefore sit on one of the horizontal lines on Maslow's diagram, and are working to satisfy the next one up. To motivate a worker, know which level he/she needs to satisfy next and be the agent of that satisfaction. If you do so conditionally, you are transactional. If you do so unconditionally, you are transformational, but the key is to be working on the right level for them – not for you.

A key in this was explained very well by Blanchard & Zigarmi (2011) or before that Blanchard & Johnson (2000). The 'golden rule - *do as you would be done by*' is not correct. Treat people not as *you* would want to be treated but as *they* want to be treated. (Consider accessing the Blanchard audio and AV versions; they are usually pretty energising to watch or hear.)

Hertzberg's health and hygiene

Hertzberg, built upon Maslowe's idea, observing that higher level motivators are capable of positive motivation, without limit to what can be achieved (Hertsberg 1987). These he called 'Health' factors. Lower level motivators, which he called 'hygiene' factors, are commonly used punitively in threatening or bullying, theory X management style. These can coerce workers to achieve the required minimum, in order to continue to receive those rewards, but cannot be used to encourage higher results.

A worker can be bullied by threats to withdraw physiological and safety needs by threatening job security to such an extent that he/she will work hard enough to avoid dismissal. It will not encourage a worker to more than the minimum to avoid that dismissal. Self-actualisation and esteem as motivators can result in extremely high levels of commitment and contribution.

Simple bullying may be seen as a threat to basic needs, by making workers generally uncomfortable. This can achieve a basic level of performance, but cannot achieve the loyalty and dedication that make us all 'go the extra mile'. That is only encouraged by the higher level motivators. Of course, this closely mirrors McGregor's theory X theory Y notion (1960). It is this convergence from different information sources, similar to research 'triangulation' that makes the ideas particularly persuasive.

Distributed Leadership

Distributed and shared leadership sometimes offered as a new notion, in reality having long history in education and health, refers to the recognition that a team intentionally contains individuals with diverse abilities such that each may offer leadership when the situation demands. The baton may be passed according to expertise and need at any moment. The team may achieve leadership by collective action. This gives a very high degree of 'ownership' and acceptance of responsibility throughout a team and collective responsibility can ensure a very reliable and creative output.

Distributed leadership can feel different and imprecise because it is not something 'done' by an individual 'to' others.

It is a set of individual actions through which people contribute to a group or organization; a group activity that works through and within relationships, rather than individual action. (Bennett *et al.* 2003, p. 3)

Power and Politics

In Newtonian Physics, power is the ability to do work. The more power available the greater the rate of work. In the workplace the same applies, Power is the ability a manager or leader has to get things done (Handy, 1993). Politics is manipulation in order to enhance our power (Handy, 1993).

Power is rarely held in just one place within the team. Rather it may be identified in a range of forms distributed among a number of players. French and Ravens (1959) identified five sources of power in a model actively employed today. Each confers an ability to lead. These can all sometimes converge in one person, but more commonly are distributed around the team giving each a responsibility to offer a degree of leadership.

Legitimate power is that power conferred simply by position in the organisational chart. The manager holds power.

Reward power is that obtained by being able to confer reward or benefit on others. We do as requested because we want the reward. This may come from being 'the boss' but may come from many other means of reward. The caretaker and receptionist may have power because we want their help with parking, visitors, access to resources, etc. To hold the key to the stationary cupboard is a position of power. A simple habit of noticing and praising success in colleagues gives us an ability to rewards and a measure of power.

Expert power exists within each team. It may be in the hands of the leader if there is only one profession and he/she is the most experienced member. However in a multidisciplinary enterprise many types of expertise exist and in a well-run team each expert moves into a position of power according to the topic under considerations.

Referent power exists where an individual has respect because of long experience, special qualification, general social skill, etc. This may occur where a player is an expert, but although the expertise is not relevant to the topic we respect him/her nonetheless. For example a doctor may have power in the meeting even where the discussion bears no relationship to matters medical.

Coercive power involves deploying the power to punish as a means of gaining co-operation. This fits with theory X thinking as described by

McGregor (1960), and would be indicative of a manager in a very poor situation.

Conclusion

A range of ideas have emerged and been tested to varying degree s in order to explain and predict leadership success. Although each is in part superseded, none is entirely discarded. Each is integrated into a whole which leads to the next step in a continuum of ideas. Therefore, each can retain some value in understanding a subtle and sometimes counterintuitive system by which we all influence the results in our collective endeavour.

The Practice

or how you might go about it

Leadership is clearly crucial, but that statement is an unhelpful generalisation until you have some idea how you personally will deliver good leadership. Over a century, different notions have been believed and then superseded be newer ones. However, each historical notion had some merit and can be seen to have been integrated into the new rather than simply replaced. Therefore, you can address each notion and draw lessons from it to enhance your ability as a leader.

Great Man or Trait Theories clearly show some qualities that clearly do predict leadership success. While we no longer accept that these are inborn as a right of social class, there are many behaviours and qualities that you can develop in yourself. Stogdill (1974) researched and demonstrated that leaders are: Adaptable, Alert to social subtlety, Ambitious, Assertive, Cooperative, Decisive, Dependable, Dominant,

Highly active, Persistent, Self-confident, Tolerant of stress, Tolerant of Paradox and Willing to assume responsibility.

Some of these 'traits' are more apt to your setting and your personality than others, but there is much to be gained by selecting the most promising and developing them in yourself. You can do the same with Stogdill's list of skills, developing abilities to suit your such as: the ability to visualise, to be creative, diplomatic and tactful You could seek to develop fluency in language, knowledge about group tasks, administrative ability, persuasiveness and social skills. In this, you are taking an evidence based approach to enhancing your leadership abilities.

You might represent these skills as a profile, noting your current skill level, your ideal skill level considering your ambition and then devise a plan to bridge the gap:

Minimum standard

Skill	1	2	3	4	5	6
Persistent	✶✶✶	✶✶✶	✶✶✶			
Adaptable	✶✶✶	✶✶✶				
Social skilled	✶✶✶	✶✶✶	✶✶✶	✶✶✶		
Ambitious	✶✶✶	✶✶✶				
Assertive	✶✶✶					
Cooperative	✶✶✶	✶✶✶	✶✶✶	✶✶✶	✶✶✶	
Decisive	✶✶✶	✶✶✶	✶✶✶			
Dependable	✶✶✶	✶✶✶	✶✶✶	✶✶✶	✶✶✶	
Dominant	✶✶✶					
Highly active	✶✶✶	✶✶✶	✶✶✶	✶✶✶		

Considering psychological leadership theories, you do not need to ask whether you want to be an X or Y leader (McGregor, 1960), but may have a complex journey to move an existing theory X culture to a theory Y. This intersects with moving from a Transactional to a Transformational leadership and employing health rather than hygiene motivators.

To achieve this involves sensitive and intricate effort but can be done. Consider what motivators are at work in each team member and endeavour to create a work environment that contributes to satisfying that level which the individual needs next. Consider making this benefit unconditional where you have a dedicated worker who will respond to good will with hard work and make the maximum contribution. Only where you have a totally uncommitted worker, will you need to make reward contingent (conditional) upon satisfactory performance. And remember from your clinical knowledge that reward is better than punishment. Blanchard & Johnson (2000) describe this, saying 'catch people doing it right – not wrong'. Wherever possible, notice and reward best performance, rather than seeking out and criticising poor performance. We know that we change behaviour more successfully by rewarding desirable behaviour, than by punishing undesirable behaviour and this works equally well with work performance.

Consider Adair (1973) and (Blake & Mouton, 1964). Every task must be achieved to the very best level possible, but each can also be considered an opportunity to enhance the individual workers and the team as well. For example, allocate tasks in a way that also benefits the individual by giving the right learning opportunities to each person according to his/her development needs. Perform tasks in such a way that the team achieves them collectively, thus enhancing cohesion in the team. Sometimes an individual may be capable alone, but better team development is achieved by collective effort.

Consider Hersey & Blanchard (1996) in conjunction with Feidler (1967) and you can analyse the people as well as the context in order to decide how you might address different situations in different ways to achieve the very best outcomes. How favourable is your situation? and how well developed are your workers? Should you be directive or affiliative as a result and will you apply an approach that amounts to directing, coaching, supporting or

Conclusion

There is considerable space to analyse and make calculated efforts to enhance your leadership skill and practice. Keep in mind that Power to lead does not reside in one person, but is distributed among a range of people. French and Ravens (1959) in a model actively employed today offer you five power sources and you can seek to develop and exploit one or several of these as part of developing your leadership capability.

References

Adair, J. (1973) *Action-Centred Leadership*. New York,:McGraw-Hill.

Alimo-Metcalfe, B. & Alban-Metcalfe, J. (2006) More (good) leaders for the public sector. *International Journal of Public Sector Management.* 19(4), 293-315

Amitay, M., Popper, M. & Lipshitz, R. (2005) Leadership styles and organizational learning in community clinics. *The Learning Organization.* 12 (1), 57-70.

Badaracco, J.L. *(*2001*)*. We don't need another hero. *Harvard Business Review,* 79*(*8*), pp.* 120–126. Barry, D. *(*1991*).* Managing the bossless team: lessons in distributed leadership. *Organizational Dynamics,* 20*, pp.* 31–47.

Barr, J, and Dowding, L. (2012) *Leaders in Health Care* (2nd Edition) Sage Publication. London

Bass, B. (1985) *Leadership and Performance Beyond Expectations*. New York: Free Press.

Bass, B.M. & Avolio, B.J. (Eds.). (1994). *Improving organizational effectiveness through transformational leadership*. Thousand Oaks, CA: Sage Publications.

Bass, B.M. (1999) Two Decades of Research and Development in Transformational Leadership. *European Journal of Work and Organizational Psychology*. 8(1), 9-32.

Bass, B.M. and Valenzi, E.R. (1974). Contingent aspects of effective management styles. In J.G. Hunt and L.L. Larson (eds.) *Contingency Approaches to Leadership*. Carbondale: Southern Illinois University Press.

Bass, B.M., & Avolio, B.J. (1994) *Improving organizational effectiveness through transformational leadership*. Thousand Oaks, CA: Sage Publications

Beerel, A. (2009) *Leadership and Change Management*. London: Sage

Belbin, R. M. (1993) *Team Roles at Work*. Oxford: Butterworth-Heinemann.

Bennett, N*., Wise, C., Woods, P.A. and Harvey, J.A. (*2003*). Distributed Leadership.* Nottingham: National College of School Leadership.

Bergmann, H., Hurson, K. and Russ-Eft, D. (1999) *Everyone a Leader: A grassroots model for the new workplace*. New York: John Wiley and Sons.

Blackler, F., and Kennedy, A. (2003) *The Design of a Development Programme for Experienced Top Managers from the Public Sector*. Working Paper, Lancaster University.

Blake, R.R., and Mouton, J.S. (1964). *The Managerial Grid*. Houston: Gulf.

Blanchard, K.H., Zigarmi, P., & Zigarmi, D. (2011) *Leadership and the One Minute Manager: Increasing Effectiveness through Situational Leadership*. New York: Morrow,

Blanchard, K.H., & Johnson, S. (2000) *The One Minute Manager* New York: Morrow,

Bolden, R., Gosling, J., Marturano, A. and Dennison, P. (2003) *A review of leadership Theory* Exeter: University of Exeter.

Burns, J. M. (1978) *Leadership*. New York. Harper and Row

Cabinet Office - *Senior Civil Service Competence Framework*. Online at: http://www.cabinet-office.gov.uk/civilservice/scs/competences.htm

Centre for Leadership Studies (2011) *Situational Leadership.* Available at: http://situational.com/about-us/situational-leadership/ (Accessed on 09/04/14).

Clark, C. (2009) *Creative Nursing Leadership and Management.* Boston: Jones Bartlett Publishers

Covey, S. (1992) *Principle-Centred Leadership.* Simon and Schuster.

Cowley, W.H. (1931). The Traits of Face to Face Leaders. *Journal of Abnormal and Social Psychology.* 26(3), 304-313.

Daft, R. L. (2005). *The leadership experience* (3rd Edition.) Mason, OH: Thomson, South-Western.

Department for Education and Skills (2003) *Management and Leadership Attributes Framework.* DfES Leadership and Personnel Division, April 2003.

Department of Health (DoH) (2011a) *Clinical Leadership Competency Framework.* NHS Institute for Innovation and Improvement: Coventry: Department of Health.

Department of Health (DH) (2011b) *The Leadership Framework.* NHS Institute for Innovation and Improvement. Coventry: Department of Health.

Employers' Organisation for Local Government – *Compendium of Leadership Competencies.* Source: *http://www.lg-employers.gov.uk/skills/leadership_comp.*

Engestrom, Y. (1987) Learning by Expanding: An activity theoretical approach to developmental research. Helsinki: Orienta-Konsultit.

Federal Express - *Leadership Qualities.* Source: *http://www.geocities.com/gvwrite/9faces.htm*

Fiedler, (1967) *A Theory of Leadership Effectiveness*. NewYork: McGraw-Hill.

Fiedler, F.E. (1969). Leadership: A new model. In C.A. Gibb (ed.). *Leadership*. Harmondsworth: Penguin, 230-41.

French, J. R. P., Raven, B. (1959) The bases of social power. In D. Cartwright and A. Zander. (1959) *Group dynamics*. New York: Harper & Row,

Gill, R. (2011) *Theory and Practice of Leadership.* London: SAGE.

Goleman D (2000) *Leadership That Gets Results.* Harvard Business Review. Mar-Apr 78-90.

Goodwin, N. (2006) L*eadership in Health Care*. Abingdon: Routledge.

Gosling, J. and Mintzberg, H. (2003) *Mindsets for Managers*. Working paper, Centre for Leadership Studies.

Greenleaf, R. (1970) *Servant as Leader*. Centre for Applied Studies.

Greenleaf, R. K. (1977, 2002). *Servant-Leadership: A Journey into the Nature of Legitimate Power and Greatness*. Mahwah, NJ: Paulist Press.

Grint, K. (2000) *Literature Review on Leadership*. Cabinet Office: Performance and Innovation Unit.

Gronn, P. (1995) Greatness Re-visited: The current obsession with transformational leadership. *Leading and Managing* 1(1), 14-27.

Hamlin. R. (2002) *Towards a Universalistic Model of Leadership:* a comparative study of British and American empirically derived criteria of managerial and leadership effectiveness. Working paper WP005/02, University of Wolverhampton. Online at:

http://asp2.wlv.ac.uk/wbs/documents/mrc/Working%20Papers%202002/WP006_02_Hamlin.pdf

Handy, C. (1993) *Understanding Organisations* Oxford: Blackwell.

Handy, C. (1992) 'The Language of Leadership' in *Frontiers of Leadership* (Eds Syrett and Hogg) Oxford: OUP.

Hartley, J., and Benington, J. (2010) *Leadership for Healthcare.* Bristol: The Policy Press

Hay McBer (1999) *School Leadership Model.* Source: http://www.ncsl.org.uk/index.cfm?pageID=haycompletechar

Heifetz, A. (1994) *Leadership Without Easy Answers.* Cambridge: Belknap Press.

Hersey, P., & Blanchard, K. (1996) Revisiting the Life-Cycle Theory of Leadership. *Training and Development*, January, 42-47

Hersey, P., and Blanchard, K.H. (1977) *Management of Organizational Behaviour.* Englewood Cliffs NJ: Prentice Hall.

Herzberg, F.I. (1987), 'One more time: How do you motivate employees?', *Harvard Business Review*, Sep/Oct87, Vol. 65 Issue 5, p109-120

Hooper, A., and Potter, J. (1997) *The Business of Leadership.* Aldershot: Ashgate Publishing Company.

Institute of Chartered Accountants in England and Wales - *Ethical Principles for Members.* Source: *http://www.icaew.co.uk*

Institute of Chartered Management - *Chartered Management Skills.* Source:

http://www.managers.org.uk/institute/content_1.asp?category=3&id=37&id=30&id=14

Investors in People - *Leadership and Management Model.* London: HMSO

James, K., and Burgoyne, J. (2001) *Leadership Development: Best practice guide for organisations.* London: Council for Excellence in Management and Leadership. Online at: http://www.managementandleadershipcouncil.org.

Katzenbach, J., and Smith, D. (1994) *The Wisdom of Teams.* New York: Harper business.

Lewin, K. (1935) *A Dynamic Theory of Personality.* New York, McGraw Hill.

Lewin, K., Lippit, R. and White, R.K. (1939). Patterns of aggressive behaviour in experimentally created social climates. *Journal of Social Psychology, 10,* 271-301.

McGregor, D. (1960) *The Human Side of Enterprise.* New York: McGraw Hill.

Maslow, A.H. (1943). A theory of human motivation. *Psychological Review* 50 (4) 370–96.McGregor, D. (1960) *The Human Side of Enterprise.* New York: McGraw Hill.

Millward, J. and Bryan, K. (2005) Clinical leadership in health care: a position statement. *Leadership in Health Services.* 18 (2) 18-25

Mullins, L.J. (2008) *Management and Organisational Behaviour* Harlow: Pearson

NHS Leadership Academy (2011) *Clinical Leadership Competency Framework.* Coventry: NHS Institute for Innovation and Improvement

NHS Leadership Centre (2002) *NHS Leadership Qualities Framework*. Source: http://www.NHSLeadershipQualities.nhs.uk

Northern Ireland Civil Service - *Senior Civil Service: Core Criteria*.

Northouse, P.G. (2012) *Leadership: Theory and Practice* (6th edition). London: Sage

Perren, L.m and Burgoyne, J. (2001) *Management and Leadership Abilities: An analysis of texts, testimony and practice*. London: Council for Excellence in Management and Leadership. Online at: http://www.managementandleadershipcouncil.org/reports/r30.htm.

Phillips, A. (2001) -*The Philips Leadership Competencies*. Source: http://ad.chinahr.com/jobads/philips/leadership.asp

Raelin, J. (2003) *Creating Leaderful Organizations*. San Francisco: Berrett-Koehler Publishers Inc.

Scottish Executive (2000) - Scottish Executive Framework. London: HMSO

Shell (2000) *Shell Leadership Framework*. Source: http://sww-general.shell.com/hr/leadership

Stogdill, R. (1974) *Handbook of Leadership* (1st Ed.). New York: Free Press.

Storey, J. (2013) *Towards a new model of leadership* NHS Leadership Academy.

Tannenbaum, R., and Schmidt, W. (1958) How to choose a leadership pattern. *Harvard Business Review* 36(2), 95-101

Tappen R M (1995) *Nursing Leadership and Management* (3rd edition) Philadelphia: F A Davis

Tappen, R. M., Weiss, S. A., and Whitehead, D.K. (2004) *Essentials of nursing leadership and management* (3rd edition) Philadelphia F A Davis

Tichy, N., and Devanna, M. (1986) *Transformational Leadership*. New York: Wiley.

United States Office of Personnel Management (2006) - *Senior Executive Service Leadership Competencies*. Source: http://www.opm.gov/ses/competent.html

Walshe, K., and Smith, J. (2006) *Healthcare Management*. Maidenhead: Open University Press.

Youngs, H. (2009). (Un)critical times? Situating distributed leadership in the field. *Journal of Educational Administration and History,* 41, *pp.* 377–389.

Yukl, G. (1989), Managerial Leadership: a review of theory and research. *Journal of Management* 15:2, 251-89.

Devlin, K, (1993). *The Joy of Sets* New York: Springer Verlag,

The NHS

Introduction

The NHS was established in 1948, assuming responsibility for a diverse range of already existing facilities. This constituted a major strand of the Labour Government's post-war drive to create a welfare-state in which individuals would receive essential help and services irrespective of their ability to pay (DoH,1947). Since that time it has been highly political and although all governments are committed to maintaining its excellence, it is inevitable a focus for reform whenever a new government or minister takes responsibility. The difficulties in running such a large organisation with such diverse aims while accommodating several diametrically opposed principles means that there will not be a perfect fit management solution. Reforms seek to move slowly forward and steady progress can be seen since the service's inception. Some difficulties emerge however when nativity leads new managers nationally or locally to believe that they can *'finally get the NHS right'*.

The NHS was founded on a number of principles, the most fundamental of which was that health care should be free of cost at the point of service delivery and accessible to all regardless of their resources. In addition to the treatment of illness, the new service was to make an active drive for health promotion through environmental improvement and disease prevention. It was believed that there was a backlog of need as a result of previous poor access to services and that once this was overcome, demand would decline. Therefore, it was expected that the cost of the service would tail off (DoH,1947).

A number of themes quickly emerged, which have been consistently present thereafter (Ham,1991).

1) Funding has never been adequate to meet demand. The anticipated tail-off of demand did not occur, and in fact, demand has increased to exceed supply throughout the life of the service, with initial NHS costs of 4%, rising to 8% - over £100Bn by 2010. Although some illnesses have been eradicated as was expected and the associated costs saved, overall demand has increased. This is attributed to a number of factors:
   a) Demographic change, with average life expectancy increasing has changed the ratio of consumers to taxpayers.
   b) Technological advances have resulted in many incurable diseases becoming treatable with the resultant new treatment and aftercare costs.
   c) Increased resource reduces treatment barriers such as waiting times and increases demand.
2) Co-ordination of the disparate services has been difficult throughout the life of the NHS and is addressed in every reform since its inception.
3) Equity of access, a driving factor in the creation of the service remains unacceptable, with poor distribution and social fairness. Again, this is addressed in every reform of the service.
4) The tension between central government control and local management has been a consistent issue, although there is an evident trend towards decentralisation discernible in each NHS reform.
5) The interrelationship between the centrally funded NHS and local government funded Social Services has always been an area of discussion and the relationships have been altered repeatedly.

6) The relationship between clinical freedom and hegemonic managerial control has been an area of contention throughout the life of the service, although a general trend towards managerialism and the restriction of clinical freedom is discernible culminating in the National Institute for Clinical Evidence, Evidence Based Practice and National Service Frameworks.

The Knowledge base

Primary/Secondary/Tertiary

UK Health services are divided into primary, secondary and tertiary provision (Ham,1991).

Primary health services are those provided by the General Practitioner (GP) and the primary care team. Secondary health services are those provided by the General Hospital NHS Trusts and Community NHS Trusts. Tertiary health services are those provided at centres serving more than one DHA and are highly specialised. Private sector health service providers are particularly active in the secondary and tertiary service sectors.

The UK NHS is unusual in allowing patients direct access to Primary Care only. Access to Secondary Care, e.g. hospital, is only on referral from a GP. (The exception to this rule is Accident and Emergency Services) Access to Tertiary Care is only achievable through referral by a Secondary Care service Clinician. Tertiary services cannot generally be accessed directly by GPs. This rule even holds for most areas of private practice. Access to a private practitioner in secondary care generally involves referral from a GP.

The NHS

The NHS was set up in 1948 under The NHS Act (DoH,1947). It assumed ownership of pre-existing charitable and Local Authority facilities and evolved a plan for development to achieve comprehensive coverage. Services were managed in three strands: Community and Environmental Health services, General Practitioner Services and Hospital Services. This "Tripartite" management system had difficulties of horizontal co-ordination and the regional variances of service quantity and quality that were very difficult to resolve. These issues were well described in the 1950s and continue to be cited as drivers for reform in the 1990 "The NHS and Community Care Act".

NHS reorganisation Act (1970)

In 1974, the first NHS reorganisation saw the introduction of tiered management with the Government department, Regional Health Authorities (RHA), Area Health Authorities (AHA) and District Health Authorities (DHA).

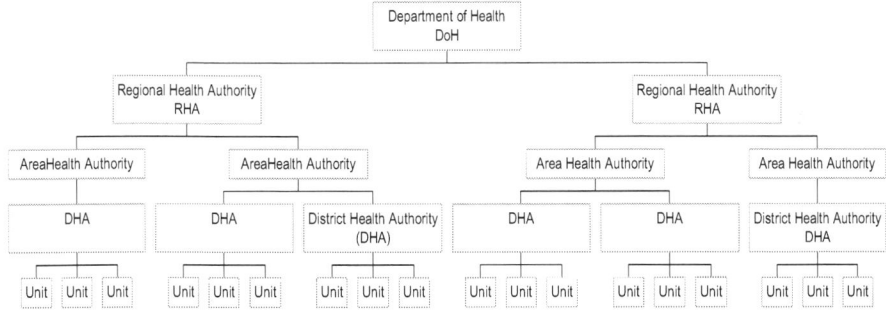

Broad policy was set by the DoH and passed, with budgets, to Regional Health Authorities (RHA)s. Policies were interpreted by RHAs and passed, with budgets, to Area Health Authorities (AHA). Policies were interpreted by AHAs and passed, with budgets, to Districts s who made local interpretation and passed instruction and funds to Units (Hospitals and Community service managers). The amount of funding passed from the DoH to each RHA was decided by the Resource Allocation Working Party (RAWP). The RAWP devised a capitation-based formula to allocate resources. According to this formula, RHAs received funds relating to the size of the population, weighted for: demographic profile, morbidity and, later, social deprivation.

Some services that were too specialised to be justified in a District (large town) were managed directly by the AHA (county) or RHA (about six counties). AHAs also had administrative and payroll responsibility for General Practitioners, through Family Practitioner Committees (FPC)s.

In 1982, AHAs were abolished, under 1980 legislation, making the newly created DHAs directly accountable to RHAs, and removing an unnecessary tier of bureaucracy. In a few years, by amalgamation, many DHAs reverted to the boundaries formerly held by AHAs. They continued to manage Units and to administer FPCs

The NHS and Community Care Act (1990)

In The NHS and Community Care Act (1990) under the Conservative government, the managerial relationship between Districts and Units was severed and the Units were allowed to apply for NHS Trust status. The control of NHS Trusts by DHAs was to be through contracts in which DHAs passed funds to NHS Trusts in exchange for their agreement to treat patients for the diseases that historical knowledge and epidemiological study suggested would be encountered. The primary function of the DHA, therefore became to assess the population's need for health care and contract with the health care providers of their choice for services. Contracts were one of three possible types:

"Block Contracts" in which the NHS Trust or other provider agrees to treat all comers for a fixed total price, rationing by waiting list if necessary

"Cost and Volume Contracts" in which a NHS Trust or other provider agrees to treat a fixed number of patients for a fixed total price

"Cost Per Case Contracts" in which a NHS Trust or other provider agrees to treat as many patients as are referred at an agreed price per patient.

Where a patient attended a NHS Trust with whom his/her DHA of residence has no contract, then a Fee for Service was payable and he/she was known as an Extra-Contractual Referral (ECR).

GPs were expected to refer patients to those NHS Trusts with whom the DHA had arranged contracts. However, some larger GP practices were allowed to hold the budget for their patients' secondary service needs and contract directly with NHS Trusts. These practices were known as General Practice Fund Holders (GPFHs). Although there was a limit to the range of services for which a GPFH could hold a budget, there were some experimental sites where large groups of practices held funds for all of their patient needs, known as Total Fund-holding Schemes. These experiments were to provide information for the reforms of 1998 "The New NHS - Modern and Dependable".

FPCs were re-designated Family Health Service Authorities (FHSA) and became independent Authorities administering GP contracts.

As a result of the 1990 reforms "The NHS and Community Care Act", the DHA had a choice of NHS Trusts and other hospitals with whom to contract and the NHS Trusts had a choice of DHAs and other health purchasers with whom to contract. It was intended that this competition would constitute a market place that would be able to regulate service cost and quality through competition. This exercise was in part successful, but the costs of the market place infrastructure were considerable and some of the savings were lost.

The RHAs were abolished as Authorities and converted into DoH Outposts, effectively reducing the structure to a greatly enlarged DoH, operating centrally and regionally, and DHAs who contracted with NHS Trusts and other providers of services.

The NHS Trusts were allowed considerable business autonomy, particularly regarding financial management, but they remained owned by the DoH and a regulatory system was established in which NHS Trusts were directly accountable to a section of the DoH.

The 1990 reforms "The NHS and Community Care Act" removed local government and other representation on Health Authorities, and established Boards of Directors for Authorities and NHS Trusts. A board consists of five Executive Directors, who are the managers of the Trust/Authority and five Non-executive Directors, who are local business managers, etc who contribute to the strategic management of the services. One of the Non-executive Directors is appointed Chairman and it is the function of the Chairman to appoint the Chief Executive Officer and other Executive Directors. In this, the Authorities and Trusts were to mirror the normal picture in industry. However, the DoH retained a strong influence over board membership, and the Secretary of State has to approve the appointment of all Non-Executive directors.

The New NHS - Modern and Dependable (1997)

In The New NHS - Modern and Dependable (1998), under the Labour government the purchasing functions of DHAs are progressively transferred to locality based Primary Care Groups (PCG), constituted from members of the Primary Care Team, Unitary Local Authorities and officers of the DHA. Boards were created which included the above and non-executive directors from the community served. These groups assume responsibility for purchasing from NHS Trusts and other health and care providers on a schedule chosen by their board. If the PCG chooses, it can become a Primary Care Trust (PCT) and provide direct services of the type formerly provided by Community NHS Trusts and take full responsibility for contracts and commissions with secondary NHS Trusts. This transfer of commissioning responsibilities to primary care teams is an important focus of these reforms, continuing the trend initiated in 1990, but the legislation also brought about a number of other important changes.

Contracts for services were to become longer. Three, four or five-year contracts were to replace the one-year contracts common after the 1990 reforms "The NHS and Community Care Act". Co-ordination between purchasers was to be made easier by the agreement of local Health Improvement Programs that would guide purchasing practice. Variations in practice were to be reduced by the issuing of National Service Frameworks that would set out the norms to be expected by patients. The National Institute for Clinical Excellence would collect, appraise and promulgate evidence about the various approaches to health promotion and treatment available with a view to standardising around the proven best. Quality of services would be subject to more-rigorous tests and poor practice would be more easily uncovered. The business mentality that had increased efficiency in NHS Trusts was also to institutionalise secrecy and poor co-operation. A transparency and co-operative spirit was to be established.

Primary Care Groups (PCGs)

A number of pilot exercises, such as locality commissioning groups and total GP purchasing groups had tested the possibility of groups based around the primary care team taking responsibility for delivering or commissioning all secondary and tertiary services for the patients in their catchment. The establishment of PCGs brought clear responsibilities to larger groups of primary care staff for service commissioning. PCGs were expected to cover patches of in the region of 100,000 patients, but considerable variances were permitted in the first wave of PCG creation. In order to remove concerns about differentials between fundholding and non-fundholding practices, PCGs cover the entire population.

PCGs were given four levels at which they may operate:

1) As the minimum, PCGs may advise the DHA in its commissioning for their population.

2) PCGs may take a devolved budget and purchase, acting as a part of the DHA
3) PCGs may become independent bodies, accountable to the DHA for their commissioning practice
4) PCGs may become Primary care trusts (PCTs), remaining accountable to the DHA for their purchasing, but acting as a service provider for a range of community services.

The movement of responsibility for purchasing from DHAs to PCGs advanced a trend to empower the primary care clinician, which had been evident in a number of NHS Reforms:

1) The further involvement of clinicians in management was achieved. This development amalgamated the manager and the clinician and partially removed an insoluble tension between the two, by giving budgetary control to the GP who has always been the biggest spender in the NHS. No longer would GPs be at odds with DHA purchasing decisions because GPs would directly experience the constraints of budgetary limitations, make decisions according to their appreciation of priorities and then be expected to accept the consequent opportunity costs.

2) A continued devolution of service was achieved. Major decisions were to be made ever nearer to the patient and his/her clinician.

3) The shift of power from acute services towards primary care was furthered. This was initiated in the 1990 reforms "The NHS and Community Care Act" and considerably furthered by this 1998 development.

As PCGs become PCTs and take direct responsibility for service delivery, the range of services formerly delivered by Community NHS Trusts is diminishing to include only services to people with learning disabilities and mental illness. It is anticipated that these NHS trusts will amalgamate to form super-county providers.

Quality and efficiency management

The reforms from 1946 seek progressively to improve the quality and efficiency of the service together, thereby eliminating difficulties where a tension is perceived between these two imperatives.

The 1998 reforms "The New NHS - Modern and Dependable create the National Institute for Clinical Excellence (NICE). This has the remit to promote excellence through audit and guidance. The institute was to critically examine the available evidence for effectiveness and efficiency, and encourage research in areas where insufficient evidence exists. This allows it to advise on best practice, where a number of possibilities exist. This is not intended to remove clinical freedom, because it is recognised that every case is different, but, it is intended that practice will narrow down onto a small range unless there is a good reason for divergence. The available range of treatments is based on achieving value for money with the restricted resources available to commissioners. Methodologies employed include examination of the Quality Adjusted Life Years (QALYs) that can be purchased by following a particular clinical approach. This is explained further in the Managing Finance chapter

The Institute also publishes National Service Frameworks (NSFs) that, based upon a detailed analysis of the evidence, can set out what a patient within a major care area can expect.

Clinical Governance is introduced to set tangible controls on service quality. CEOs must report to the Board about the targets and achievement of quality standards and these reports are intended to attract the same attention and rigour as financial reports. I.e. NHS Trusts are to make the same efforts to ensure that quality is up to the mark as they currently do to ensure financial balance. Professions are expected to enhance their self-regulatory machinery to ensure that recognised standards are addressed. Additionally, they are to increase lifelong learning initiatives for Continuing

Professional Development (CPD). These requirements were reinforced by the Health Bill (1999), altering state registration requirements for the professions to make CPD an essential requirement for continued registration.

Adherence to the quality requirements was to be monitored by the Commission for Health Improvement (CHI). This body was removed from government and could report on the extent to which quality machinery is being established, its effectiveness and the general impact on care. The Commission was to carry out local reviews to assure as well as monitor quality of service provision. This CHI was discontinued in 2004 when its functions were taken over by the Commission for Healthcare Audit and Inspection.

Health Improvement Programs (HIMPs)

The DHA is responsible for leading and co-ordinating HIMPs for the residents in their catchment. The program involves input from PCGs, service providers (NHS Trusts), the local Authority and other agencies with an interest in public health. The HIMP will describe the major health needs of the population, the consequent service needs and set out the three year strategic commissioning plan that will bring service provision into line with this agreed requirement. The program will take account of national targets for improvements in services, morbidity and mortality.

The HIMP is a resource that can be used to validate commissioning plans made by PCGs, now CCGs thereby fulfilling the DHA's responsibility to supervise purchasing practice. It will also assist with HR planning to identify future workforce needs in order to commission training of health professionals. (See "The Management of People")

NHS reorganization: The Health and Social Care (Community Health and Standards) Act (2003)

This Labour Government legislation sought to address weakness in NHS Trusts, first established in the 1990 reforms. Trusts were considered to be hampered by restrictions regarding how they may manage financial and other resources. These limitations were restricting the efficiency and creativity with which services could be delivered. This was addressed by the creation of NHS Foundation Trusts. Trusts were required to demonstrate exceptional levels of performance after which they were promoted to Foundation Trust status and allowed increased flexibility and some reduction in monitoring. This proposed a situation much like the 1990 reforms with two tiers of provider organisation. Foundation Trusts were envisaged as elite in the same way as were NHS Trusts following the 1990 reforms. Just as in 1990, this inequality was to be resolved by the eventual elevation of all NHS Trusts to NHS Foundation Trust status.

The legislation created Monitor' to act as regulator for Foundation Trusts. The function of Monitor was to be changed by the 2010 legislation to become an economic regulator.

The act also brought into existence the Commission for Healthcare Audit and Inspection to monitor quality in NHS provision and the Commission for Social Care Inspection which was to monitor Social care quality.

These were combined and merged with the Mental Health Act Commission to form the Care Quality Commission in 2009.

The White Paper, *Equity and excellence: Liberating the NHS* (2010) and Health and Social Care Bill (2012)

This was Conservative Government legislation moving DoH functions into a politically independent NHS Commissioning Board. This envisaged the abolition of Strategic Health Authorities and assumed overall responsibility for service commissioning through Clinical Commissioning Groups (CCGs).

The Board was responsible for the establishment of 211 CCGs as well as Commissioning Support Units (CSUs), which would provide technical and other support as required by the CCGs. In 2013, the NHS Commissioning Board became known as NHS England and has 4 regional Branches with 27 local branches.

The act redirected Monitor, the supervisor of Foundation Trusts created in 2003 to become an economic regulator for the service. In this they were to address any examples of anticompetitive practice and inefficient service models.

Conclusion

The UK NHS, although imperfect, has earned a good international reputation. It has consistently sought to provide high quality care with equity of access. A number of issues have been present throughout the ½ century of the NHS, including an inevitable resource shortfall against demand, a constructive, dynamic tension between clinical autonomy and managerialism and ambiguity between central and devolved control. Debate around these issues is continually resulting in re-examination of provision and the high public interest will ensure that the UK NHS is a volatile and dynamic public service.

References

DoH (1947) *NHS Act* London: HMSO

DoH (1949) *NHS (Amendments) Act* London: HMSO

DoH (1951) HMSO London *NHS Act* London: HMSO

DoH (1952) *NHS Act* London: HMSO

DoH (1973) *NHS Reorganisation Act* London: HMSO

DoH (1979) *Patients First* London: HMSO

DoH (1982) *NHS Reorganisation* London: HMSO

DoH (1989a) *Working for Patients* London: HMSO

DoH (1989b) *Caring for People Community Care in the Next Decade and Beyond* London: HMSO

DoH (1990) *The NHS and Community Care Act* London: HMSO

DoH (1997) *A New NHS - Modern and Dependable* London: HMSO

DoH (2003) *NHS reorganisation: The Health and Social Care (Community Health and Standards) Act* London: HMSO

DoH (2012) The White Paper, *Equity and excellence: Liberating the NHS (2010) and Health and Social Care Bill* London: HMSO

Donne,J. (1986) ; *Better Management Better Health* Bristol: NHSTA

Enthoven,A.(1985) *Reflections on the Management of the NHS* Nuffield Provincial Hos. London: HMSO

Grice,D. (1994) in Wheeler (Ed) *Whither the Professions Now: Conference Proceedings* Oxford: Oxford Brookes University:

Ham, C. (1998) *Boards of directors : are there any lessons for Health Authorities* Birmingham: National Health Service Training Authority

Ham,C. (1997) *Health care reform : learning from international experience* Buckingham : Open University Press,

Ham,C. (1994) *Health Care reforms* Macmillan, London.

Ham,C. (1991) *The New National Health Service: organisation and management* Oxford: Radcliffe Medical Press

Pettigrew,A.M., Ferlie,E., and McKee,L.(1992) *The leadership role of the new health authorities* Public Money and Management ,April 39–43.

Maxwell,R.(1989)) *Reshaping the NHS* Oxford: Policy Journals,.

Stewart,R.(1996) *Leading in the NHS* London: Pan Business Books

Wheeler,N. (1990), **'***Working for Patients' and 'Caring for People' The Philosophy* British Journal of Occupational Therapy 53 (10) 409-14

Collaboration

Introduction

Professionals and managers in technical organisations such as the NHS and social care can almost never work in isolation (Huxham & Vangen 2005). Our lives today are set within a greater web of connections than any previous generation would recognise (Lank, 2006). Success therefore, requires effective working with colleagues.

Collaboration may be seen as a purely personal relationship between practitioners or a major relationship between large organisations. However even inter-organisational collaboration is not achieved by managers alone. In the collaboration between an NHS Trust and Local Authority Social Services the tone may be set by managers. However, much of the valuable collaborative effort is made by clinicians and junior managers, who effectively direct resources and ultimately are responsible for success or failure of the enterprise.

Collaboration benefits from Synergy, the notion that two activities put together boost efficiency and effectiveness and Gestalt, the notion that the whole is greater than the sum of the parts.

Collaboration is easier for some than others, but consideration of some principles will improve success for everybody.

As clinicians or managers, we think about achieving independence. We set out on a career as a novice (Benner, 1984) highly dependent on more senior colleagues (Hersey & Blanchard 1996) and strive over time to achieve a state of independence where we can manage our duties without seeking help. However there is a far more sophisticated state of development where we start to be dependent upon others in a collaborative condition of equals. Since this dependence is mutual, it is

better called interdependence. Thus, as observed by Covey (1999) we have a developmental continuum of:
Dependent ➔ Independent ➔ Interdependent.

This interdependent stage is not achieved by all practitioners, but is the foundation of collaborative practice.

Collaboration might be considered along a four point continuum, as described by Himmelman (2002). We might begin by: **Networking**, progress to **Co-ordination** of our enterprise, **Co-operate** with others to mutual benefit and then finally progress to full **Collaboration** to produce a mutual product and improve the overall performance and competence of each participant.

Networking == Co-ordination == Co-operation == Collaboration

Networking

This is described by Himmelman (2002) as exchanging information for mutual benefit. It is commonplace between organisations such as NHS Trusts and Social Services Departments. It requires a degree of trust and an assumption that the organisations have similar and compatible goals. It also accepts that success for one organisation in achieving these goals is in the interest of the other. For each organisation to be aware of the actions and intentions of the other is clearly valuable since it allows each to act so as to avoid conflict and overlap and, where possible to reinforce the actions of the other.

Co-ordination

When the exchange of information leads to an alteration of plans, by agreement, then Himmelman (2002) describes this as co-ordination. Plans may be co-ordinated to better serve a customer, such as a patient/client. They may also be co-ordinated to reinforce the goals of the organisations. Co-ordinated activity requires a clear compatibility of organisational goals and an explicit adoption of a win/win model between the organisations.

Each needs to be seeking ways of operating that is engineered to be helpful to both organisations. This requires a notion of synergy rather than compromise.

Co-operation

Where the organisations are willing to go beyond changing plans to sharing resources, then Himmelman (2002) describes co-operation as working. Sharing may be of personnel physical plant, such as premises or skills and contacts. This requires that the organisations see an outcome, such as patient/client care, that is paramount. Therefore they are able to seek benefit of the client through means other than their own action and apply resources accordingly.

Collaboration

Collaboration is described by Himmelman (2002) as taking the further step of enhancing the other's organisation for the good of the user. Thus the collaborator is not simply assisting the colleague to achieve more, but enabling that colleague to become directly more able. This requires a particular type of trust and good will since it allows the possibility that the collaborator is enabling another not simply to do better, but to become better that him/her. This may be as a result of altruistic concern for the client or in the belief that this is a reciprocal relationship in which both parties can expect to grow.

These terms are in common parlance, but it is helpful for the reader to develop an explicit understanding of each. There is a clear progression form networking to collaboration and it may be that in healthcare all professionals and managers should strive for the highest level. However, it may equally be that consideration should be given to the differences and conscious choice made about the level of collaboration that is appropriate at each juncture.

1) Huxham (1996) offers us a similar progression, but with greater ramifications:
2) **Independence == Networks == Alliances == Federations == Fusion**
3) These terms may apply to interconnection between organisations but can equally relate to interrelationships between individuals.

Independence

Fast, flexible and easy to control.

As described by Covey (1999), we strive to be able to leave our novice phase and operate without constant reference to a more experienced supervisor, becoming independent. This initial step is challenging and in some settings can be an adequate end in itself. Independent contractors in many industries find this a most comfortable and manageable existence seeking to maintain it as far as possible. Some measure of collaboration is inevitably required, but this can be conducted on a contract basis such that the autonomous independent practitioner retains total control. For example the independent delivery driver manages his/her own business autonomously. Although he/she needs technical (mechanical) support, that can be kept entirely under his/her control.

For practitioners and managers in Health and Social care this must be a rarely afforded luxury.

In progressing further independence is not discarded but rather integrated and transcended in order to progress to working as a part of a network.

Networks

When individuals and agencies begin to network, they start to take advantage of benefits that each can bring to the other (Huxham 1996). A network of management consultants continue to work independently, but are able to call upon the support of each other to magnify the expertise and skills that they can offer to customers. They are able to accept larger briefs by executing them collectively and pass excess work to one another, so that they never disappoint a customer and maximise their individual; business.

Where the network is proven successful, then it may be formalised into an alliance

Alliances

Formalised mechanisms can be drawn up and set into contracts. This will establish a collaborative partnership where each individual retains independence and autonomy but benefits from explicit rights to receive aid and support and clear duties to offer such to other members (Huxham 1996).

If they further develop this alliance in order to make closer links, relinquishing or sharing some autonomy they can form federations.

Federations,

Federations have more formal, legal interconnections as organisations. They have shared, collective responsibility for overall service delivery, rather than simply each discharging its contribution independently. They may decide to laterally delegate functions. For example, rather than each having separate administrative support there can be overall administration carried out by one party on behalf of all. A degree of federation between NHS Trusts occurs when one maintains a telephone service on behalf of all, or one runs a large laundry for many others. The responsibility is laterally delegated.

Federations may also set up a super-agency over all parties managing functions such as HR. However, it is a feature of federations that this is a power passed from the lower body to the higher - Reverse Delegation (Handy, 1993). The lower bodies seek to maintain control of the higher, rather than the usual model where the opposite applies.

Fusions

In the final instance, full interdependence may be recognised by a total fusion of organisations. This requires a full revision of loyalties and identity. At a macro level this can take the form of a merger between two NHS Trusts into one far larger one. This tends to lead to greater efficiency because scale economies can reduce costs and duplicated functions can be discontinued. It is noticeable, however, that these savings are also available to organisations in a federal relationship, but this can be hampered by a difficulty in achieving total trust.

Mergers are frequently a misnomer. *There is no such thing as a merger* (Galpin and Herendon, 2014). There is always only one 'surviving' CEO, etc and one culture will be dominant in the new organisations. Most mergers of NHS Trusts amount to a 'takeover' of one by the other.

At a micro level this merger can amount to the OT, the SW, the PT, the Nurse, the psychologist and the Psychiatrist being 'fused' together into a Community Mental Health Team, which holds a greater loyalty for them than their original professional team.

Drawing Notions together

These notions might be drawn together in an exercise of 'Critical Analysis' (Aveyard, 2011) to give support one to another through an exercise similar to Triangulation (Aveyard, 2104) and to create a longer progression in an exercise of synthesis (Aveyard, 2011).

Covey (1999)_	**Huxham (1996)**	**Himmelman (2002)**
Dependence		
Independence	Independence	
Interdependence	Networks	Networking
Interdependence	Alliances	Co-ordination
Interdependence	Federations	Co-operation
Interdependence	Fusion	Collaboration

This allows us a longer progression as people and organisations become more sophisticated in working together:

Dependent== independent== Interdependent: through networking== Interdependent: co-ordinating through Alliances== Interdependent: co-operating through Federation== Interdependent: collaborating through Fusion.

Co-operate or assert yourself?

Collaborative playing can raise a tension between individual desire to assert ideas and a desire to co-operate and satisfy the concerns of others.

Rollinson and Broadfield (2002) address this issue, but consider that these cannot be treated as alternatives but need to be drawn together. Successful collaboration needs players to be constructively assertive regarding their own beliefs and insistent on fulfilling the needs of all other players at the same time. Rollinson and Broadfield (2002) do not allow that this needs to be a compromise of drives, but that for full collaboration players must peruse each to full effect.

They offer a grid to show the result of high and low levels of assertiveness and co-operation.

Co-operation Assertion	Low	Medium	High
High	***Competition***		******Collaboration******
Medium		***Compromise***	
Low	***Avoidance***		***Accommodation***

This model surprises by suggesting that Compromise is not necessarily a desirable thing. The compromising player is neither sufficiently assertive nor sufficiently co-operative. '*Must try Harder*' on both fronts. If the player is too accommodating, he/she is falling short on Assertiveness. If he/she is too competitive, he/she is falling short on Co-operation. Finally if he/she is avoiding all issues, he/she is insufficiently Assertive or Co-operative.

The Practice

or how you might go about it.

Aims, objectives, purpose, vision

Any type of collaboration becomes an entity, separate from those of the participants, or from which the participants are drawn. You will need to decide collectively exactly what your collaboration is about. This can initially appear an exercise in stating the obvious, but the assumption that all members have the same expectation can lead to endless difficulties if it is not true.

It is helpful to agree on:

Mission – the purpose of the collaboration. This is an expression of why you set it all up. If the collaboration did not exist, would it be necessary to create it. If 'Yes' then 'Why'. The 'Why' is the mission for the collaboration. The **Vision** is usually taken to be an image of how the service will look once you have it in place. '*I see a service where any one team member makes immediate contact with each client and assess the needs for services from the full range of team skills and then….*' This gives your team an identity.

The mission and vision give a guide to the overall Aim.

Aim – a general statement of what is to be achieved, eg *to address the health care needs of people with learning difficulties in the catchment of..*'

This aim is too broad to be actually discharged so it needs to be divided into a list of objectives.

Objectives - behavioural and SMART (Specific, Measurable, Achievable, Relevant, Time bound) statements of what will be achieved.

eg Objectives:

- To assess the healthcare needs of clients within one week of referral.
- etc.

Team considerations

Team types

As is explained in detail in the chapter Managing Human Resources, a team of people can have a range of player types. Belbin (1981) suggests that a collaborative team needs:

Company Worker, Chair, Shaper, Plant, Resource Investigator, Monitor Evaluator, Team Worker and Completer finisher.

It will assist you in establishing collaboration if you can work towards having a good range of these roles covered. Most members of the team will be capable of fulfilling a number of these roles and might therefore take on a role according to need. It may be necessary to ensure that there is no competition for roles such as 'Chair'.

Personality types

Psychometric Tests such as the Myers Briggs (1989 + 2104) Personality Types analysis explained by Pearman & Albritton, (2010), are useful for bringing to the surface different ways of seeing things and preventing conflict. Understanding difference in personality types allows you to value diversity rather than seeing it as a source of conflict.

This same benefit can be achieved by swift analysis of Learning Types, using devices such as VARK (2104) and Honey & Mumford (2004).

Team life cycles

Collaborations and Teams are not formed in finished state.

A range of writers have formed opinions about the stages that are experienced. Jaques (2000) has collated four authors, showing how ideas converge to form very similar conclusions. This is another example of critical appraisal and synthesis (Aveyard, 2011)

	Phase 1	Phase 2	Phase 3	Phase 4	Phase 5
Schutz (1958);	Inclusion	Control	Affection		
Bion (1961);	Flight	Fight	Unite		
Golembiewski (1962);	Hierarchy	Conflict	Growth	Structure	
Tuckman (1977)	Forming	Storming	Norming	Performing	Adjourning
Napier (1981);	Testing	Confrontation	Compromise	Reassessment	Resolution

You can usefully ask how your collaboration stands on this journey and contribute to its progress to a functional state.

Trust, Power & Leadership

Trust

It is essential that there is trust within the newly collaborative team. This may be a measure of the maturity of the team, and the degree of interdependency to which the team aspires. If there is inadequate trust, then you might carry out a diagnosis based on assessing the fit between the image of the team held by each member.

You might address whether there is a match between member perceptions of the collaboration's place on the continuum: do members see themselves as dependent, independent, Interdependent: through networking, Interdependent: co-ordinating through Alliances, Interdependent: co-operating through Federation or Interdependent: collaborating through

Fusion. If players see themselves at different points on this journey, then you have identified a point conflict which you can begin to resolve.

You might also use Rollinson and Broadfield's (2002) grid to assess whether you have adequate assertion and co-operation present in the team. Reading the grid 'backwards', you can ask whether you are seeing: Collaboration, Competition, Compromise, Accommodation or simple Avoidance. This can give you a good guide to the assertion and co-operation contribution of each player.

Power

Power within the group, defined as the ability to get things done, may derive from a number of sources. French and Ravens (1959) identified: Legitimate power, Reward power, Expert power, Referent power, and Coercive power, in an analysis that is still followed today.

You can give thought to how you may enhance your own power, and whether use of power in the team is constructive or causing conflict. Where there is unhealthy conflicts over power, eg between legitimate power and referent power, making these hidden issues visible can make a valuable contribution to correcting them.

The exercise of 'politics' in the workplace amounts to manoeuvring in order to enhance your own power. This may be legitimate or destructive. You can examine practice and identify possible areas of difficulty. Once made explicit, these areas of potential conflict can usually be resolved. Where they remain unrecognised they cause failures in collaboration which are resistant to correction.

Legitimate power is that power conferred simply by position in the organisational chart. The manager holds power.

Reward power is that obtained by being able to confer reward or benefit on others. We do as requested because we want the reward. This may come from being 'the boss' but may come from many other means of reward. The caretaker and receptionist may have power because we want their help with parking, visitors, access to resources, etc. To hold the key to the stationary cupboard is a position of power. A simple habit of noticing and praising success in colleagues gives us an ability to rewards and a measure of power.

Expert power exists within each team. It may be in the hands of the leader if there is only one profession and he/she is the most experienced member. However in a multidisciplinary enterprise many types of expertise exist and in a well-run team each expert moves into a position of power according to the topic under considerations.

Referent power exists where an individual has respect because of long experience, special qualification, general social skill, etc. This may occur where a player is an expert, but although the expertise is not relevant to the topic we respect him/her nonetheless. For example a doctor may have power in the meeting even where the discussion bears no relationship to matters medical.

Coercive power involves deploying the power to punish as a means of gaining co-operation. This fits with theory X thinking as described by McGregor (1960), and would be indicative of a manager in a very poor situation.

For more details on this see the chapter Leadership.

Leadership

Leadership in a collaborative team is likely to be distributed rather than focussed in one place.

Distributed leadership may result from different power sources or may be through an active process where each member takes the lead according to the topic currently under consideration.

There is a chapter on Leadership much of which will be relevant to this discussion. In particular, a collaboration needs leadership that is distributed, grounded in McGregor's Theory Y, Transformational in nature and follows a contingency approach. (See the Leadership Chapter.)

Conclusion

Collaboration is almost inevitable in a complex industry such as health and social care. Exactly where your service lies on a collaborative continuum as described above will depend on context and organisational maturity. Wherever you sit in the organisational hierarchy, you have a responsibility and opportunity to advance collaboration to the benefit of patients and clients.

To progress your own thinking and behaviour by embracing interdependency will benefit your practice and your career. This is not easy; not a step that you can make quickly, but it will be an ever growing feature of performance given the escalating web of connections that constitutes professional practice.

References:

Aveyard, H. (2011) *A beginners guide to critical thinking and writing*. Maidenhead: OUP

Aveyard, H. (2014) *Doing a literature review*. Maidenhead: OUP

Belbin, R.M. (1993) *Team Roles at Work.* London: Butterworth Heinemann

Belbin, R.M. (2004) *Management Teams: Why They Succeed or Fail* 2nd ed., London: Butterworth Heinemann.

Belbin. R.M. (1981) *Management Teams: Why they Succeed or Fail.* London Penguin

Benner, P. (1982). *From novice to expert*. American Journal of Nursing, 82(3), 402-407

Benner, P. (1984). *From novice to expert: Excellence and power in clinical nursing practice*. Menlo Park, CA: Addison-Wesley.

Benner, P., & Wrubel, J. (1982a). Skilled clinical knowledge: The value of perceptual awareness. Part 1.*Journal of Nursing Administration*, 12(5), 11-14.

Benner, P., & Wrubel, J. (1982b). Skilled clinical knowledge: The value of perceptual awareness. Part 2.Journal of Nursing Administration, 12(6), 28-33.

Covey,S. (1999) *The Seven Habits of Highly Effective People.* London: Simon

French, J. R. P., and Raven, B. (1959) The bases of social power. In D. Cartwright and A. Zander. (1959) *Group dynamics.* New York: Harper & Row,

Handy,C. (1993) *Understanding Organisations.* London: Penguin

Hersey, P., & Blanchard, K. (1996) Revisiting the Life-Cycle Theory of Leadership. *Training and Development*, January, 42-47

Himmelman (2002) *Collaboration for a change.* Minneapolis:The Hummelman consulting Group

Honey, P., & Mumford, A. (1982) *Manual of Learning Styles* London: P Honey *http://www.belbin.com/*

Huxam,C (1996) *Creating Collaborative Advantage*. London: Sage

Huxham,C & Vangen,S (2005) *Managing to collaborate.* Abingdon: Routledge

Iles,V. (1997) *Really managing health care.* Buckingham: OU Press

Jacques, D. (2000) *Learning in Groups,* London: Kogan Page

Lank, E. (2005) *Collaborative advantage: How organisations win by working together*. Basingstoke: Palgrave McMillan.

Mulins,L. (1989) *Management and organisational Behaviour* London: Pitman

Myers, I., & Briggs, M. *(1985) Manual: A Guide to the Development and Use of the Myers-Briggs Type Indicator* Palo Alto: Consulting Psychologist Press

Myers Briggs (2014) *http://www.myersbriggs.org/*

Payne,M. (2000) *Team working in MP care*. Hampshire: Palgrave

Pearman, R., and Albritton, S.C. (2010) *I'm Not Crazy, I'm Just Not You: The Real Meaning of the 16 Personality Types,* 2nd edition. Boston and London: Nicholas Brealey

Rollinson,D., & Broadfield,A. (2002) *Organisational Behaviour and Analysis* Harlow: Prentice Hall

VARK (2014) *http://vark-learn.com/the-vark-questionnaire/*

Project Management

Introduction

Project Management (PM) involves the achievement of clear objectives, against a timescale and within agreed cost constraints (Meredith & Mantel 1999). The process of project management relates closely to the management of change. See the chapter Managing Change.

PM depends upon many of the characteristics and principles of effective line management and functional authority, integrated with a range of skills and techniques that have been developed to meet the needs of the project situation - a multi-skilled discipline.

There has been a widening of the concept of project management from the traditional approach developed to support major construction projects from the 1950s to the 1970s, to what may be described as '*total project management*' which places the same value on leadership, teamwork and communications as it does on the techniques of planning and control (Meredith & Mantel 1999).

It is intended that the project management chapter will build on the concepts covered in earlier chapters, while providing an opportunity for you to explore what is becoming an increasingly important aspect of management practice.

Evolution and Applications

Projects apply wherever organizations can identify a goal and then plan and control its achievement.

It was principally through military projects such as the US Navy's Polaris program, and NASA's Apollo and shuttle programs that the disciplines of project management have been developed (Meredith and Mantel,1999).

These concepts and techniques are now successfully applied in all sectors of private industry and the public and volunteer sectors.

Examples include: Civil engineering and construction, Installation of production facilities, Defense development programs, Software and systems development, Development/launch of new products, Publishing, Engineering design, Organization of plant shutdown or relocation, Development of scientific equipment, Organization of special events (e.g. conferences, sporting events, concerts, charity functions).

The range of applications for the skills and techniques of project management are so diverse that project management has become industry independent, existing as a discipline in its own right. Nonetheless many industry specialists will consider that their requirements for project management are different from everyone else's. While some special issues do exist, none more than in health & social care, most principles are generalizable.

Characteristics of Projects

There are societal demands that have led to the development of project management activity.

Meredith and Mantel (1999) point to a number of these, to include:

- The growing demand for complex, sophisticated, customized goods and services,
- The expansion of human knowledge, and our ability to apply a number of disciplines to the development of goods and services
- Intense competition among organizations and the demand this makes for ever faster results
- Society's assumption that technology can achieve anything
- The increasing size and complexity of projects being undertaken.

Principal Project Objectives

The major requirement of any project is to deliver. However, project outcomes or 'deliverables' are not only defined in terms of product and performance. There are other considerations, equally important to the overall success of the endeavor.

It would not be considered to be a success to achieve the project outcome on time but at an unaffordable cost. It is equally of little use to develop an innovatory product, within the agreed budget limitations, only to find that project delays have meant that the product has been beaten to the market place and missed its market opportunity. So, all projects have specific objectives for:

- Time
- Cost
- Performance.

These three objectives must be achieved simultaneously, with the added difficulty that a change to any one of them may affect the likelihood of achieving the others as planned (Frigenti, & Comninos, 2002).

Meredith and Mantel (1999) confirm this with its composite target including: performance, time and cost. The performance objective is indicated by the 'required performance' (or product specification). The time constraints are represented by the time schedule for the project activities, and in particular by the 'due date' for project completion. Lastly, the objectives for cost are represented within the project budget, and principally by the 'budget limit' set for the overall project.

Naturally each of these factors has an effect on each of the others. For instance, putting workers on overtime in an attempt to bring activities back to schedule has a cost implication for the project. Thus, success is defined as achievement of all three conditions. To achieve two at the expense of the third is an easy task, good management requires all three. This mirrors the quality observation that to achieve better quality with more resource is easy. Good management requires improved performance while also containing cost.

In the final instance, one or two of the principal objectives can become more important than the other,

particularly towards the termination of the project. Under such circumstances, it is the project manager's responsibility to manage these trade-off's and to ensure that the project achieves an acceptable outcome.

A Budget

A Budget will be set for the project, by the project sponsor. This is an exercise of top-down budgeting.

Top-down Budgeting

Overall cost estimates are broken down in stages by less senior managers into budgets for specific work packages.

The budget is broken down in stages by progressively junior managers into successfully finer detail, resulting in **The Project Budget**

Bottom-up budgeting (the alternative approach)

Estimates are made of man-hour and material requirements for all activities, based on the work breakdown structure and converted into financial costs

Indirect costs, contingency reserves and profit margins are added Estimates are improved by applying analytical and statistical method resulting in **The Project Budget**

Both of these approaches are valid but have different results. Ideally, in a sound project both approaches are used and if the two approaches can reach similar conclusions that amounts to a triangulation which gives confidence that the figures are valid.

Characteristics of Projects

'A project is a human activity that achieves a clear objective against a time scale.' (Reiss,1992)

There are some distinctive features of projects, encompassed within the above definitions that you may have included within your own. For instance: Projects have a beginning and an end, They are planned and controlled, They are non-routine, unique undertakings, They create some form of change, They involve a variety of human and other resources, They involve activities that cross functional boundaries, They have time, financial and performance goals.

Some aspects of a project may have been undertaken before, or the project may be generally similar to another that has already been completed. Yet in some significant aspect the project will be unique, and will take those involved across new ground.

Project Life Cycle

the project life cycle is a means of describing the typical, organic way in which projects progress from conception to completion (Reiss,1992). They describe most projects as passing through similar stages,

1) A slow start as people and resources are brought together.
2) Momentum rapidly builds as progress is made
3) Slowing towards the finish as the results are brought together, then
4) The team is disbanded.

They also propose that most projects would fit a regular pattern if the level of effort (measured in person-hours or resources expended) were plotted against time throughout the project life cycle (Meredith and Mantel, 1999)

While minimal effort is normally required in the early stages, insufficient attention during the planning phase may lead to problems later in the project. Equally, it can be important to bring the project to completion and avoid any unnecessary time spent during the wind up phase. Many projects go over budget and schedule because of insufficient control of time spent in the activities leading to completion.

Project Stages

All writers and PM models indicate some of the phases through which projects pass. The degree of rigidity reflects the nature of the projects involved. There is a spectrum in methodologies from the relatively safe and prescriptive models such as PRINCE2 (2014) or more agile methodologies such as Scrum (Schwaber, 2004). Aggregating a range of approaches, it is possible to distill four phases, each with a number of sub-phases or stages:

Phase	Principal Stages	Meaning – Purpose
Identification	Conception	Generating the idea for a project
	Selection	Choosing which project(s) to implement
	Definition	Clarifying goals and targets
Planning	Preparation	Preliminary research and clarification
	Planning	Deciding what is to be done, when, by whom and at what cost
Organization	Organization	Putting support and resources into place
	Monitoring and control	Checking progress and taking any remedial action
Implementation	Evaluation	Appraising project performance against plans
	Termination	Bringing the project to a close

While these stages may be considered to be distinct for the purposes of discussion, inevitably they overlap. In some cases they may take place in a different order. For instance, once the project has been completed and the project team disbanded other parties may undertake project evaluation.

Also, activities such as project definition and the establishing of clear objectives may not effectively take place until the project progresses, in an emergent manner. However, this might reflect a lack of communication at management levels and would tend to impact on the smooth running of the project.

Context

The project may have been formulated by senior management or could be in response to a request from an external client. However it was conceived, it's successful completion will depend on the activities and efforts of a number of people who together make up the project team, coordinated by the project manager assigned to the project.

This section examines the interrelationships between the parties concerned with the outcome of a project. It concentrates particularly on the role and responsibilities of the project manager as the centrally important figure, and looks at what makes a successful project manager. Finally, it considers the different ways in which projects may be supported within organizational structure.

Stakeholders and Other Parties

roles:

- **Project Initiator**: the Project Manager's line manager
- **Project Manager**: the team leader
    - **Project Team Members**: those individuals who complete the project tasks.

The Project Manager: Role and Responsibilities

- Understanding the project objectives and then maintaining and communicating a vision of what the project must achieve
- Coordinating the availability of resources and the activities of team members
- Achieving the project's objectives in terms of cost, time and performance
- Satisfying the client and/or the company.

It can be helpful to distinguish between functional management and project management (Meredith & Mantell, 1999), because different a different set of skills will apply when a manager is moved laterally to lead a fixed-term project and these need preparation.

.Project Managers	Functional Managers
Usually generalists	Usually specialists
Have a wide background of experience and knowledge	Have specific knowledge of the area they manage
Use a systems approach	Use an analytical approach
Skilled at synthesis, i.e. creating a coherent whole	Skilled at analysis and providing administrative responsibility
A facilitator	A direct, technical supervisor

(Meredith & Mantell, 1999)

A project manager ideally has experience of managing some form of complete enterprise. Project management has much in common with running a business — but without the ultimate authority and many of the rewards!

Project Responsibilities and Demands

The project manager's responsibilities include planning, organizing, staffing, budgeting, directing and controlling the project.

Depending on the stage at which the project manager is appointed to the project and the organization's attitude to devolving responsibility, one or more of these responsibilities may be taken by other managers. For instance, it is not unusual (particularly in organizations relatively unfamiliar with project management or when the project manager is considered relatively inexperienced) for budgetary responsibility to be held by a more senior manager.

The PM's Responsibilities towards the organization would include:
- The competent management of the project and its resources
- Keeping senior management informed of progress and problems
- Developing proposals for overcoming such problems
- Keeping in touch with the wider issues surrounding the project (the 'big picture' referred to by Briner et al.).

Senior management has responsibilities for the project is concerned and support by top management will be crucial to its success. The project manager is dependent on senior management to clarify the boundaries of each individual's level of authority and areas of responsibility for the duration of the project.

The PM's responsibilities towards the project include:
- Maintaining the support of senior management and the motivation of team members towards the project
- Setting project milestones
- Maintaining the integrity of the project despite the conflicting demands made by all
- Resisting any unnecessary change to the project specification
- Constantly reviewing progress and taking appropriate action to bring the project back on course
- Achieving the composite project objectives for time, cost and performance in the face of adversity.

The PM's responsibilities towards the project team include:

- Defining roles and responsibilities
- Setting individual performance targets
- Providing work schedules and activity lists
- Maintaining the cohesiveness of the team
- Effectively communicating plans, progress and the outcome of decisions
- Providing suitable development activities to meet individual and team needs
- Giving constructive feedback on individual performance.

The Characteristics of an Effective Project Manager

General assertion and negotiation skills are required to help the PM in:

- Acquiring adequate resources for the project
- Acquiring and motivating project personnel
- Dealing with obstacles to progress
- Making trade-off's between project goals
- Coping with the risk and fear of failure
- Negotiating and communicating at all levels.

To handle the variety of project demands effectively, the project manager must understand the basic goals of the project, have the support of top management, build and maintain a good information network, and remain as flexible as possible. This calls for both technical and administrative credibility, political sensitivity and effective leadership skills.

In researching project leadership Pozner (1999) found that project managers themselves identified communication skills, such as listening and persuading, most often used among the various attributes that make a difference in successfully managing projects. This was followed by a range of other abilities:

Communication skills	84%
Organizational skills	75%
Team building skills	72%

Leadership skills	68%
Coping skills	59%
Technological skills	46%

What is striking in this research is that leadership related skills are being used far more frequently than the technical skills relating to the project topic. This tends to support the notion, expressed above, that project management can be seen as a profession, independent of any area of industry. It is not enough to be a skilled engineer, when leading an engineering project. Leadership, negotiation and communication skills will play a far greater part in project success. If these skills are not found in the same individual, then a more complex project team will be required.

Pozner (1999) also found critical problems that PMs have to face. Once again, he found that these were issues requiring leadership rather than technical skills for their resolution:

Resources inadequate	69%
Meeting unrealistic deadlines	67%
Unclear goals/direction	63%
Team members uncommitted	59%
Insufficient planning	56%
Breakdowns in communications	54%
Changes in goals and resources	42%
Conflicts between departments or functions	35%

Project Organization

When a project is initiated, a decision must be made about how it will be housed within the organizational structure of the parent firm. Secondly, it must be decided how the project itself will be organized.

It might be assigned to a unit of a functional organization, as a self-contained unit within a project organization or as an integral part of a matrix organization.

As discussed in the chapter Managing People, The matrix organization combines some of the advantages of the pure project organization with the more desirable features of the functional organization, and avoids some of the disadvantages of each.

Building the Project Team

Whatever the organizational structure, there will be a need to identify those individuals who will undertake the project activities and build them into an effective project team.

Selection of the key team members will depend on a number of factors such as:

- Roles and responsibilities to be assigned
- The technical and project experience required
- The availability of individual staff.

Belbin (1993) and others have identified different working roles that people adopt when working together as a team.

Implementer	A practical organizer
	Turns decisions into action
	Hard working/likes stability
Coordinator	Maintains the team performance
	Strong sense of purpose
	Co-ordinates the activities of others
	Self-disciplined/inspires others
	Good communicator/listener
Shaper	Self-motivated/focuses on objectives
	Makes things happen and others follows
	Challenging style
	Seeks patterns, decisions, urgency
Plant	Source of original ideas
	Creative, intelligent
	Unorthodox, unconcerned with detail
Resources Investigator	Brings outside ideas, opinion and information into the group, Creates networks
	Gregarious and sociable
Monitor/Evaluator	Intelligent, rational, good evaluator
	Both feet on the ground
	Clear headed/hard nosed
Team Worker	Perfect team member
	Loyal and supportive
	Stable personality
	Holds team together, helps resolve conflict
	Listens and builds on others' ideas
Completer/Finisher	Concern for detail and meeting targets
	Helps maintain a sense of urgency
	Dislikes careless work

Belbin (1993) proposes that we all have preferred team roles, and that a well-balanced team requires all of the above, but not in equal measure.

More than one 'plant' may cause friction, whereas multiple 'implementers' and 'team workers' are needed to form the majority of the team. Typically, the project manager is more likely to be a 'shaper' than a 'coordinator' by nature. In coping with the human problems of managing the team, the project manager will rely on a combination of their personal characteristics and their management methods and procedures. Management by Objectives (MBO) (Druker, 1993) has particular relevance to the highly participative project situation, as have the skills of being able to manage and resolve issues of conflict.

Project Evaluation and Selection Resulting in a Project Initiation Document (PID)

It is the responsibility of senior management to try to ensure that the project represents the most effective means of achieving what the business is striving to achieve.

An evaluation of options should assure: optimizing investment in development activities, development of clear project objectives, the avoidance of unacceptable levels of risk, and matching project deliverables with business goals

By conducting a formal process of evaluation there are additional benefits, particularly if the relevant statistics are made openly available. Members of the management team should be better able to appreciate the reasons for decisions taken. Also, the process will give a clearer understanding of the outcomes and risk associated with approved projects.

This will result in a contract for the project in the form of a PID. (Gov,2014) With the PID in place, the project can be executed. This leads into 'How you might do it'.

The Practice

or how you might go about it.

Project Identification

Here, be clear and detailed about what is going to be done. Set the Aim and a list of detailed, SMART Objectives.

Identify the scope of the project, indicating what is included in the work content, making clear what is outside of the scope as well as what is within it. Scoping the Project is best achieved through some form of hierarchical approach to planning. The project is broken down into a number of major activities, each of which is further subdivided into tasks and sub-tasks. Care should be taken to ensure that the tasks listed at any level of the hierarchy are given in matching detail.

When listing the activities involved in a project it is necessary to show which are logically dependent on the completion of other activities before they can commence. In some cases an activity may not start until another has also started. There may be more than one immediate predecessor to some activities, and in other cases the completion of one activity may enable several other activities to take place this might appear at this stage or as part of the planning stage in Gantt or Critical Path diagrams.

Clarify the way in which the organization as well as the project team will achieve the outcomes and

Make entirely clear the milestones which will constitute stage boundaries. Staging and stage teams will be defined as part of 'Planning'.

Set accountability for the project and make explicit the managerial relationships by which it will be supported executed and evaluated.

Make a detailed analysis of stakeholders:

Stakeholder analysis

Stakeholder	Involvement High/med/low	Interest High/med/low	Influence High/med/low	Attitude Positive/negative
1				
2				
3				
4				
5				

This will initially ensure that you overlook nobody and then guide you in managing the necessary relationships.

In analysing stakeholders, Iles (2006) suggests that they can be further categorised according to whether they are likely to be vociferous in their opinions, stubborn in their objections, or will follow the general consensus. These types she describes as *Mules, Lions and Sheep*.

Of course a stakeholder may be a Lion in an area dear to him/her and a sheep in an area where he/she has no strong view. So people are Mules, Lions or Sheep in specific relation to your project.

Lions must be in support your project, or it will not succeed. These are people worthy of detailed attention. Keep visiting them until you believe you have gained their support. Do this ahead of any decision-making meeting.

Mules must not be against you. These are people worthy of detailed attention, too, but only until you are confident that they will not oppose you. Keep visiting them until you believe you have removed any objections that they might have. Also do this ahead of any decision-making meeting.

Sheep will follow the group. You will not need to spend extensive time persuading this group.

Option Appraisal

In selecting a project, the usual fixed points are as above: cost, time and product.

However, there will always be a great many ways in which that product might be achieved and as part of the project identification the options must be identified, weighed up and the best option selected. For example, if the product required is a telephone exchange system for a major NHS Trust, then at first examination it might appear that the task is to set one up at the best cost/benefit ratio, as described in the Chapter Managing Finance. However other options need to be considered, such as: outsourcing the service to a dedicated telephony company, or becoming an adjunct to the telephone service already existing at a nearby NHS Trust.

Thus there are three options to consider:

1) set up a free-standing telephone exchange
2) contract with a specialist telephony company to deliver the service
3) enter into a federal partnership with another NHS Trust, private hospital or LASSD to create a service for all.

Each of these options should be considered and the best option recommended. In each case a project management team will be required, but if in one of the partnership schemes, this will take on a different form.

The option appraisal document will take the following form:

1) Introduction and Background, including Organisation Strategy and Policy
2) Issues, priorities and analysis of the current position
3) Aim and Objectives
4) Options List with explanations
5) Benefits needed/measures/weightings/ratings
6) Option costs
7) Cost/Benefit analysis & preferred option
8) Clear specific recommendation
9) Implementation and evaluation plan
10) Conclusion/summary
11) References
12) Appendices

Introduction and Background, including Organisation Strategy and Policy

This will set the context in which the project is proposed. It will address issues including:

Policy: The Trust, The DoH, The WHO, Mind/Age UK/etc

Strategy: Stated direction for the organisation's long term development,

Organisational analysis, such as SWOT, TOWS, PEST, (See the chapter on Marketing)

Market analysis: Demographic analysis, morbidity/mortality, societal analysis, etc.

Issues, priorities and analysis of the current position

List your development issues and priorities. You can analyse this current position and present it very effectively in a table showing your situation as part of a time continuum:

Criteria	Past	Present	Future
Clients	*What **were***		
Environment	*............ things like?*		
Demographics			
Health policy		*What **are** things*	
Legislation		*like now?*	
Technology			
Facilities			
HR			
Finance			*What do you*
Constraints			*...want things*
Access			*.......... to be like?*

Aim and Objectives of project

It is important to distinguish between:

a single, overaching Aim which states what is to be achieved, but is not sufficiently specific to be actualised and

a list of Objectives, which can be SMART and once executed are amenable to evaluation.

Options List with explanations

Here list explicitly at least three options, giving details of how each can be achieved and what would be involved in taking that route.

Benefits needed/measures/weightings/ratings

Here it is necessary to state the benefits that the product is to deliver to the organisation and its clients. This is derived from detailed consultation with the stakeholders, listed above.

Benefits need to be listed and then weighted to show which take priority. This weighting is a subjective exercise, but takes on some validity if all stakeholders are involved in the process. Ideally, once the benefit list is set, rather than simply consulting, the option appraisal will take one of two approaches to compiling a representative list of weightings:

1) ask all stakeholders to weight independently and average the scores.
2) Ask all stakeholders to work collectively until they can agree a scoring by consensus.

A weighted benefits list for our telephone service might be as below:

	Weighting	Means of assessing
Speediness of response	25	*From studies of similar provisions*
Patient accessibility	15	*Ease of patient use considering impairment, etc*
Carer convenience	20	*Times of day access for working carers, etc*
Reduced error and lost calls	40	*From studies of similar provisions*
Total	100	

Here, the stakeholders have agreed on four benefits. They have then decided which is most important to them and by how much.

Note this is only a benefit weighting exercise. Cost is factored in later, so 'cheap' is not a benefit for this purpose. To include it here would amount to double counting.

Next a stakeholder panel, supported by technical data can rate each possible option according to each criterion:

	Weight	Rating #1	Score #1	Rating #2	Score #2	Rating #3	Score #3
Speediness of response	25	5	125	6	150	4	100
Patient accessibility	15	6	90	8	120	9	135
Carer convenience	20	7	140	7	140	7	140
Reduced error & lost calls	40	8	320	9	320	6	240
Total	100		675		730		615

This shows that option #2 is the best quality, with option#2 as second best and option #3 as third.

Option costs

Each option must be costed in order to assess best value. This might be according to a full absorption costing method, which includes a share of all overhead, fixed costs, or might be on a marginal costing basis simply reflecting the additional expenditure involved in the implementing the project. This will depend on the protocol preferred by the Trust or Organisation. For explanation of costing methods, see chapter 5 Managing Finance. This is an exercise of bottom up budgeting, because the cost is established by aggregating expenditure. This related to Zero-based budgeting, as in the chapter: Managing Finances.

Option	Cost/£K
Option # 1	110
Option # 2	120
Option # 3	99

Cost/Benefit analysis & preferred option

Option	Cost/£K	Benefit	Cost/benefit	Benefit/cost
1	110	675	0.163	6.13
2	120	730	0.164	6.08
3	99	615	0.161	6.21

This analysis shows that the option 3 is cheapest, and although it delivers commensurately lower benefit, the reduction in benefit is less than the reduction in cost, so that it is the best value for money option.

Clear specific recommendation

From the option appraisal, it is possible to make a clear recommendation of option 3.

To read more about option appraisal and economic appraisal, see chapter 5 Managing Finance.

Having identified the preferred option it is necessary to enumerate any risks associated with the project.

Conduct risk analysis.

The NHS's preferred risk assessment matrix (DOH, 2014) makes a good device to quantify and articulate risk associated with the project.

Catastrophic					
Major					
Moderate					
Minor					
Negligible					
	Rare	Unlikely	Possible	likely	almost certain

Conclusion of Project Identification

So, before agreeing to progress to the planning stage ensure that you have explicit agreement from above you in the organization and throughout your project team on the following key issues,:

- Project priorities
- Key tasks
- Alternative methods
- Internal communications
- Reporting requirements
- Standard procedures
- Staff availability
- Skills and attitudes required

- Training and development needs
- Areas of responsibility and authority
- Contractual aspects
- Methods for project evaluation.

Planning

Here you will set the duration and cost of the project. You will also agree the membership of your team with allocation of work to individual members, with accountability and monitoring/reporting procedures.

Duration of the project will include explicit agreement of stages in the execution with clear definition of stage boundaries and mechanisms for agreement that a stage has been completed. Processes for moving on to each next stage can be set at this time.

Project mapping

This duration and the precedent arrangements are most easily shown of a GANTT chart and/or a Critical Path diagram.

Gantt Chart 1

	Description	January	February	March	April	May	June	August
Stage 1		=======	=======					
Stage 2				======	======			
Stage 3				======	======			
Stage 4				======				
Stage 5						====	====	
Stage 6							====	
Stage 7							======	======

In GANTT Chart (1) stage 1 is a prerequisite for the commencement of stages 2, 3 & 4. Stages 2 & 3 are prerequisite for stage 6. Stage 4 is prerequisite for stage 5 and stages 5 & 6 are prerequisites for stage 7.

In this diagram, all stages are critical, indicating that any delay on any of those stages would result in delay to overall completion.

Gantt chart 2

	Description	January	February	March	April	May	June	August
Stage 1		======	======					
Stage 2				======				
Stage 3				======				
Stage 4				======				
Stage 5						======	======	
Stage 6							======	
Stage 7							======	======

In GANTT chart 2 stage 1 is a prerequisite for the commencement of stages 2, 3 & 4. Stages 2 & 3 & 4 are prerequisites for stage 6. Stage 4 is prerequisite for stage 5 and stages 5 & 6 are prerequisites for stage 7.

In this diagram, stages 1, 4, 5 & 7 are critical, indicating that any delay on any of those stages would result in delay to overall completion, but some delay on stages 2, 3 & 6 could be tolerated without delaying the overall project.

In agreeing the team, it is not essential that each stage has the same team. You might enlist different expertise at different stages. You might be able to enlist different 'general' workers for different teams if that helped with the logistical problems involved in releasing team members from their normal duties. This might also be useful in accommodating holidays, etc.

The GANTT chart, above will show which stage team is required at which month in the year. It is essential that this is entirely explicit from the beginning of the project so that team members can make arrangements for cover to their normal duties and to ensure that this does not clash with holiday arrangements. It is essential that this availability is agreed early rather than trying to replace gaps when a member fails to be ready as required.

The GANTT chart allows you to make plans for the availability of materials, premises, etc on a *Just in Time*, basis to allow the project to progress

Stage time analysis

For each stage or task within a stage, there is an earliest start time and a latest allowable finish time. There is an activity duration time. The amount of 'float time' is the difference between the overall window from earliest possible start and latest acceptable finish time and the activity duration time. This measure shows your allowance for slippage and variance without impinging on the completion date.

However, as shown above human and other resources must be made available at exactly the right moment for the activity to occur and allowing slippage or imprecision can result in either wasted resource or delay because of absence of resource. A *'Just in case'* supply model will accommodate slippage' whereas a *'Just in time'* supply model will not. However *'Just in time'* is a far more efficient approach to deploying manpower and other resources. So, where resources are crucial the use of float time should be minimized by following a precise project plan.

Resource requirement

From the GANTT chart it is clear exactly which resources are required at each period in the plan. This is used to order material deliveries, free up time for team members, reserve technical expert attention, reserve use of plant, etc. Although the plan can have scope for timing adjustments in readiness for the unexpected, the more flexibility you write into the plan, the more difficulty you will have in scheduling this wealth of resources.

Resource smoothing

The GANTT chart shows demand on human and other resources and where a number of resource intensive stages overlap, then for that period you need a larger number of people to execute it. Then you might have low intensity periods when few people are needed. This makes staffing the project very difficult. A solution can be to manipulate stages so the demand on people is as smooth as can be achieved. If there are options regarding the timing and ordering of stages, then this should be exploited to make manpower demands as steady as can be achieved. It is easier to deploy a fixed team steadily than to work with many people one week and none the next.

The same concern may apply to use of roads, parking etc. If deliveries all occur at the same time, then traffic problems will be caused. Resource smoothing could be deployed to make steady use of access points and avoid bottlenecks.

Organization

Once the plan has been created, agreed and resourced, the execution can be comparatively straight forward. It falls to the Project Manager to organize people and monitor to ensure that the plan is rolling out as intended. As a result the planning stage is the most demanding, critical and interesting. If planning is sound then the execution is routine. This is counter-intuitive. Project Managers and members of the Project Team, are usually eager to 'get started' and can be frustrated by endless questions and demands for detail about the plan, but if it is appreciated that the plan is the key to success, the hard work and the interesting piece, then the mere execution becomes the lesser part. This mirrors the student's greatest project, his/her end of course thesis. He/she is always itching to get on with data collection, thinking that that is when the project has really got going. However, that is the easy piece; the methodology and method discussion are far more difficult and more important. Nonetheless there is a feeling that we have not got started until stage 1 is initiated and the Project Manager has to counter that misconception.

Organization of the project, therefore involved deploying resources in line with the plan, monitoring to ensure that the results are as required in terms of Time, Cost and Performance. Making changes to correct in the case of variance presents some interest for the Project manager, who will alter practice or outcome goals in response to issues that emerge during this execution of the plan.

Implementation

Implementation stage refers to the initial running of the service that was commissioned as a result of the project. This is then subject to evaluation against the criteria set in the initiation stage.

At this stage, any necessary modifications can be undertaken and the project team disbanded. In many cases the evaluation will be undertaken by the project sponsor or the functional manager who is to be responsible for the ongoing running of the service.

Accountability around the time of the handover can be ambiguous and it is useful if this has been made explicit at the PID stage. A degree of overlap may be beneficial, but this needs to be clearly defined to prevent an open-ended commitment on the part of the Project Manager and a possible conflict between him/her and the functional manager.

Where a Project Manager is employed on a fixed-term contract, then he/she may be looking for the next project while concluding the current one. To ensure that this does not lead to poor project performance, it can be appropriate to allow a period of employment after then end of the project to smooth this transition.

Lean thinking

Lean thinking is an approach to reorganization and project management designed to deliver high quality and cost effectiveness. Lean is unusual because it disputes the popular notion that, ultimately, quality can only be improved by allocation of further resources.

Lean thinking seeks to improve quality by reducing 'flow' (patient throughput) and reducing waste in all forms. This has the effect of reducing costs and increasing quality.

Lean thinking has periodically been presented as the new wonder cure for the problems of the NHS (The Conversation Journal, 2014) but lean is not new, having been in operation since the 1960s, when it encompassed the unpopular 'Time& Motion' movement. Lean was initiated in Japan, by Taiichi Ohno who lived 1912-1990, and is best known for its use in Toyota manufacturing, where it has been credited with much of their success.

Lean sets out to eliminate waste, by refining systems and processes with as little human, resources and time as possible whilst maintaining quality. Waste is divided into unavoidable waste and immediately avoidable waste. Lean sees no excuse for the latter and improvements can be delivered as soon as the project commences, rather than at some time in the future.

A lean project will usually follow five stages:

1) Define *'value'* from the perspective of the user (Patient, client, carer and commissioner)
2) Understand and standardize the Value stream by which this value is delivered.
3) Examine 'flow' of goods or users through this value stream and eliminate any waste.
4) Repeat, accepting that Perfection can be the only goal.

Define *'value'*

Value is anything that the customer, consumer client, etc sees as a benefit of the product or service. Activity that the customer does not consider to add value to the service or product can be seen as a waste of time. A patient values a drug because it is therapeutic. He/she may also value the fact that it can be easily swallowed, so putting into a capsule adds value. He/she may value that it is in an easy access container, so this adds value. He/she would not value the drug being florescent, so to do so would be a waste.

A university student values learning. He/she also values good quality assurance and even examinations, because that makes the degree better respected and supports using it to apply for a job. Fairness and equity in granting variances to rules, such as deadline extensions are also adding value, so this should be subject to guidance. Was a major committee to be convened to assess each such claim, that might not add value for the customer since a simple decision could be made by a course leader, following standard guidance. This move would delay decisions, thus removing value and waste resources in convening the committee. This would be seen as waste.

Understand and standardize the value stream

There are a great many steps in the chain that produces a product or service. The Lean examination asks of each step, whether it is really necessary. Ie, does it add value to the product? If it does not, then consideration is given to discontinuing it.

When a piece of waste is identified, it is useful to ask 'Why?' The answer is rarely definitive so we ask 'Why?' again. If sufficient 'Why?'s are asked we track back to a root cause of the problem, which can be remedied. Attempting to remedy a symptom rather than the root cause can be less effective. This is referred to as a *root cause analysis*. This can be shown diagrammatically when it becomes known as a *fishbone diagram* because of the appearance of the finished diagram, It is generally found that the root cause is unearthed by asking five sequential 'Why?' and this tracking back gives the analysis its other name of *the 5-'Why? s'*. These analyses were devised in the first place by Prof Ishikowa, (Radnor 2006). (George & Maxey 2005).

There may be many reasons for waste appearing in a value chain, restricting flow. Unnecessary loops in the process may have been accepted because that is how it has always been done and nobody has noticed that it is essentially redundant. An example of this might be the repeated collection of biographical information from patients in hospital. This cannot be shown to add value to the treatment experience and consumes resources; it is waste. Where no possible means of sharing that data is possible then this would be 'unavoidable waste', but if a solution is available then it would become immediately avoidable waste and lean thinking would want it discontinued.

Waste may also have been introduced to please and reassure those delivering the services failing to recognize that they consume resources without adding value. In the case of unnecessary bureaucratic procedures, they can actually decrease value as well as consuming resources. In an attempt to alleviate this the UK Government has a major initiate to 'Cut Red Tape' (Cameron, 2014)

Examine 'flow' of goods or users through this value stream and eliminate any waste.

Having identified the value stream by which goods and services are delivered, it is incumbent on the assessor to watch it happen and identify wasteful activities and variances in its execution. This may involve a wide range of tools as described by Radnor (2006). George & Maxey (2005). In particular, *six-sigma* offers a series of metrics that allows the lean project manager to evaluate efficiency and to demonstrate improvement through the application of lean principles.

Repeat, accepting that Perfection can be the only ultimate goal.

Success in any industry only continues as long as the organization is ahead of or up with the competitors. Lean exercises are a part of getting ahead, but since all organizations are constantly improving, to stand still is to fall behind. Therefore, Lean principles require perfection as the only standard. This means that improvement must be constant.

Overriding principles

It is considered that a lean thinking exercise requires:
1) That is a continuing program and culturally ingrained, and is not a fad or flavor of the month.
2) It has the continuing support of the highest level of management in the organization
3) Staff are empowered to study their work streams, identify areas of waste that can be eliminated
4) Resources are dedicated to supporting and driving the necessary changes
5) Focus on the system not blaming operatives, studying the flow that creates values and applying the lean tools
6) Rapid results by deploying rapid improvement events

Lean thinking is not new but does have the potential to offer improvement to the user experience and save resources.

Chapter conclusion

Project management is a major way of working, either for professional project managers or for functional managers faced with a one-off piece of development activity. The execution phases are important, but far less important than the Identification and Planning phases. These are the stages that predict success. Similarly, the skills of leadership, negotiation and communication are shown to be better predictor of success than simple technical skill in the subject area. A wide range of HR & leadership skills, collaboration, quality change management and financial skills are required. Other chapters of this book will be relevant to your project management practice.

References

Adair, J. (1973) *Action-Centered Leadership*, London: McGraw-Hill,

Fayol, H. (1971). *General and Industrial Management*, London: Pitman,

Adesse Consulting (2005). *Applying Lean and Reducing Waste (Excess Processing)*:
eprints.whiterose.ac.uk/86334/1/lean_tea_euram.19.04.15.final.pd

Badiru, A. B. (1988) *Project Management in Manufacturing and High Technology Operations,* London: John Wiley and Sons

Belbin, R.M. (1981).*Management Teams: Why They Succeed or Fail,* London: Heinemann,

Belbin, R.M. (1993) *Team Roles at Work*. London: Butterworth Heinemann

Benton,P. (1990) *Riding the whirlwind* Oxford: Blackwell

Bevan, H et al (2006). Lean Six Sigma: Some Basic Concepts: NHSSIST001

Briner, W., Hastings, C, and Geddes, M. (1996) *Project Leadership,* $_2$nd edition, Aldershot: Gower Publishing Limited.

Burbridge, R.N. G. (1990) *Perspectives on Project Management,* London: Peter Peregrinus Ltd

Cameron,D (2014)*red tape challenge*
http://www.redtapechallenge.cabinetoffice.gov.uk/home/index/

Culpin, M. F. (1989) *The Management of Capital Projects*, London: BSP

DoH (2014) *Lean principles*
http://www.institute.nhs.uk/building_capability/general/lean_thinking.html

DoH (2014) Risk assessment approach
http://www.nrls.npsa.nhs.uk/resources/?EntryId45=59825

Druker,P. (1993) *The practice of management* New York: Harper Business

Frigenti, E., and Comninos, D. (2002) *The Practice of Project Management*. London. Kogan Page

George,M & Maxey,J. (2005). *The lean, six sigma tool book*. London: Mcgraw Hill

Gov (2014) PIDs http://www.dfpni.gov.uk/content_-_successful_delivery-project_initiation_document

Graham, R. J. (1985) Project Management: Combining Technical and Behavioral Approaches for Effective Implementation, Amsterdam: Van Nostrand Reinhold

Guthrie, J (2006). *The joys of a health service driven by Toyota*: Financial Times.

Handy, C. B. (1993) *Understanding Organizations,* , London: Penguin Books Ltd, ISBN: 0140156038

Harrison, F L (1992) Advanced Project Management, 3rd edition, Aldershot Gower

Hines, P. (2002). *Lean Profit Potential*: London: Lean Enterprise Research Centre

Iles,V. (2006*) Really Managing Healthcare*. Maidenhead: OUP

Jones , A., & Mitchell, B. (2006). *Lean thinking for the NHS*: Bristol: NHS Confederation.

PIP (2007) Lifting the Lid on Lean Solutions *Pathology in Practice*. 8(1) www.pathologyinpractice.com

Lock, D. (2001) *Essentials of Project Management*, Aldershot: Gower

Lockyer, K., and Gordon, J*. (*1991) *Critical Path Analysis and Other Project Management Techniques*, London: Pitman,

Mathieson, S. (2006). *Wait Watchers*: Health Service Journal Intelligence.

Meredith, J. R., and Mantel Jr, S. J… (1999) *Project Management:* London: Wiley

Murman, A. (2002). *Lean Enterprise Value; Insights from MIT's Lean Aerospace Initiative.* New York: Wiley

Pozner,J. in .Meredith, J .R., and Mantel Jr, S. J. (1999) *Project Management:* London: Wiley

Prince (2014) *https://www.prince2.com/what-is-prince2*

Radnor, A. (2006). *Evaluation of the Lean Approach to Business Management and it use in the Public Sector*: Edinburgh: Blackwell

Reiss, G (1992) *Project Management Demystified:* Today's Tools and Techniques. London: E & FN Spon

Richman, L. (2002) *Project Management Step-by-Step* New York: AMACOM

Schwaber, K. (2004) *Agile Project Management with Scrum* Washington: Microsoft press

Sharp, J., & Howard, K. (2002) *The Management of Standards for Research* Project Aldershot: Gower

Shenhar, A. (1992) Project management style and the Space Shuttle Program (Part 2): A retrospective look, *Project Management Journal*, Vol.XXIII, (1)

The Conversation Journal academic rigor and journalistic flair, (2014) *http://theconversation.com/nhs-turns-to-the-car-industry-for-management-ideas-but-it-wont-save-2-billion-33961*

Wall, A.J. *Project Planning and Control Using Micros*, NCC Publications, 1988.

Womack, A. (1990). *The Machine that Changed the World.* Rawson Associates: New York.

Womack, A. (2005). *Going Lean in Healthcare* London: Institute for Healthcare Improvement.

Managing Information

Introduction

The 21st Century may be described as the Information Age (Naisbit, 1982). Up until the 18th Century, the majority of human endeavour was expended on agriculture. The 19th century the industrial revolution saw most of human effort moving to manufacturing industries, with mechanisation enabling the agricultural industry to maintain and increase output with only a very small segment of the human workforce. The 21st century has seen manufacturing industry able to increase output and dramatically reduce the need for a human workforce through the information revolution. The segment of the total population employed in manufacturing has shrunk and will continue to do so. This has been made possible by the process of intelligent automation. Human labour is shifting towards the management of information as the major means of generating wealth. Information and knowledge have become the dominant product underlying a large proportion of industrial activity and being the sole product of a long list of professions from Law to Stock-broking. Thus, it has become essential for all employees active in any industry to be skilled at handling information. As agricultural skill moved from being essential for survival to being unnecessary for most of the population, so the ability to manufacture also becomes unnecessary for most people. Whether manufacturing develops into a hobby activity, as agriculture was modified into gardening, remains to be seen. What is clear is that "Knowing things" is replacing "Making things" as a way of earning a living. Alongside the shift in production from food through goods to information, is the steadily growing service sector made possible by increasing wealth and leisure. This chapter examines the management of information in health care, the largest of the service industries.

Managing information includes the development of computing skills, but equally important is the management of information in other formats. It is essential in health care that information is held, is accessible and is recognisable where and when it is required. This chapter considers making that possible by considering the principles that apply to all storage media.

The Theoretical Framework

Storing and Retrieving Information – A Personal Database for Life

The amount of information that will be necessarily collected by a new health or social care professional throughout his/her career is massive. Having the information is of no value, however, unless it can be retrieved when it is needed. Therefore, information must be locatable. Further, information must be *easily* locatable because anything less will be an inefficient use of time. It is essential for every new professional to devise a system for storage of information of all types that is robust enough to see him/her through a lengthy career. What is not practical is to wait until enough material has been accumulated to realise the need, because by then the exercise is almost wholly impossible. (Mokhof, 2014)

It is necessary that storage systems are logical and transparent because, although in early years a quixotic system may be made workable by a good memory, once it has grown large it will be progressively difficult to track items at need. When it begins to be a time consuming exercise to find a particular item, then that is the time to revise and update a system.

However, if no system exists at all, it will be nearly impossible to impose one on a mountain of accumulated information. Material will be lost.

It is essential, therefore, to be scientific in information storage as early as possible and to build a database that manages information from every source. The professional always notes the source of any useful reading. A report into internal communication carries more weight if the author can say, "According to Swansburg (1990), *75% of a manager's time is spent talking and listening*". This is more persuasive than if it said, "*Most of a manager's time is spent on talking and listening.*" Equally, the author will be believed more easily if he/she can say, "*A study reported by Swansburg...* ", instead of, *"I read somewhere.."* or the non-attributed and never believed *"Research has shown... ".* Therefore, it is essential that professional clinician or manager record sources for information held and make note of content and source from books they have read. Additionally, this referencing system will allow additional research when necessary. In early years of practice, good memory may allow the individual to go to the book in question with a little effort, but as the material accumulates (and memory deteriorates!) this becomes less possible. Notes from reading should be integrated into a unified information system rather than a vast array of card indexes, each compiled for a different purpose. The notes from an inspiring book should be filed alongside the instructions for patients following Total Hip Replacement, if they relate to the same subject area.

The system devised will hold all of the information collected in a lifetime's study. However, that is of no value unless the recorder knows broadly what is there in order to initiate retrieval. Again, a sound and logical ordering will allow a comprehensive grasp of content.

A good information system, therefore, has a number of qualities:

1) It is unified, carrying all of the collected information from a lifetime of endeavour. It is even difficult to achieve demarcation between work and domestic life, and therefore it may be advantageous for the system to cover all areas of life. Information will be in paper and electronic format, but this need not result in two systems. Rather there should be a single system evident across both media. Thus if the nurse wishes to collate all that he/she has on a chosen subject he/she will interrogate the same heading(s) in both media as different branches of a unified information system
2) The system must be transparent. Where any piece of information is to be found must be self-evident and unambiguous. This will prevent information loss and reduce the time involved in accessing it.
3) It must be flexible and infinitely expandable to accommodate new information and new categories of information
4) Sources must be clearly identified so that they can be attributed and so that when further research is indicated, this can be done with maximum efficiency.
5) The professional clinician or manager must know, in broad terms, what the system holds in order that when an opportunity to benefit from what is held it can be quickly exploited.

It should be noted that information of many types might be needed at a future time as legal evidence Therefore in some situations, the manner of storage is critical because it may, one day, be read aloud, by a hostile advocate, to a coroner or judge. See the management of people – accountability

Different media

Information may be recorded in a variety of media, and there is currently no system that meets all needs. Each has benefits, and can play a part in a unified information system Paper records remain important legal documents and this has not been entirely superseded by IT systems (DOH, 2013). Card index systems have the benefit of portability, accessibility and ease of sorting for small records. IT based systems are almost infinitely expandable, flexible and are potentially very easy to interrogate. IT systems are being devised to mimic the benefits of other systems. E.g. single write CD ROM systems allow a record to be dated and to have unchangeable permanence, thus replacing the evidence value of a written record. However, they cannot match the portability and instant access of some paper systems.

Recording patient/client information

Separate/Unified case notes

There is a long running aspiration for the unification of case records

Traditionally each professional group has kept records about each patient or client treated. These records serve a number of purposes. They are primarily to enable the clinician to plan monitor and communicate treatment interventions. They also allow a colleague to take over a case if necessary. Secondarily, records allow quality audit and serve as evidence in judicial enquiry.

Where the clinician considers that the treatment and progress needs to be known by colleagues he/she will write a summary in the medical case notes and/or nursing records. However, this practice has many shortcomings:

1) There is significant duplication of effort.

2) It allows the risk that the clinician omits information that a colleague would wish to know.
3) Biographical patient data is collected repeatedly which duplication of effort places unnecessary strain on clinician and patient/client.

Minimal biographical data may be more easily managed by making centrally printed labels available to all clinicians. This eases the burden on patients/clients but, in the interest of confidentiality, it covers only the minimum data.

Many hospitals and services have developed a unified case record that carries the detailed notes of all of the clinicians involved with a patient/client. This avoids duplication of effort and ensures that all clinicians have access to all information. However, there are various ways of devising unified records, each having its pros and cons.

Currently this applies within an NHS Trust, with only summaries passed to other Trusts and GPs on discharge. However, with the controversial central uploading of GP patient records these would become available to clinicians wherever a patient is admitted. This has clear benefits and use of data for research can only be good. However, health records are very sensitive and confidentiality concerns are leading to debate about scope and speed of this innovation. (DoH, 2013b)

Continuous or sectional

Unified case records may carry continuous entries in chronological order regardless of author, or there may be a section for each profession involved with the patient/client. The chronological order system allows the reader to follow the experience and progress of the patient holistically, but requires careful skip reading if the reader is to track a specific event such as wound care. The profession specific approach, more widely found, allows each profession to monitor their own area, but requires constant flicking between sections to put together the nursing, physiotherapy and occupational therapy interventions that might constitute the intervention package after a surgical intervention. This demarcation process might encourage clinicians to be parochial in what they read when faced with a heavy caseload and can result in important information being missed.

The physical location of unified records may also present difficulties. Generally, records are kept on wards so that they can be accessed in the presence of the patient. However, that may be inconvenient when accessing records to record information and later for departmental audit If the unified record is part of a ward round, case conference, etc, then it is not available to the clinician for an extended period. Additionally, there can be a need to access records in department to audit quality or enact supervision This has resulted in a variety of devices to achieve a unified record and a department record simultaneously. This partially defeats the object of a unified record, and demonstrates an inadequacy of the unified record notion. Attempts to overcome this inadequacy include photocopying records in order for them to be in two locations. In settings where the IT services allow, records are held on a central computer server and accessed at terminals at all clinical settings. This requires extensive security measures to protect confidentiality and may involve stepped access so that levels of authority only allow access to restricted levels of data. Thus, for instance, managerial and administrative authority might allow access to information about category, length of stay and location, but not diagnosis and social situation. Additionally, the system has to allow a distinction between read-only access and the right to change or add information. The central server based system, once security has been ensured, has considerable potential benefits. Access terminals need not be in the same building or organisation as the server. Ever since the publication of "A New NHS" (1998), trials have been conducted into allowing Health Centres and GP Practice Surgeries to access central NHS Trust records and receive instant and reliable information about investigations and treatments concerning their patients. The amount of information made available in this way is limited, but the opportunity for growth is clear.

System, in recording ensures that records will be read

Once information becomes freely available across organisational boundaries, the volume, already great, is likely to increase rapidly and the time taken in reading will become the limiting factor. A clinician who wants his/her records to be read by colleagues should set them out in the most accessible and transparent way possible. Records in chronological script, while logical , can be insufficiently rewarding to justify the time needed to read them. The reader may either attempt to skip read the paper and risk missing important material or decide not to look at the work at all, because time does not allow. If there is a consistent system in the way records are made, with headings and sub-headings then the reader can rapidly find the areas that concern him/her and gain essential information at minimal cost. A good system is logical, transparent, consistent, comprehensive and universally employed.

In a *logical* recording system, information is given in causal sequence and such as Presentation, Examinations, Interventions, Outcomes and Aftercare. This will mean that the reader is able to anticipate each step in the information chain and will more easily absorb the material offered. Additionally, if the reader is to skip read the paper, it is more likely that he/she will find the pertinent material.

To achieve *transparency* the system requires its logic to be easily identifiable and well sign-posted. This may be best achieved by the clear use of headings and subheadings.

To achieve *consistency* the reporter must always adopt the same order and presentation in report writing. He/she must resist variations wherever possible. This is more difficult than may appear. It requires considerable forethought, because the system that seems logical in the first instance may not be sufficient when an unusual case arises. To change order to meet emerging conditions will set back the reader who has become accustomed to an established style. Therefore the system adopted should be tested in the abstract in order to ensure that it is truly robust. The general rule "Adopt and adapt a proven method" applies to recording systems, however simple the job may appear to be at first sight. It is advisable to adopt an existing recording and reporting methodology, with adaptations if necessary, because it will have been developed over time to meet all eventualities. Two popular systems are the Subjective, Objective, Assessment and Planning (SOAP) approach and Problem Orientated Medical Recording (POMR) systems.

To be *comprehensive*, a recording/communicating system must have one methodology that meets the whole need. There must not be a string of other communiqués needed alongside the central record in order for the picture to be complete. Rather, a recording/communicating system must be devised that comprehensively meets the need. It should seek to sweep up the functions of the plethora of forms and notes that arise in unplanned practice.

Uniformity in a recording/communicating system requires that the same system be employed by all members of a profession who are involved with the same client group, and if possible on a much wider basis.

Legal Documents

Medical records are legal documents, and NHS Trusts are required to keep them, in their original paper form, throughout an episode of care and thereafter for many years according to a complex schedule (DoH,2013). A

Trust can be required to produce these records by a coroner, or a judge in criminal or civil proceedings. Recognising that all clinical-records might become designated "Legal Documents", the clinician should systematically employ content and language in the recognition that it may be read aloud in a court by an adversarial advocate. This caution encourages the clinician to be thorough and accurate in record keeping, but it should not place a burden greater than that required by good clinical practice. The best defence against embarrassment in a court is not the so-called "Defensive Medicine" but consistent good practice.

In addition since the Access to Medical Reports Act (1988), patients and relatives have access to these records, which has modified the language and ideas expressed considerably.

The definition of a Medical Record is imprecise but can encompass a wide range of clinical documents. However, the NHS Trust has the power to designate some records as "transient" and destroy them after an episode of care has ended. Transient records are those notes made to facilitate treatment and communication but not necessary to establish the rationale or progress of the treatment involved

Over recent decades, most NHS Trusts have copied old medical records onto Microfiche, read-only CD-ROM and other digital stores. This results in a very significant saving in space, and leads to records that are more durable and easier to access or search. However, although these records are often accepted in court, it is uncertain that they completely discharge the responsibility on the Trust to keep the original documents. This can only be finally decided by case law, which is an emerging and evolving commodity. Consequently, most NHS Trusts make the transposition onto digital devices, but arrange for the original papers to be stored at a low cost location.

Right of Access

Data Protection legislation initially gave individuals access to any information identifiably referring to them held and on a computer. This rarely included medical records since they were primarily paper-based documents. Medical Records legislation was adjusted to close this loophole (Access to Medical Reports Act, 1988). Any patient in a hospital has the right to obtain, on demand a photocopy of his/her hospital and other medical records. Each NHS Trust has a procedure by which application may be made and the information must be made available within a reasonable time-scale. The Trust is entitled to charge for this service at a rate necessary to defer costs incurred. The rate of charges may be the marginal costs i.e. photocopying etc, or full costs which include staff time, and overhead costs Thus, the charges can vary considerably. Trusts are also expected to arrange to restrict some information where it is deemed clinically damaging to the patient, or to support the patient when he/she receives unpleasant information through this right.

Revisions made to Data Protection legislation in 1999, extend rights of access to personal information on paper as well as computer databases. This gave patients access to all of their records upon demand and effectively superseded access to medical records legislation.

Duty of confidentiality

All employees of a NHS Trust and others contracted to carry out work for the NHS or Social Services are bound by a duty of confidentiality. They may not divulge that a named person is receiving or has received treatment or care without the consent from that individual. Failure in this duty is a gross misconduct frequently resulting in dismissal. This duty is reinforced by the codes of conduct of all health and care professions, where failure can result in removal from a state register. This requirement is self-explanatory and it is very rare that a clinician will knowingly breach it. However, clinicians are at risk when they discuss a case in a place where they fail to realise that a member of the public may overhear them. There is also an expectation that patients are not named in management meetings where this information is not necessary for a decision to be made. It is the case that all managers and administrators are bound by confidentiality rules, but personal information should not be communicated to, or sought by, any individual who does not need to know that information.

Government information collection

The NHS is centrally controlled and locally managed through progressively independent provider units (NHS Trusts). This has made it extremely difficult to know how much activity is taking place, whether that activity addresses the highest priority need locally and whether it represents the best value for the public money consumed. Prior to the 1983 general management reforms "The Griffiths Report", responsibility for ensuring priority provision and value for money was entrusted to local managers and clinicians. They were considered the best judges of local need and priority. However, professional loyalty, known as Tribalism and self-interest, presenting as empire building were possible distractions from balanced judgement. During the 1980s, the DoH developed machinery to collect data about the productivity of service providers. Activity data is collected in three categories: individual patients/clients, service productivity and individual use of time. Health Authorities are required to submit information about morbidity and mortality within the catchment and the plans to improve the health of the local population.

Morbidity = illness/accidents

Mortality = deaths

Individual patient data is collected in the form of Minimum Data Sets including; referral route, biographical data, residence, diagnosis, treatment, length of stay and outcomes. This data was formerly used to track patients for payment, and more recently for quality assurance purposes.

Service productivity data involves identifying and counting events. Events identified are contacts (initial or follow up) and episodes of care. This collection may take one of a variety of forms.

Individual use of time may be recorded through an annual time sampling exercise. This requires clinicians to record, retrospectively, how each unit of time was spent, by placing it into a predefined category. These time segments are aggregated allowing an understanding to emerge of the detailed practice of each profession. Time sampling was described in detail in The Management of Time.

This data is collected and passed to the DoH. The results are collated and each provider is shown where they appear in comparison to the national and regional norms. This feedback loop helps managers to know when changes are required. It is intended that this collection of data should be of primary benefit to local managers as near as possible to the workforce and the supply of data to the DoH should be achieved as a by-product of this local good management practice. Therefore, the data should be easily available to managers at department and ward level for their immediate action and NHS Trust or DoH should be incidental beneficiaries of information collected to meet the needs of immediate managers.

The data collected, however, has not proven to be robust and if applied inflexibly provides a perverse incentive to good practice. Clinicians pressured to increase episodes of care and/or reduce length of stay in hospital may find it disadvantageous to accept complex cases. This would result in cases that show a good prognosis being accepted for treatment in preference to those who are in circumstances that are more difficult. For example, a patient needing a prosthetic hip, but otherwise fit and living with supportive family can be treated and discharged in little more than a week. However another patient for a similar procedure living alone in poor housing and with other joint pathology will need far longer rehabilitation. The latter patient is a higher priority for treatment, but to treat that patient may result in apparently inefficient practice, if the returns are treated insensitively. The use of Diagnostic Related Groups (DRGs) to assess workload and payment is convenient but needs to be modified to reflect Case weightings if the data is to be valuable.

Where a department, such as physiotherapy is crudely assessed according to number of patient contacts, they could feel pressured into improving their figures by offering more treatments in groups, delivered by non-professional HCAs or simply offering treatments of a shorter duration. This practice may result in a reduced care but give the impression of higher productivity if raw data is examined insensitively.

Importing notions of productivity into health care is good but presents difficulty because of the unique nature of every episode of care. However, it is necessary to maximise the amount of care that is achieved with the finite resource available and, for this reason, statistics about treatment are necessarily collected. The duty upon managers is to look dynamically at this data and use it intelligently, not mechanistically, to maximise the care achieved with the resource available.

In patient-data collection a number of other statistics are important. These may be defined as below:

Terms

Midnight Bed State

Midnight Bed State = the number of heads on pillows

This is a physical count of the number of patients sleeping in NHS beds at midnight, conducted by nurses.

Bed Occupancy

Bed Occupancy = Number of patients/Number of beds X 100

This is a percentage of beds occupied on any given day. Ideally, this should stand at around 90 - 95%, meaning that 90 to 95 out of every 100 beds are occupied. This figure indicates that beds are not lying idle and therefore being wasted, but there are some beds available for emergency admissions. Higher than 95% occupancy is rare because of the time between discharge and admission (Turnover time).

In some mental health settings, patients are discharged on trial. In this case, a bed will be reserved to ensure that they can be rapidly readmitted at need. This bed will show as occupied. Where a number of patients are on leave pending discharge it may be unnecessary to retain a bed for each of them. Five patients on leave might require only two beds reserved. This can result in more patients being technically in hospital than there are beds. This situation gives bed occupancy of more than 100%.

"Hot Bedding", in which beds are filled on the same day as the previous patient was discharged may also result in the appearance of double occupancy.

Length of Stay

Length of Stay = Number of days or part days between Admission and Discharge

Length of stay (LoS) figures are known for every Hospital or NHS Trust. However, this statistic can be misleading. To compare LoS between hospitals can tell little unless the case mixes are matched, the use of day surgical units is similar and the socio-economic and demographic profiles of the populations are well matched.

Turnover Interval

Turnover Interval = Number of days/part days from Admission of one patient to Admission of the next

The turnover interval is greater than the length of stay because of the turnover time - the time from discharge of one patient to admission of the next.

Communicating Information

Information frequently becomes important only when it is communicated.

Communication is a process involving transmitter and receiver. The transmitter encodes information and transmits it, and the receiver receives and decodes it. Error can be introduced at any of these four stages.

Encode: Transmit: Receive: Decipher.

It cannot be assumed that material transmitted is received as intended. However, it can be assumed that what is received is based upon what was transmitted. Walton (1997) describes this as **The Arc of Distortion.**

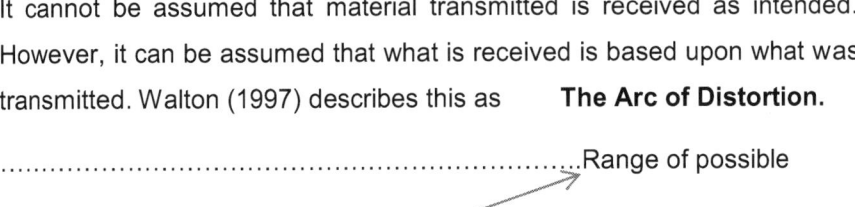

....Range of possible

Message transmitted

....messages received

The task of the parties to the communication is to minimise the depth of the arc. However, it should be understood that distortion cannot be entirely eliminated and therefore the system must allow for a degree of misinterpretation. The communicators cannot know that the exact message has been received, but can be confident that understanding is somewhere within this arc.

One and two way communication

Communication can be seen as a one or two way process. One-way communication such as Radio or Newspaper communication lacks an opportunity for checking accuracy of understanding, where two-way communications allows checking by both parties. However, one way communication is under the control of the transmitter, whereas two-way communications allows the message to be diverted by the questioning process so that the planned message is not adequately covered during a conversation.

The NHS and Social care organisations use 1-way communications to be absolutely sure that a message has been conveyed with speed and clarity. These include Team Briefing, Information bulletins and newsletters.

They use 2-way communications to test understanding and to receive feedback on information. Devices used include Roadshows, Suggestion boxes, Virtual conferences, etc.

Selecting the best media

All communication media have strengths and weaknesses. Qualities to consider include Immediacy, Permanence, Reciprocity, Control, Accessibility and Plausibility. Each quality will be important in different settings.

Immediacy

Immediacy is achieved by telephone, or verbal communication with people in the near vicinity. This may be paramount where timeliness is the dominant requirement. However, it has the disadvantage that little planning can be applied to precisely what is communicated. For this reason, much legal advice is given in the written form. Verbal communication also has the disadvantage of impermanence. This information will suffer from distortion of memory as well as communication distortion.

Permanence

Permanence is achieved by paper communication and emails This is necessary, when either the sender or the receiver is expecting to refer back to information later. Verbal communication is frequently followed up with a written record thus achieving both immediacy and permanence. This need for enduring information might also be considered when giving public presentation. Where visual aids to communication are by Photographic Slide, PowerPoint Data Projection then once the slide has been changed it is no longer available. The speaker and the audience are denied the opportunity to refer back to that information as the presentation proceeds. Posters or Flip Charts, however, achieve a useful reference throughout a presentation.

Reciprocity

Reciprocity allows communication to be two-way, thus ensuring accurate reception. This means that better understanding is achieved by conversation. The principle is employed in public presentations by encouraging discussion from an audience. Reciprocal information giving is generally verbal, but consideration should be given to written reciprocal communication by letter, with Electronic Mail via the Internet (Email) offerings a swifter substitute. Reciprocity allows practitioners to comment on and improve communicated plans which will make a change more likely to succeed. This is addressed in detail in the chapter on Change Management.

Control

Control is achieved by planning and is easiest to achieve in the written form. This results in sensitive matters being resolved by letter in preference to telephone communication Where a sensitive issue arises in conversation, it is advisable to seek time to check the correctness of any response. It is for this reason that adjournment is so common in industrial negotiation. Where sensitive material is to be transmitted in a public forum, it is normal to use visual aids and personal briefing notes not just to better convey the message, but also to maximise control over information conveyed.

Accessible

Making communicated information accessible requires careful consideration of the receiver. Communication must be conducted under conditions to suit the recipient, not the communicator. Material must be available at a time and place where sufficient receiver attention can be given. This means that conveying essential information to patients/clients who are distressed by any aspect of care may be unsuccessful. It may be impossible to convey details of treatment in the same interview in which the diagnosis has been revealed, or to give health promotion advice in a session including uncomfortable treatment.

Information must also be in language accessible to the recipient. Technical language (jargon) presents a known bar to understanding that clinicians strive to avoid, but it is easy to use such inadvertently. Additionally, many clinicians overlook difficulties caused by language that is culturally specific. A receiver from a different culture, social class or locality may apply different meanings to the words used. Material delivered in written form must consider reading age. It is usual to set language to be accessible to people of a fairly low reading age. Commonly 8-years old. This is not assuming that the reader has only that level of attainment, but it is possible for a highly able reader to read material intended for a less able person but not the other way around.

Language must be planned from the perspective of the recipient rather than the communicator.

Plausibility

Plausibility is essential in communicating information. Research has shown that audiences are persuaded by three factors in a communication

(Mehrabian, 1971). Least persuasive are the words spoken. More persuasive is the intonation and voice quality when presenting. Of greatest importance are the body communications given when speaking. Mehrabian observed the relative importance of these three factors in persuading an audience to believe a message and, more critically, he pointed out that maximum effect is achieved when all three devices are in harmony. Therefore, it is important to ensure that the spoken message is correct, then voice qualities support the message and finally demeanour, eye contact, etc are compatible with the message that is being delivered. This convergence best ensures understanding and co-operation.

The Practice

or how you might go about it
Storing and retrieving

The difficulty in exploiting information is finding it when you need it. The common complaint of new post-holders in any profession and at any grade is the difficulty they find in "Coming to grips with the predecessor's filing system". The worst filing system is one without logic. This occurs more commonly than might be expected, because information storage starts small with the owner knowing what is where. The stored information incrementally grows until it is unmanageable and the system collapses. Once collapse has occurred, retrieval is a very difficult task and procrastination ensures that it is not achieved. The lesson is that you must establish your information storage systems early in your professional life, with a natural home for all types of information created ahead of need. This requires you to have a measure of discipline, because it involves you proactively planning to create efficiency that will only pay off at some indeterminate future time.

Case example

A student comes across a paper describing research in which human arousal is shown to derive from sources often not consciously recognised by the subject (we nowadays say *participant*).

He/she then looks around for something to explain this arousal and frequently hits on the wrong explanation.

In this research, female interviewers approached male participants and *vice versa*. At the termination of the interview the interviewer gives contact details, lest the interviewee think of more to report on the topic of interview. Naturally, the covert point of the study was to measure the percentage of participants who initiated further contact seeking a social meeting.

The hypothesis was that if an interviewee is in an arousing environment he/she may attribute that arousal to the person with whom he/she is conversing. Wrongly thinking that he/she found that person exciting.

The results were that a statistically higher percentage of people made contact with their interviewer when the interview was conducted near a waterfall, on a high bridge, etc.

This is further supported by the number of relationships initiated in fairgrounds, night clubs and other energising settings.

This is very memorable research, being useful in a professional and social setting. However, the student does not make an academic record, in particular failing to write and store the reference. As a consequence she was unable to use this very valuable knowledge in future essays, or general argumentation.

A simple habit of recording knowledge in a systematic and retrievable form magnifies manyfold the amount of information that is available to us all.

To say *'research tells us...'* is completely worthless if you do not have the reference. Next time someone says to you *'the research tells us...'* to you say *'that's really interesting. What's the reference? I'd really like to read it'*. Just sit back and watch them splutter.

Approaches to cataloguing

Information is commonly stored according to one of three logics. Each may be appropriate according to the data stored. They are:- alphabetical order, chronological order and a category-sub-category decision tree.

Alphabetical storage

Alphabetical storage is very common but rarely satisfactory. This involves attaching a title to every item and storing every new piece of according to that title. Difficulty arises because it requires absolute consistency of designation. "Personnel" information may also appear as "Human Resource", "Welfare", "Pay & Conditions" etc. Is Neurodevelopmental technique to be filed under Stroke, CVA, TIA, or Hemiplegia? If they are all condensed into CVA, does that include TIA or is that separate? If TIA is separate, it will be a long way from CVA which is most unhelpful. So, with such a system, you are faced with a wide range of different directories that may hold information relevant to your enquiry. And, information correctly categorised and filed is separated by the vagaries of the alphabet. Information on "Dressing Materials" could be in an entirely different place from information on "Post Amputation Stump Bandaging".

Alphabetical categorising is appropriate for information that is essentially homogenous, such as patient/client records. Therefore, where there is no categorical logic to follow, title is unambiguous and no interaction between data is needed, then an alphabetical system will enable your individual records to be easily found.

The same can be true where all data is subject to a unique number. If everything has a number then simple numerical order will work well. See the Dewey system favoured by libraries. (Dewey, 1876) *{This challenges for the record for the oldest reference in a modern textbook –still available!, Ed}*

Chronological Storage

Some records are best categorised by when and in what order they occurred. Thus, we record diaries sequentially, rather than having a section for work, another for domestic and a third for amorous encounters. The chronological logic makes retrieval possible and is very helpful for identifying cause and effect relationships. Case records contain information in time order tracking patient progress, but it would be illogical to store accumulated knowledge according to the date on which it was acquired. None-the-less much information is so stored. Undergraduate study is in one place, sporadic continuing professional development follows and the MSc/ PhD learning is in another quite separate place, categorised according to when it was gained, not according to what knowledge it contains. Equally, students frequently keep knowledge gleaned on placement in a separate file from that gained in university albeit that it relates to the same clinical condition. In addition, they can have a 'personal profile' from placement that is different from their 'personal profile' at university. Unless they have multiple personalities this is very strange.

When you want information it will be subject specific, not specific to what course you learned it on. Rarely will you need to know 'what did I learn in 2014 or at OBU; frequently will you want to know what do I know about Osteochondromatosis. Therefore, it follows that you need a storage system that follows content, not the time the material was gained.

Category - Sub-category Storage

Much of the information collected at work and domestically would benefit from being stored, not simply according to its defining title, but according to the category in which it sits. Categories at the initial stage can be very large and clearly defined. By a series of sub-categorising, it is easy to reach some very specific definitions by which to store data. The right category is easily located by answering a small number of clear questions, with the result that items are reliably categorised and related items are close together. Mobilisation after Stroke lies beside Unilateral Transfers, although they are distant on an alphabetical scale.

This is the basis of the very successful Read Code Classification System for disease and treatment that enabled dramatic improvement in the classification of disease and NHS interventions. Internationally the International Classification of Diseases (ICD) uses a similar approach.

Question	Answer
Information needed. Is it: domestic, work or social?	Work.
Is it clients, treatments or colleagues?	Treatments.
Is it CVA, RA or etc?	CVA

Above, shows an embryonic system for storing information. By answering three unambiguous questions the searcher has reliably navigated to stroke treatment and can access all information on patient transfers. There is no ambiguity about the description and location of the material required. Had he said Stroke in preference to CVA or Care in preference to Treatment, the result would have been the same. It is the idea that navigates the searcher, not the actual word chosen. This minimises the possibility of mistake or duplication. The exercise required no memory about what was where or knowledge of other than the elementary fact that the system works upon a decision tree notion.

The above system lends itself to management of a filing cabinet or the files on a computer. In both cases, it is essential to decide the logic of the categories as soon as the system is started. In paper, or electronically, this system allows for near infinite expansion, devising new categories and sub categories as the need arises. What is essential is that nothing is stored that has not been categorised according to the system. In paper systems, the practice is to keep items in a "To be Filed" tray until time allows its correct categorisation. Many people fail to use the same discipline with computer storage of files and file carelessly because of lack of time. The consequence is that much material that is known to have been filed yet is irretrievable. The solution to this problem is to have the electronic equivalent of a "To be Filed" tray. You could keep a directory on the computer called "Temporary" or "To be filed" into which new files are placed if time does not allow for their immediate careful allocation. These can sit until time allows you to correctly store them.

It is important to have only one filing system through all aspects and phases your life. The same decision tree that defines your filing cabinet sections should govern choice of computer directories and one directory set should carry files from all of the software you use. There will be a CVA Treatment section in your personal filing cabinet, and on your computer. A search for CVA Rx information will involve looking in both of these places, but in each case you will be looking under the same chain of headings.

Personal Organisers

Personal Organisers still come in paper forms but are primarily in digital forms. Both can revolutionise your effectiveness by ensuring that you always have fundamental information to hand. Alternatively, they can be reduced to the level of very expensive and clumsy diaries. In addition to diary pages, the PE system has a number of useful components to dramatically increase your effectiveness. These include items below. Use them as a start point, but you should be continually adding to the list.

Contacts Directory

This should far exceed a telephone number list, by including simple information gleaned about each of your more regular contacts. If they mention the progress of their children in one conversation, then there is great advantage to be gained by enquiring about the same at future meetings. All contacts should be in this book, domestic, social and work and the book should never be out of your reach. Do not make the mistake of having one address book in at home, another at work, etc. This will inevitably lead to your needing a critical number and offering the weak excuse, "It's in my other book".

This contact management is a major component of networking and networking is a major component of Emotional Intelligence (Salovey, Mayer &Caruso, 2004).

"To-Do" lists:

Whenever a task emerges it can be captured instantly, ready for review according to whatever prioritisation schedule you favour. See "Time Management". This list will always be complete and up to date, and will prevent you from collecting a plethora of small lists and yellow notes that are lost or time consuming to collate. Since the Personal Organisers is always with you, nothing can be missed and there is always a record of current workload to hand.

Your To-Do list might have two sections. The first is the sheet showing the tasks that have been through your prioritisation process and that you are working on at present. The second list is for collection of emergent tasks, that you will consider alongside tasks from all other sources in your next prioritisation exercise.

Meeting planners

Where you are chair or a member of a meeting, it is good to give it a page in your Personal Organisers. Whenever an item occurs that is relevant to the meeting it can be immediately noted and by the time the call for agenda items comes out, you have a ready-made list. Additionally, it will make useful reference during the meeting.

Interview Planners

It is good to give a full section to each of the most critical contacts in your life. As items emerge, it is easy to note them and when you next meet, either by chance or for a planned meeting, you have a ready-made agenda for discussion. If you do not do this, then you will be unable to control the relationship with your boss/subordinate/peer. Additionally, brief notes about previous conversations will allow you to create continuity in your discussions and remember any personal information that they might have chosen to disclose.

Project planners

If you are responsible for part or all of a project, then contacts will pass you helpful information and suggestions about it at opportunistic moments. If each project has a page in your Personal Organiser, then you can capture them as they occur. Additionally, you will always be in a position to report the current position of any project when challenged.

Back it up

Data is always vulnerable. Personal organisers in paper or digital form are notoriously easily lost and may be stolen. There have even been cases of personal organisers held for ransom. This system, like all data systems needs to be subjected to a back-up system. In the case of an electronic organiser, computer copying by system synching is straightforward, and this should happen frequently. Paper systems are difficult to back up, but many people keep two systems with a desk organiser held by a secretary to mirror the personal portable one. Contact list and allied information might be periodically photocopied.

One comprehensive organiser

You will only carry one organiser with you. Therefore have just one, and use it for all functions. If necessary, have one with a password lock so that you are happy to store personal information alongside work information. You will know that the system is working when you cease to find the need for other systems and, above all, when you stop leaving yourself messages on sticky yellow notes.

Databases

You will collect data on many things, particularly patients/clients and subordinate staff. You will find that you want to use this data for a wide range of purposes and, for some, the data collected will be in the wrong form. Much analysis and research is performed using secondary data, i.e. data that already exists because it was collected for another purpose. If a database is created with the broadest consideration of its potential uses, then the data collected can be ordered and stored in such a way that its retrieval will be simple and unambiguous. Attempting to discover whether air quality affects patients' sleep, a researcher may want to correlate recorded pollen counts with Nurses' records about patients' sleep. However, although records cover this information most reliably, it is frequently not in a form that makes it good for this purpose. The difficulty arises in two areas;

1) Sleep information is not always recorded in the same place on the sheet/computer, and is therefore prohibitively time consuming to collect, and
2) The expressions used to describe sleep can vary and are therefore difficult to find. Additionally, it is an assumption that two expressions such as "Slept well" and "Had a good night" mean the same, which may not be correct.

If, however, the data had been collected with research analyses in mind as a possible use, then the terminology could have been standardised and the structure of reports made accessible by strict ordering and headings. When information is so clearly a valuable commodity, it is sensible to collect it in a way such as to maximise its value. This need cost no more, but requires creative thinking at the outset of any data collection exercise. Indeed careful consideration about order and terminology at the outset of a data collection exercise will reduce the long-term cost of collection and recording as well as increasing the eventual value.

Where it is likely that a type of data will be wanted in the future for any purpose it is helpful to place a signal that can be found by a researcher or computer search. This might involve consistent use of sub headings etc.

Ideally, you will have one database for any subject. All information about clients will be on one system, rather than one for their medical needs, another for their care arrangements and a third for their schooling. If these three types of data are stored separately, then the opportunity to interact the data is lost, and the danger of data being lost between two homes is considerable.

Collecting information

It is necessary to build up a body of information and there are a number of disciplines for doing that. All of the following are well used in health care settings:

Observation

Observational data usually refers to the scientific data collected by professionals such as nurses and therapists. It is according to recognised protocol and follows a standard checklist format. The procedure is well proven and reliable. It offers a useful model that can be transferred to a range of other situations.

Questionnaires

Questionnaires are used throughout the health care industry, but are not always conducted to a very high standard. A basic protocol, as follows, might be helpful.

1) Identify the purpose or overarching question to be answered by the questionnaire. I.e. devise a form of research statement for your enquiry. Questionnaires appear rambling and intrusive, when wide ranging data is requested because the enquirer asks everything "just in case". The purpose of your enquiry should be placed on a real or virtual poster in front of the questionnaire designer and used to ensure that questions are focused and justified at all times.

2) Search the archives to find an existing questionnaire that could be used or adapted. This gives the benefit of using a proven tool and the opportunity to correct errors reported by the previous researcher. Creating your own questionnaire is time consuming and there will be errors that would not be present in a previously tested device.

3) Modify the questionnaire or devise from scratch if necessary, and challenge the right to ask every question against your research statement. To ask a question that is not necessary to meet your purpose is unnecessarily intrusive and may result in a reduced response rate.

4) Order questions logically. Cluster questions on one subject together, and tell the respondent when you are about to change the subject.

5) Intersperse closed questions with open text invitation, allowing an opportunity for explanation. This reduces frustration on the part of the respondent and increases the response rate. Put an optional, free text question after each series of closed questions to allow the respondent to elaborate if he/she wishes. However, do not open

with a free text question, because that may give the impression that the questionnaire is challenging to complete and will reduce the response rate.

6) Start with easy questions and build up to more searching or intrusive ones if necessary.
7) Consider the analyses that are to be conducted and ensure that the data collected will be suitable. For example most regression and some correlation tests require continuous or interval data where other tests can manage with categorical data.
8) Check for leading or pejorative language that might guide the respondent to a particular answer.
9) Check for double questions, such as "Was your ward clean and tidy?" If it were clean, but untidy, how would you answer? If you needed to ask for this information, then two questions would be required.
10) Format the questionnaire to look as professional as possible. This improves the response rate.
11) Write detailed instructions to the respondent or the staff member who is to administer the questionnaire.
12) Pilot the questionnaire, make changes in response, re-pilot, make further changes and only then administer the questionnaire.
13) Over-personalised questionnaires eg to individuals by name, are not proven to gain a good response rate, but small incentives such as competitions or free pens do help.
14) It is important to report and publish questionnaire work in order to become a resource to others collecting similar data.

Interviews

You may wish to interview informants to gain information. Interview data is capable of delivering very rich information, but is time consuming and subject to interpretation by the interviewer. Therefore much that can be learned by interview, but it is important to recognise limits regarding the extent to which opinions expressed may be generalised to a wider group. It is also important to ensure that since the interviewer must selectively report what was said, what is reported does derive from the interviewee and is not projected by the interviewer.

Again, a sequence of events should be followed:

1) Identify the purpose or overarching question to be answered by the interview(s) write a research statement. Interviews may appear rambling and intrusive, when wide ranging data is requested because the enquirer asks everything "just in case". This might again be placed on a real or virtual poster in front of the interviewer and used to ensure that questions are focused and justified at all times.

2) Search the archives to find an existing interview protocol that could be used or adapted. This gives the benefit of using a proven tool and the opportunity to correct errors reported by the previous researcher. Creating your own schedule is time consuming and, again, there will be errors that would not be present in a previously tested device.

3) Challenge the right to ask every question against your purpose statement. To ask a question that is not necessary to meet your purpose is unnecessarily intrusive and may unnecessarily distress an interviewee.

4) Order questions logically. Cluster questions on one subject together, and tell the respondent when you are about to change the subject.

5) If the interview is a highly structured one, involving closed, questions, intersperse the closed questions with opportunity for open discussion.
6) Start with easy questions and build up to more searching or intrusive ones.
7) Guard against leading or pejorative statements and language that might guide the respondent to a particular answer.
8) Write detailed instructions for the interviewer, even if you are to conduct the interviews yourself, this is essential as a discipline for your thinking and as a permanent record.
9) Pilot the interview process and make changes as a result.
10) It is important to report and publish interview exercises in order to become a resource to others collecting similar data.
11) With due consents, record and transcribe the interviews and analyse by looking for themes in respondent comments. E.g.. three out of the four interviewees observed that financial constraints were playing a part, R1 said "*I thing that…* " etc.

Group interviews

A small group of respondents may be more revealing in their comments because they can respond to and build upon each other's contributions. This cannot happen in individual interviews. It may be helpful to interview between two and six respondents together. The protocols for this are as for individual interviews.

Focus groups

In order to learn something about the views of interested parties a group of stake holders might be brought together and asked to have a free ranging discussion in the general area of your interest and seek to achieve some consensus about their wishes. This provides information about what people might think, given information and the chance to discuss the matter in depth. It is better than interviews and questionnaires in that it allows respondents to give a very considered view after discussion and subject to negotiation with other interested parties. However, it is important not to make false assumptions about the honesty of members or the generalizability of the conclusions.

The part played in a focus group by the researcher is to collect a representative sample of participants and facilitate the event. Facilitation involves assuring confidentiality, thereby encouraging honesty, leading brainstorming and negotiation discussions and supplying relevant information, where requested. By this means, health authorities have sought to collect informed public opinion about priorities for committing limited resources.

Sociological observation

A different kind of observation is conducted in sociological and anthropological enquiry involving being present when interactions occur and making interpretations about the meaning thereof. This is a valuable but highly skilled activity. Managers seeking to employ this means of data collection would need expert tutelage and assistance.

Participant observation

It is recognised that it is not always possible to observe social interaction without affecting that interaction with your presence. Participant observation therefore allows that the observer is a part of the group and data is collected on that premise.

Ethical considerations

If your data collection may be considered research, then it might be necessary to ask your local ethical committee to examine your plans. If in doubt, it is helpful to consult the committee chairperson, who will often reassure you that you do not need committee approval.

Research needs consent; audit is a standard responsibility for you as a clinician and usually does not require the same protocols.

Conclusion

Information is not just a tool of industry, but a major product. In health and care, an important part of the service that you provide will be what you know or what information you can access and deliver at short notice, rather than what you do. The sheer volume of information that you will acquire in your career will be massively more than in previous generations, and you need to be highly efficient in how you handle it. How well you can acquire, manage and communicate your information will be a major determinant of how valuable you are to your clients or patients.

References

Dewey, M. (1876), *Classification and subject index*. Project Gutenberg eBooks

DoH (2013) *Essential Guide to Medical Records* London: HMSO

DoH, (2013)b *Summary Care Records* London: HMSO

http://www.nhs.uk/NHSEngland/thenhs/records/healthrecords/Pages/servicedescription.aspx

Mehrabian, A (1971) *Tactics of Social Influence* London: Prentice-Hall

Mehrabian, A. (1971). *Silent messages*, Wadsworth, California: Belmont

Mehrabian, A. (1972). *Nonverbal communication.* Chicago: Aldine

Mehrabian, A., and Wiener, M. (1967). Decoding of inconsistent communications, *Journal of Personality and Social Psychology,* 6, 109-114

Mehrabian, A., and Ferris, S.R. (1967), Inference of Attitudes from Nonverbal Communication, *J Consulting Psychology*, 31(3) 48-258

Mokhov, O. (2014) *http://www.hongkiat.com/blog/5-effective-ways-to-keep-your-files-under-control/*

Naisbitt,J. (1988) *Megatrends: Ten New Directions Transforming Our Lives* New York: Grand Central Publishing

Oppenheim,A,N.(1982)*Questionnaire design, interviewing and attitude measurement* London: Pinter

Salovey,A., Mayer,B., & Caruso, D. (2004), Emotional Intelligence: Theory, Findings, and Implications, *J Psychological Inquiry:* (12) 197–215

Swansburg,RC.(1990)*Management and leadership for nurses* Philadelphia: Lippincott

Taylor, M.C. (1999) *Evidence-based Practice for OT.* Oxford: Blackwell

Walton,M. (1997) *Management and managing – leadership in the NHS.* Cheltenham: Nelson Thornes

Managing Financial resources

Introduction

The NHS and Social Services can never, arguably, be adequately funded. Demand is potentially unbounded and resources are inevitably finite. Financial demands escalate because of the progressively ageing population, technological progress and increasing consumer expectation. In every case, when a new solution is created for a formerly terminal illness, the patient continues to live and will therefore consume further healthcare resources. Technical healthcare advances are entirely beneficial, but in each case, they result in increased services demand rather than decreased.

Available funds have steadily increased from 4% GDP (Gross Domestic Product) at the inception of the NHS in 1945 to 8% GDP, in 2014 (Rivett, 2014). However, although advances during that period are remarkable, the service has not moved any nearer to 100% satisfying demand.

There is a responsibility on any society to make as much resource available for health and care as is possible, and then upon managers and clinicians to obtain the maximum benefit for patients and clients from this resource. Since only clinicians and some managers can know the real priorities in health and social care, they have an ethical duty to engage with the efficient management of resources. This function cannot be delegated to management accountants alone. Clinicians cannot demand a particular episode of care for an individual patient without taking some responsibility for other pieces of care that will not happen because resources are consumed in this case. This is Opportunity Cost, see below.

Managing the balance sheet for an organisation such as an NHS Trust is a remarkably difficult exercise. The Trust is required to achieve the simple task of spending the same amount of money as it attracts in contracts. On the surface this is easy and whenever a Trust fails to do so newspaper headlines are scathing. However this task is made difficult for two reasons:

1) at the outset of the year, The Trust does not know how much money it will earn, because contracts are not yet in place and when they finally are agreed many have a variable component. Thus income cannot be known.

2) at the outset of the year, The Trusts does not know the cost of things. For example, in the middle of the year, an outside body will change the salary paid to doctors, nurses and clinicians, which represent about 80% of The Trust's spend.

Therefore to set a plan to make these two figures match is problematic. In spite of newspaper headlines, many Trusts underspend against income rather than overspend. What is remarkable is that Trusts frequently do achieve the required balance, not that they sometimes do not.

Of course, problems 1 and 2, above are not unique to health and social care. The same is true of Marks & Spencer or BUPA. These organisations resolve the problem by including a flexible component in the balance sheet known as 'profit'. If the costs are higher than predicted and income lower, then profit is reduced. If things deviate in the other direction, profit is increased. This variable profit outcome absorbs fluctuations in a way not available to NHS Trusts.

(BUPA is a non-profit organisation in that there are no shareholders. However, profits are made and these are reinvested in future years' activities.)

The Theoretical Framework
The Financial Channels

The NHS is funded by central taxation. This comes in part from National Insurance payments, collected through payrolls. The balance comes from the general national taxation pool.

Funds are passed to Strategic Health Authorities (SHA), (now being replaced by NHS England regional branches NHS E) according to a formula that takes account of population size, demographic makeup and social deprivation. SHAs or NHS E apportion resources to Primary Care Trusts (PCT) (now being replaced by Clinical Commissioning Groups, guided by NHS E local branches). PCTs or CCGs work with those groups to enter into contracts (commissions) with NHS Trusts and independent sector providers to deliver care to their population. Commissions are set for one or more years. The nature of services to be purchased and the number of patients expected are based upon knowledge from previous years. If insufficient treatment is commissioned in this way, then waiting lists will be held until the DHA and PCG can fund further treatments, subject to central government constraints on waiting, for example as outlined in The NHS Constitution (DoH, 2009). SHAs have also acted as payroll for General Medical and Dental Practitioner services.

NHS Trusts receive moneys in exchange for agreeing to provide services to patients through commissions. The transformation of NSH Trusts into NHS Foundation Trusts, has released them in some measure from financial constraints, but not the requirement to perform in relation to contracts set.

Social Care is funded in part from central taxation passed to local authorities through Social Services Grants and partly through local taxation: Community Charge or *'Rates'*. Local Authority Social Services Departments (LASSD) receive funds from the District or County or Unitary Council according to the council's assets and as far as possible in line with "Ratepayers' wishes". Social Services departments employ staff such as social workers and occupational therapists, to deliver services, but a minimum of 80% of their resources must be spent through contracts with independent contractors. This usually accounts for the provision of residential care and domestic home care.

Both the NHS and Social Services Departments add to their available resources by making means tested co-payment charges. The burden upon the consumer in Social Services is generally far higher than in health care, although there is a trend to increase the contributions in both fields. Co-payments in the NHS include: prescription charges, Ophthalmic and dental charges, car parking charges, charges to insurers for treatment of road traffic accidents and further charges as are periodically discussed. Co-payments in Social Services are levied on residential services, day care services and home care services. These co-payments can amount to 100% of the total cost and as with Home Care may even exceed the market cost leading consumers to elect to pay for private provision as a cost saving exercise. Means tests seek to ensure that patients and clients are not prevented from receiving care on financial grounds, and government initiatives seek to 'cap' the total bill that a service user can contribute (DoH, 2013).

Income and Expenditure

NHS Trusts gain income by entering into contracts with SHAs, PCGs and other agencies, such as BUPA to provide treatments to those patients who are the responsibility of the commissioner. An NHS Trust is required by statute to match its expenditure exactly to its income. A NHS Trust is not permitted to run in deficit or to make a profit. This rule is moderately relaxed for NHS Foundation Trusts, where a small surplus is permitted provided that it is part of a planned exercise to bring about service development. However, since there is no notion of 'profit' the general principle remains the same. This means that a NHS Trust is required to calculate how much it will cost to provide a service sought by a purchaser and this must be the price at which the service is offered. The NHS Trust is not permitted to cross-subsidise services. I.e. it may not make an accountancy loss on one service and make it up on another. Each contract must operate in balance. The calculation of cost, however, is a very complicated exercise, and a degree of interplay between the costs of different services can be observed influencing apportionment of overheads, etc. Synergy between services will affect the cost and viability of services provided.

Direct & Indirect Costs

Provision of a service will involve some expenditure directly on the service and some expenditure indirectly spent in order for the service to be provided (Howarth and Gruen, 2005)

For illumination, this section will explore X-ray assessment services.

Case Example: X-ray Costs

Direct Costs include:	Indirect Costs include part of the costs of:
Radiographers & Receptionists	The Management Board
Consumable materials	General premises such as Reception,
(Formerly film, now less so)	Car Park, etc
Dedicated X-Ray premises	Support services such as Portering
Maintenance of machinery	Public Relations Department.
	Building and grounds maintenance.

The direct costs can be established with a reasonable degree of accuracy, but the percentage of the indirect costs that should be attributed to X-Ray are open to considerable discussion. This makes it difficult to agree on a 'fair' cost for X-Ray services. There has always been an opportunity for a degree of disguised 'cross-subsidisation' in these calculations.

Fixed and Variable Costs

Fixed costs will be payable regardless of the amount of work to be done. Variable costs will depend upon the amount of work to be undertaken, i.e. they increase with every unit of production. (Howarth and Gruen, 2005)

Case Example: X-ray Costs

Fixed Costs may include	Variable Costs include
Radiographers & Receptionists on salaries Dedicated X-ray premises General premises such as Reception, Car Park, etc The Management Board Public Relations Department	Film where used and other consumed materials. Maintenance of machinery Support services such as Portering Staff on sessional contracts

Clearly some items described as fixed may be variable in some circumstances. E.g. if the radiographer is employed on a session basis to attend only when needed, then he/she would constitute a variable cost. Alternatively, if the machinery was serviced and replaced at regular intervals rather than after a fixed number of treatments it would become a fixed cost.

Full and Marginal Costs

The full cost of a service is that calculated to account for all direct, indirect, fixed and variable costs in total. However, if a certain number of treatments were planned and a price agreed that recovered all of the fixed costs as well as the variable costs associated with those treatments, then thereafter the cost to the Trust would only be the variable costs, because the fixed costs had already been recouped (Howarth and Gruen, 2005). The marginal cost is defined as the additional cost of producing one additional unit of productivity It would be appropriate, in that case, to offer further activity to the purchaser at the marginal cost, i.e. the cost of production. A difficulty arises if the additional activity is sold to a different purchaser. In this case, one purchaser may appear to be subsidising the other. I.e. the two purchasers purchased the same service at different prices. If this happens, more than very rarely, it must be a failure of planning in that the Trust failed to accurately predict the volume of activity for the year. An accurate prediction of activity would allow for apportionment of the fixed costs over all of the activity and thereby achieving a consistent unit price.

This same situation explains why hotels will sell late rooms for reduced prices and airlines sell empty seats very cheaply. It can seem paradoxical that it is in the interest of the hotel to sell a room for the marginal cost only for the last few rooms but if they sold all rooms for that price they would become bankrupt. In some cases a cheap room makes good financial sense but if that was extended to all rooms, the hotel would not be viable.

Apportionment of overheads

Each service provided by a Trust must be priced at the true cost. This requires fair apportionment of overheads (Indirect Costs) to each service (Gapenski,1994).

How much of each overhead the X-ray department should bear may be calculated according to one of several methodologies. The simplest methodology is to apportion overhead costs according to the ratio of direct costs. If the X-ray direct costs amount to 5% of the direct costs for all of the Trust's services' direct costs then the X-ray department would bear 5% of the costs of the car park, the management board, the reception, portering services, etc. This system is simple to calculate and therefore commonly applied. However, the drawback is that it carries no incentive to be frugal in the use of these services. If the charge were proportionate to use, then there would be an incentive to control usage and allow the overhead to reduce thus releasing resources for other purposes. The alternative, therefore, is for x-ray to bear overhead costs in line with usage of each. Thus, the portering service overhead might be apportioned to X-ray according to the amount that they use it. A general reduction may be achieved, because it is not seen as "free", so users moderate their demand leading to savings on that service which can be redeployed into direct patient services.

How Trusts apportion overheads will affect the prices charged for each service, and could be manipulated to reduce the prices in a competitive service area and load price where the Trust enjoys a monopoly. This, however, would constitute subtle cross-subsidisation. Internal and external auditors will examine the apportionment of overheads to seek to prevent this practice.

Capital and Revenue

Money consumed in producing a good or service, and the income earned by selling that good or service is referred to as revenue. Money spent on an asset, such as a building or machine, is referred to as Capital (Howarth & Gruen, 2005)

Revenue is consumed in making a product or service and can only be retrieved by sales. Capital expenditure is matched by asset increase and the capital could be released by sale of the asset. Revenue purchases are generally recurrent, where capital spends are generally a series of one off events.

The distinction between of capital and revenue is indistinct at the margin. Is a treatment couch that is replaced every five years a capital asset or is it consumed in delivering care? Accountancy procedures in each organisation define capital and revenue for their own purposes leading to artificial but consistent boundaries. The NHS and Social Services define capital spends by amount. Any single item purchase more than an agreed limit is taken to be capital spend.

Capital Charges

Holding capital has a cost. If the capital is loaned to an organisation then there will be interest to pay. If the capital is owned by the organisation, then by using it for purchase of assets means forgoing interest income. In order for this cost to be reflected in service prices, the NHS requires Trusts to pay a capital charge for the assets they hold. This makes fair competition with private sector service providers and encourages them to be frugal in their capital holdings.

Capital charges include a number of elements. These are a "rent" on the money, a depreciation repayment and an inflation adjustment. The rent on the money is represented by a 3.5% payment to the DoH on the total value of the assets held by the Trust per annum. The depreciation component is calculated by assessing the life of the asset and requiring a payback to the DoH such that it will be fully repaid by the time the asset is completely depreciated and needs replacing. This calculation is made assuming straight-line depreciation. I.e. an asset with a ten-year life is deemed to lose one tenth of its value each year. In reality most assets depreciation is on a curve, but at the end of its life, the effect is the same. Rather than paying the DoH an additional component of money to compensate for inflation, as is the case with a bank loan, the value of the asset is periodically reassessed and debt increased accordingly. Thus, capital charges include a 'rent' component and a depreciation component. Inflation is managed by revising the debt to reflect the changing value of the currency. This revaluation will also adjust the debt to reflect considerations such as fluctuating land values.

(Your mortgage interest involves: 'rent' on capital + repayment + correction for inflation.)

The detail of the calculation may be of only passing interest and subject to revision (or see DoH: Capital Charging) but the net effect is to make service providers see capital as having a cost. If they can minimise use of capital, then they pay less capital charges and release funds for other purposes, or reduce prices thus making it more likely that they win contracts in the future. In the private sector, this is self-evident. In the public sector capital charges lead to the same position by making capital no longer free (Wheeler, 1992).

Pricing

Price may be set as "what the market will bear". Competition keeps prices to a minimum, where there are enough suppliers, the services are comparable and information about each is freely available to customers In health and care services, there is rarely good competition and services vary in how they are packaged. For this reason, it is required that price equals cost. This seeks to minimise prices, but presents two difficulties:

1) The absence of competition in many areas fails to deliver the efficiency that was an objective of the purchaser: provider separation, ever since the 1990 National Health Service and Community Care Act.

2) The absence of a profit motive for a Trust removes a drive to increase activity.

Quality Adjusted Life Year (QALY)

Many attempts have been made to assess the value achieved by health care outcomes. A simple currency is the extension of life. Procedure "A" adds on average 5 years to life. If the procedure costs £1,000 then a year's life is 'purchased' for £200. The value for money of a procedure may therefore be measured in life years gained per £1. A clear failing of this notion is that there is no recognition of the quality of the life experienced. To extend a life but giving very poor Quality of Life (QoL) is not as good as extending life with full QoL. Also alleviating the burden of Rheumatoid Arthritis does not extend life at all, but we consider it a very valuable outcome of health care.

Quality Adjusted Life Years (QALYs) are an attempt to factor in the quality dimension (NICE, 2010) (NICE, 2014). One year of life in full health is rated at one QALY. Life with disability or chronic pain may be given a discounted rate. This is not to diminish the value of people with disabilities. However, the intent of health care is to reduce illness and disability as well as to increase life span. So, to simply measure extended life is inadequate. This methodology condenses quality and length of life into a single scale. Conceptually, a year of life with a profound disability is given a QALY value of less than 1. Thus a procedure that extends life for five years, but those years have a very poor quality achieves less than a procedure that extends life by five years and those years are in full health. A procedure that enhances quality of life but does not extend it at all may be seen as of great importance when measured in QALY values although a measure of life extension would not rate it at all.

Intervention	Life expectancy before Rx	Life expectancy after Rx	Gained	Gained
Intervention A	0 year	5 years: Full health	5 years	5 QALYs
Intervention B	0 year	5 years: Poor health (50%)	5 years	2.5 QALYs
Intervention C	5 years: poor health (50%)	5 years: Full health	0 years	2.5 QALYs
Intervention D	25 years poor health (50%)	25 Years Full health	0 years	12.5 QALYs

If a price for each intervention is given then a cost per QALY gained may be calculated and this may be useful as a measure of how much good can be done with the limited moneys available to a health or care purchaser.

Intervention	QALY gain	Cost	Cost/QALY gained	Rank order VfM
Intervention A	5 QALYs	£2,000	£400	2nd
Intervention B	2.5 QALYs	£1,500	£600	4th
Intervention C	2.5 QALYs	£1,000	£400	2nd
Intervention D	12.5 QALYs	£3,000	£240	1st

This methodology provides a structure useful in prioritising health interventions with limited resources. It has the advantage of considering the lifesaving alongside the life enhancing. Difficulties are encountered in two areas. Setting the level of discount for less than perfect health is very subjective and agreement is difficult to achieve. Allotting a reduced QALY value to a life with profound disability can imply that the person is less valued as a consequence. Although this is not the intention, the suggestion makes the measure difficult for some managers to employ.

Regulations

The management of money is highly regulated. This is particularly the case with money from the public purse. Regulation is achieved with a series of Standing Financial Instructions (SFI)s. SFIs regulate behaviour when receiving or spending moneys. Each Trust and Local Authority has its own SFIs but they have much in common. Most include the following examples.

1) Any purchase worth more than £5,000 requires receipt of at least three independent price quotes and the lowest chosen, provided the goods/services are of equivalent worth.
2) Any purchase requisition must be made by an authorised officer and countersigned by a more senior officer.
3) No employee may receive gifts of any nature from clients/patients.
4) Cash deposited by resident patients/clients must be received by two officers together and the record signed by both.

SFIs in any organisation will run to many pages and it is the responsibility of the individual to acquaint him/herself with them as appropriate. Failure to do so can constitute a breach of contract, resulting in termination of employment.

Audit

Each organisation has a legal duty to conduct audit annually. This will involve internal and external auditors at the expense of the organisation. Audit will cover three areas: audit of accounts, probity audit and value for money audit.

Audit of accounts

Each organisation is required to submit two types of accounts: *Ledger* accounts (*Cash flow*), showing the flow of moneys in and out of the organisation and *profit & loss* accounts which show cash flow and also take note of debtors and creditors, stock level changes etc. A NHS Trust is required to show both of these accounts in balance. Fluctuations from year to year are permissible, but in the long-term, there can be neither profit nor loss.

Probity Audit

Auditors will ensure that no improper appropriation or use of money has occurred. This will amount to policing of the SFIs, and thereby ensuring that the moneys passed to an Authority or Trust are used for the purpose intended (Rivett, 2014).

Value for Money Audit

Auditors will assess whether the organisation has obtained the very best value for the money that has been available to it.

Economic appraisal

Faced with a number of ways in which a service might be delivered it is necessary to decide which will represent the best value for money for clients and patients. A number of comparison devices are available for this purpose.

Cost effectiveness analysis

This refers to an analysis to decide whether a financial investment will save at least as much money as it costs. We might service a central heating boiler because service costs are less than breakdown repair costs. It is cost effective to service a boiler.

It is cost effective to immunise children because the cost of vaccines is far less that the later costs of treating illnesses.

It is cost effective to send an OT to a client's home if the cost of the visit and adaptations made is less than the cost of hospitalisation after a fall, even after allowing that only a percentage of patients have a fall.

Example

Cost of visiting and assisting in 100 homes = £100,000

Number of houses needed to visit in order to prevent one hospital admission = 10

-That is a *'number needed to treat'* analysis (Aveyard, 2014)

Average Cost of hospitalisation = £14,000

Cost of intervention per 100 homes = £100,000

Costs if no visit is made = £140,000 *(assumes 10 admissions at £14,000/episode of care)*

Therefore this OT intervention may be called cost/effective.

Economic analysis

This might be an exercise of:

Cost Minimisation – set the standards and volumes of activity and select the provider who can meet these requirements at the lowest cost. This has been used by NHS Trust and LASSDs for many years for laundry, cleaning and gardening services, but although it is also applicable to clinical services the complexity of weightings within a Diagnostic Related Group (DRG) makes it difficult to manage.

Utility maximisation – where we have a fixed budget, we can compare providers to see who can give us the most for that money. We commonly do this when we are buying a car or a holiday.

Cost/benefit analysis

Cost benefit analysis generally allows us to vary the cost and the utility and ask whether we can get more value for money at different price points. Of course if you pay more, you'll get more, but is the extra benefit sufficient to justify the extra cost? This is answered by using a cost/benefit analysis.

This requires us to have a currency for cost and also for benefit. The latter is the difficult one.

Benefit analysis involves us in identifying and listing the benefits that we value in the product and then weighting each to create a measuring tool. The second stage is to rate each option on this scale to get an overall utility figure for each option which can be set against the cost to derive a cost/benefit ratio. The best value for money is that with the best cost/benefit ratio.

eg, for a car you might value: safety, reliability MPG and appearance.

Deciding which is most important can be done by distributing ten points between these qualities, thus:

Quality	Weighting
safety	4
reliability	3
MPG	2
appearance	1

Different people rate this differently but that is OK if you rate a car for your own purchase.

There are three cars available and you can assess each to see how it scores on your scale:

Quality	Car 1 rating	Car 2 rating	Car 3 rating
safety	8	7	5
reliability	6	7	9
MPG	7	7	9
appearance	7	10	5

Apply your rating to the weighting and you can see which car is best for you:

Quality	Car 1 ratingXweight	Car 2 ratingXweight	Car 3 ratingXweight
safety	8X4=32	7X4=28	5X4=20
reliability	6X3=18	7X3=21	8X3=24
MPG	7X2=14	7X2=14	8X2=16

appearance	7X1=14	10X1=10	5X1=5
Total score	78	73	65

Car 1 is best car, no 2 is second best and no 3 is third.

Next the cost of each car is considered:

	Car1	Car2	Car3
Utility	78	70	65
Cost	£10,K	£11K	£6K
Utility/cost	7.8	6.3	10.8
Cost/utility	0.12	0.15	0.09

By this calculation, car 3 gives you best value for money, car 1 is second best vfm and car 2 is least vfm.

In comparing different approaches to delivering healthcare the benefit may be defined using QALYs, see above, as is done by the NICE. Alternatively a service commissioner could attach different values to features of the service they wish to commission, such as access, efficacy, acceptability, etc and perform the same exercise as above.

This can be used for major tasks such as commissioning care for a major illness or minor issues such as equipping a children's ward with toys.

To read more about Option Appraisal, see chapter 11 Project Management.

The Practice

or how you might go about it.

Budgetary control

NHS Trusts and Social Services departments generally work to fixed expenditure budgets, reviewed annually. Your department may be allocated a budget based upon an expected income from the contracts to which it contributes. Alternatively, it may will be given an income and expenditure targets. In either case, your annual spending allowance is derived (Atrill & McLaney, 2006).

An annual spend is not manageable as a whole. Budgetary control requires that an annual expenditure target be subdivided into manageable units. These units are known as budget lines. A line might represent a staff group, treatment materials, transport costs etc. Resources are allocated to a line and expenditures are coded to particular lines in order to ensure that actual spends accord with budgetary target spends. The next step is to divide annual spend targets into monthly targets and monthly reports will show *budget targets* and *actual spends* to allow the manager to see whether their spend is as required. In months two to twelve, there will be an accumulated effect from previous months. Therefore the statement will also show *budget to date* figures and *actual spend to date* figures so that the manager can know the emerging position. Many budget statements show the position projected to month twelve. This effectively tells the manager the anticipated *year end position* if he/she continues at the present rate of spend. The budget statement, therefore, may appear as below.

Line	Budgtotal	Budget this month	actual this month	variance this month	Budget to date	actual to date	variance to date	end of year projection
Senior Staff								
Basic Grade								
Assistants								
Admin Staff								
Total: staff								
Materials								
Transport								
Stationary								
Energy								
Telephones								
Tot:non-s'f								
Total								

This shows the proforma for a typical budget statement. Strictly speaking, the first three columns are the budget statement; the remaining columns are the expenditure statement. This statement can be expected monthly and serves to formalise the target spend and assess actual performance against that target budget. Budget statements may take a variety of forms, but the above information will always be given. The task of the reader, knowing that that information is there, is to find it.

Virement

Where there is a surplus under one budget line, the budget manager may be permitted to over spend on another line so that the totals remain in balance. This movement of resource between lines is known as virement. The rules regarding virement vary between Trusts and the manager should not assume that virement is permitted. Virement from non-staff lines to staff lines is rarely permitted because staff are a long term, recurrent expenditure commitment and cannot therefore be funded by a short term virement (Atrill & McLaney, 2006).

Virement from staff to non-staff lines (as in the case of a staff vacancy) may be permitted, but the organisation may wish to consider other priorities for the resource released by this staff vacancy. Virement between staff lines is generally permitted, because it is a necessary condition for skill mix revision. If the skill mix revision is long term, then virement will be permitted for the current year and the future year budget will show the correct target figures. Virement between non-staff lines may be acceptable, but there is a need to explain an under-spend before deciding to reallocate the resource. There may be outstanding invoices or stock reduction, both pointing to imminent expenditure. Additionally, the Trust may have greater priorities for the resource released by an under-spend than to simply move it to another line in the same budget.

Month thirteen

At the end of month twelve, there will be creditors and debtors associated with a budget year which remain to be resolved. It may not be appropriate to allow these receipts and spends to appear on the first month of the following year, because each year should be discrete. In this case the catching up of a year's accounts may be noted on a statement called month thirteen which usually runs alongside month one of the following year.

Zero based Budgeting

Budget plans for a year may be based upon the previous year with alterations to reflect inflation and the increases or decreases expected in performance (Atrill & McLaney, 2006). However, in zero-based budgeting, each budget is reconsidered annually and built up from scratch according to identified need. Clearly, some resources must roll forward from previous years, e.g. salaries and rents, but others may be reconsidered in the light of emerging priorities Zero-based budgeting is necessary to facilitate change in a volatile market Zero based budgeting also allows for correction of lines, where the actual expenditure is necessarily different from budget, such as staff who are paid more that budget because of long service or merit awards, etc.

Costings: Staff & Non-staff

Adding a new member of staff to a department requires new moneys in the budget. It is important that these costs are estimated accurately (Atrill & McLaney, 2006). The salary will, normally be subject to incremental or PRP variance. This means that the post may attract a salary anywhere between £x and £y. the normal protocol is to set the budget at the mid-point. Therefore if the scale is £25,000 – £29,000 according to experience, then the budget line will show (25000+29000)/2=27000. The assumption is that some staff will be below the mid-point and others above and that this will allow the budget to balance. However, if your department has low staff turnover, either because of the economic conditions or regional variance, then you will find all of your staff occupying the top of incremental scales. This will overspend your budget through no fault of yours. In this situation, you should argue for your staff to be budgeted at the top of the scale.

A staff member receives an annual salary, but this is not the total cost to the employer. Your budget must also allow for your employer's contribution to National Insurance, currently 6% and Superannuation (Pension) contributions. This results in an "On Cost" to salaries, usually set at 12 or 15%, but sometimes higher.

A staff member may use secretarial time, travelling expenses, stationary and telephone costs, etc. these must also be factored into the cost of a new employee.

A bid or another member of staff might, therefore, look as follows:

Item	Annual Cost/£
Salary (at mid-point):	27,000
On costs:	3,105
Secretarial support (0.1 WTE):	2,000
Travelling costs (est. 2,500m @50p):	2,250
General:	2,200
Total revenue cost:	**36,555**

This shows the necessary revenue cost, of £36,555, for a new member of staff who may draw a salary of £27,000.

The Vacancy Factor

Staff lines will show salary for twelve months' employment. However, staff move positions and it is rarely possible to replace them immediately when they leave. There will be a period when the salary is not being spent. Managers may enjoy using this resource by virement, as above (Atrill & McLaney 2008). However turnover of staff should not be treated as a surprise or as an individual event. A large budget centre is likely to have a number of vacant lines at any time. This should be seen as a standing situation where a regular percentage of revenue expenditure is not spent each year. This factor, if not allowed for, will result in repeated under-spending. A budget holder may account for this vacancy factor by including it as a line in the budget statement. The money represented by the vacancy factor might be deducted from the totals, so that it is expected that managers will spend less that the full budget may suggest. Alternatively, plans may be made annually to spend this vacancy factor on developmental work to advance the service. Finally, this may be used to pay for agency or bank cover. Agency staff can appear expensive, but the calculation above shows that an agency employee costing £36,000 is a value-for-money replacement for a staff member normally paid £27,000.

Case Examples

There follow a number of case example budgets. Each is a very small budget, but demonstrates the issues at work. Each tells a story with some exaggeration to make the point. Each should be studied and conclusions drawn. Explanations of each follow the figure.

Case example 1

Line Month 3	budget total	budget this month	actual this month	variance this month	Budget to date	actual to date	variance to date	end of year projection
Senior Staff	28000	2333	2000	-333	7000	6000	-1000	-4000
Basic Grade	26000	2167	2100	-67	6500	6300	-200	-800
Assistants	21000	1750	1500	-250	5250	4500	-750	-3000
Admin Staff	15000	1250	1000	-250	3750	3000	-750	-3000
Total: staff	90000	7500	6600	-900	22500	19800	-2700	-10800
Materials	31000	2583	60	-2523	7750	180	-7570	-30280
Energy	1990	166	150	-16	498	450	-48	-190
Telephones	2345	195	209	14	586	627	41	163
INCOME	-2300	-192	8	200	-575	24	599	2396
Tot: non-staff	33035	2753	427	-2326	8259	1281	-6978	-27911
Total	123035	10253	7027	-3226	30759	21081	-9678	-38711

This shows a budget in which all staff and non-staff lines are underspending. The failure to earn income as budgeted appears as an overspend on that line. Telephone use is overspent. The "to date" lines show that this situation has persisted for some time. There is an accumulated underspend. The projected year-end figure is one of significant underspending. The manager may have bulk or seasonal material purchases planned, which could consume the £27911 material costs. The manager may be saving staff moneys for winter pressures. The budget year is April – March. Therefore, the final three months may be expensive because of weather etc. If these explanations do not apply, then the manager needs to act to make best use of the resources available.

Case example 2

Line Month 3	budgt total	budgt this mnth	actual this month	variance this month	Budget to date	actual to date	end of year project'n
Senior Staff	28000	2333	2400	67	7000	7200	800
Basic Grade	26000	2167	2345	178	6500	7035	2140
Assistants	21000	1750	1000	-750	5250	3000	-9000
Admin Staff	15000	1250	3000	1750	3750	9000	21000
Total: staff	90000	7500	8745	1245	22500	26235	14940
Materials	31000	2583	4008	1425	7750	12024	17096
Energy	1990	166	1509	1343	498	4527	16118
Telephones	2345	195	209	14	586	627	163
INCOME	-2300	-192	-1	191	-575	-3	2288
Tot: non-staff	33035	2753	5725	2972	8259	17175	35665
Total	123035	10253	14470	4217	30759	43410	50605

This shows a budget in which there is a small overspend on staff totals this month arising from an excess of administrative staff that is partially compensated for by the underspend on assistant staff. There is also an overspend on non-staff. The failure to bring in £191 income presents as an additional overspend. The year-to-date columns show that this situation has persisted for three months. The projection is for a large overspend. It may be that the material overspend is accounted for by bulk purchasing and therefore that line will be correct by the year-end. However, There is need for a significant reduction in staff if the overspend of £14,940 is to be averted.

Case example 3

Line Month 3	budgt total	budgt this mnth	actual this month	variance this month	Budget to date	actual to date	variance to date	end of year projection
Senior Staff	28000	2333	2300	-33	7000	6900	-100	-400
Basic Grade	26000	2167	2100	-67	6500	6300	-200	-800
Assistants	21000	1750	160	-1590	5250	480	-4770	-19080
Admin Staff	15000	1250	1000	-250	3750	3000	-750	-3000
Total: staff	90000	7500	5560	-1940	22500	16680	-5820	-23280
Materials	31000	2583	4521	1938	7750	13563	5813	23252
Energy	1990	166	170	4	498	510	13	50
Telephones	2345	195	200	5	586	600	14	55
INCOME	-2300	-192	-200	-8	-575	-600	-25	-100
Tot: non-staff	33035	2753	4691	1938	8259	14073	5814	23257
Total	123035	10253	10251	-2	30759	30753	-6	-23

This shows a budget that appears to be performing correctly, when attention is given to the total columns (known as The Bottom Line). In fact, there has been an underspending on staff lines for some months, and the manager has taken advantage of the opportunity to make a large materials purchase. Although the budget is in balance (£2 underspend), the projection to end of year is misleading. In the absence of further material overspending, the budget will underspend because of the staff shortages such as Assistants. Assuming that the work of these assistants is necessary to patients, then a good service has not been provided and they need to be recruited to the level allowed by the budget.

Case example 4

Line Month 3	budget total	Budget this month	actual this month	variance this month	Budget to date	actual to date	end of year projctn
Senior Staff	28000	2333	2450	117	7000	7350	1400
Basic Grade	26000	2167	3100	933	6500	9300	11200
Assistants	21000	1750	3000	1250	5250	9000	15000
Admin Staff	15000	1250	2000	750	3750	6000	9000
Total: staff	90000	7500	10550	3050	22500	31650	36600
Materials	31000	2583	0	-2583	7750	0	-31000
Energy	1990	166	0	-166	498	0	-1990
Telephones	2345	195	0	-195	586	0	-2345
INCOME	-2300	-192	-300	-108	-575	-900	-1300
Tot: non-staff	33035	2753	-300	-3053	8259	-900	-36635
Total	123035	10253	10250	-3	30759	30750	-35

This shows a budget that initially appears to be in balance. This month's total shows an underspend of just £3. The to-date columns and projection columns support this interpretation. However, the staff expenditure lines are heavily overspent and this is masked by underspends on materials etc. Since energy, material and telephone costs will eventually need to be paid, it is inevitable that this budget will overspend before the year-end. Additionally, the budget holder appears to have vired resources from non-staff lines to staff lines, which is generally prohibited. There needs to be a swift reduction in staff expenditure on this budget.

Financial Business Planning

Business Case

Below, there is the basis for an organisation's Business Plan. A Business Case would follow a similar framework, but focus is on a specific business development, such as the addition of an additional Community Mental Health Team.

The business case would describe any developments in detail and include a full Option Appraisal showing all of the ways that the development might be achieved, with an economic analysis, shown above, to support the identification of a preferred option.

Business Plan

Your business plan shows the projected activity, income and expenditure for future years. It is common for the business plan to extend for five years with general statements of the direction to be followed during the subsequent five years. Income and expenditure projections will be based upon an understanding of the marketplace and a realistic estimate of the business that can be won. The financial plan will show the viability of the organisation, based upon that assumed activity. A business plan is commonly devised when an organisation is seeking new capital. It projects the financial position demonstrating the ability of the business to service and eventually repay the debt. (DoH, 2010)

Your business plan, therefore, shows the growth of your part of the organisation. A number of non-financial sections support the business plan. These are the implications of the planned growth for other aspects of the organisation. They show the reader how the infrastructure will be brought into place at the right time for planned developments to occur.

A typical business plan will have the following components:

Business Plan

Mission Statement

This is an unambiguous statement of the reason for the existence of the organisation.

Example Mission Statement:

"To maximise the health of the catchment population, by promotion of health and prevention, treatment or relief of illness".

Strategic Direction

This is a long-term indication of the future developments for the organisation, usually over ten years e.g.:

"To reduce dependence on institutional care business and develop community based provision for …"

Summary of current Business

This section describes any current business of the organisation. It shows what is done, how the quality is assured and what the volume of output is. It indicates who the customers are, and the nature of the consumer if these are different.

Market Analysis

Audit and analysis of the external and internal factors affecting the organisation's prospects in the market place. This analysis must demonstrate the feasibility of the planned developments. Market audit and analysis devices such as SWOT and TOWS appear in the chapter "Marketing

Assumptions and contingencies

Many assumptions are made in writing a plan. That is acceptable, if they are explicitly recognised.

Example assumption:

"It is assumed that government legislation will allow an increase in private beds in a NHS Trust."

Where appropriate, contingency plans should be shown for deployment if the assumption proves incorrect.

Example contingency plan:

"If private beds are not permitted, then the new beds described in "Developments Planned" will be:

1) offered to other NHS purchasers 2) offered to BUPA purchasers or 3) mothballed until needed.

Developments Planned

This section contains detailed description and explanation of each of the developments planned. It will show the human and other resources required, the demand, the details of the activity planned with quality and volume measures, etc.

Financial Projections

These sections show income and expenditure projections for the next five years, based upon current business and the developments (increases and decreases) above. They show viability of the organisation with adequate revenue surplus to service and repay existing and any new capital investment. Year one projections will be highly detailed and precise, subsequent years become progressively imprecise. These will be updated yearly informed by experience. In a rolling plan these pages are rewritten annually, so that the next year is made firm and a new year-five is added.

In any health or Social services business plan there will be a pro-forma for these pages. This will show exactly the form in which the information is to be given. With some additions for special details, the pro-forma will look as below.

	Year 1	Year 2	Year 3	Year 4
Income				
Income 1	1400K	2000K	2000K	2000K
Income 2	1000K	1100K	1100K	1100K
Income 3	2000K	2000K	2000K	2000K
Income total	44000K	5100K	5100K	5100K
Expenditure				
Expenditure 1	2000K	2000K	2000K	2000K
Expenditure 2	2000K	2000K	2000K	2000K
Expenditure 3	900K	900K	1900K	900K
Expenditure total	4900K	4900K	4900K	4900K
Balance	(500K)	200K	200K	200K
Cumulative Balance	(500K)	(300K)	(100K)	100k

Additional pages will be drawn up to show the detail of income and expenditure for each year.

Sensitivity Analysis

Re-run the figures with different assumptions, such as higher/lower demand, higher/lower salaries etc and see how they affect the balance sheet and at what point they become critical. Create contingency strategies for action at each critical variance level.

Human Resource Plan

This section shows the way in which any changes to the human resources will be made. It demonstrates how the necessary workforce will be in place at the best time for the developments to be achieved. The plan will include work force projections and demonstrate the expected availability of suitable recruits. There may be necessary training and/or retraining, and lead times must be adequately considered. There will also be consideration of redundancies. The costs of all of these developments will appear in the financial section.

Estates Plan

This section shows the way in which any changes to the physical resources - buildings, equipment, etc, will be made. It demonstrates that the necessary premises and equipment will be put in place at the optimum time for the developments to be achieved and that the costs are realistically reflected. It will also show the effects of disposal of plant and buildings. This section must, additionally, show the maintenance, and routine replacement of existing building and plant. Lead time for problem solving and staff training will be considered. The costs of these developmental and maintenance activities will appear in the financial section.

Marketing Plan

This section shows the marketing activity that will be employed to ensure that the planned developments and continuance of current business are achieved. It will also show ongoing market research to evaluate any developments in demand for the services/goods to be and being marketed. For operational marketing practice see "Marketing.

Overall, therefore, the Business Plan shows:

1) your market analysis that justifies your confidence that the business development is viable.

2) the detailed financial projections to demonstrate that the development is viable

3) all of the resources needed to make this happen and exactly how each will become active at the time that the plan requires it.

4) all of the actions to be undertaken to bring the business development about.

Management of your own financial resources

The above principles of budgeting and even business planning are as applicable to your own finances as they are to management of a major industry. Revenue budgeting will enable you to gain the very greatest benefit possible from your income, without need for unplanned (and very inefficient) debt or fear of financial difficulty. Sensible budgeting will ensure that you are in a position to have holidays, replace your car, etc, when necessary without feeling the pinch. Personal business planning will enable you to decide exactly how much you can afford to spend on a mortgage, car loan, private yacht, etc.

A personal budget statement might look like that below. You might take the framework and put in your own figures.

A Model of Your Personal Finances

Expenditure	2010/1	1,2	2,3	3,4	4,5	5,6	6,7
Education	5000	10000	10000	5000	2000	2000	2000
Household (Tot)	18062	18062	18062	18062	18062	18062	18062
Mortgage	10184	10184	10184	10184	10184	10184	10184
Endowments	1116	1116	1116	1116	1116	1116	1116
Phone	1200	1200	1200	1200	1200	1200	1200
Gas	1500	1500	1500	1500	1500	1500	1500
Elec.	800	800	800	800	800	800	800
Insurance	612	612	612	612	612	612	612
Rates	1650	1650	1650	1650	1650	1650	1650
Maintenance	1000	1000	1000	1000	1000	1000	1000
Other (Tot)	12984	12984	12984	12984	14484	13484	12984
Presents	1000	1000	1000	1000	1000	1000	1000
Parties	500	500	500	500	500	500	500
Visits	1000	1000	1000	1000	1000	1000	1000
Holidays	1500	1500	1500	1500	3000		1500
Groceries	3000	3000	3000	3000	3000	3000	3000
Clothes	1000	1000	1000	1000	1000	1000	1000
Cars	3000	3000	3000	3000	3000	5000	3000
Animals	500	500	500	500	500	500	500
Children's trips	500	500	500	500	500	500	500
Memberships	192	192	192	192	192	192	192
Sky	312	312	312	312	312	312	312
CPSM	204	204	204	204	204	204	204
BMA	276	276	276	276	276	276	276
Exp Tot	36046	41046	41046	36046	34546	33546	33046
Income	41700	41700	41700	41700	41700	41700	41700
1	20000	20000	20000	20000	20000	20000	20000
2	21000	21000	21000	21000	21000	21000	21000
Other	700	700	700	700	700	700	700
Surplus	5,654	654	654	5,654	7,154	8,154	8,654

Notes:

1) The figures in a projection are always given in the current year's prices. Therefore there is no allowance for inflation in the projections. This is acceptable because the income and expenditure are expected to experience inflation at roughly the same rate and the effect is thus neutral.

2) The projection shows an increase in education costs for two years followed by a decrease. Holiday and motoring costs are projected to be lower for a period and then to increase when the projected education expenditure tails off.

3) It is essential to ensure that all possible expenditures are captured on this model. Calculate monthly equivalents to these figures and assess them monthly against actual expenditures. This will enable you to ensure that your model is robust.

4) If you construct this model on a computer spreadsheet, then you can run "What If.." or *Sensitivity Analyses* to predict the effect of changes to any of these figures. You will see that some figures make little difference as they change (non-sensitive) and some figures have a large effect if they change (Sensitive). You are sensitive to some fluctuations and not sensitive to others. If mortgage rates go up radically you will be adversely affected. Ie you are sensitive to mortgage changes. Fluctuations to electricity prices in the above analysis are not important. You are not sensitive to these changes. It does not make a major impact on the bottom line.

A Personal Monthly Budget Sheet

	2010/1	Month 1 budget	Month 1 Spend	Month 2 budget	Month 2 Spend
Education	5000	417		417	
House	18062	1505		1505	
Mortgage	10184	849		849	
Endowments	1116	93		93	
Phone	1200	100		100	
Gas	1500	125		125	
Elec	800	67		67	
Insurance	612	51		51	
Rates	1650	138		138	
Maintenance	1000	83		83	
		0		0	
Other	12984	1082		1082	
Presents	1000	83		83	
Parties	500	42		42	
Visits	1000	83		83	
Holidays	1500	125		125	
Groceries	3000	250		250	
Clothes	1000	83		83	
Cars	3000	250		250	
Animals	500	42		42	
Children's trips	500	42		42	
Memberships	192	16		16	
Sky	312	26		26	
CPSM	204	17		17	
BMA	276	23		23	
Exp Tot	36046	3004		3004	
		0		0	
Income	41700	3475		3475	
1	20000	1667		1667	
2	21000	1750		1750	
Other	700	58		58	
		0		0	
Surplus	5,654	471		471	

Conclusion

The expert management of financial resources is critical to the effectiveness of health and social care. There is a constant debate about how much resource can be allocated to health and social care. However, although increases are possible, these are at the margin. There is finite revenue that can be collected through taxation because above a certain percentage tax avoidance and evasion exceeds the returns from an increased taxation rate.

How the resources are distributed between health, education law, etc may be debated, but it is agreed that all are necessary. Increase in one can only be achieved at the expense of decrease in another.

Health and social care provision is maximised by the most efficient use of the available, limited resource. The management of financial resources is not restricted to budget holders. All clinicians commit resources when they prescribe and deliver treatment and care. Seen in aggregate, these expenditures are far more important than financial control attempted by managers. It is partially for this reason that successive governments have sought to bring together clinical and financial management through Clinicians in Management initiatives. You, as an individual clinician or manager have a duty to ensure the most efficient use of resources in order to maximise the amount of care and treatment available to your patients/clients.

References

Atrill, P. & McLaney,E. (2005) *Financial accounting for decision makers* London: Kogan Page

Atrill P, McLaney E (2008) *Accounting and Finance for Non-Specialists,* London: Prentice Hall

Barrow (2008) *Practical Financial Management* London: Kogan Page

Blundel (2004) *Effective organisational communication* London: Prentice Hall

DoH (2010) *Business Planning Sourcebook* – London: HMSO

DoH 2013 *The Care Bill* – reforming what and how people pay for their care and support. London: HMSO

DoH, (2009) *The NHS Constitution*, the NHS belongs to us all. London: HMSO

Fisher,A., & Lovell, B. (2006) *Business ethics and values* London: Prentice Hall

Gapenski,L. (1994) *Healthcare finance for the non-financial manager.* New York: AUPHA

Gruen, R., Howarth, A. (2005) *Financial Management in Health Services. England* Harlow: Pearson Education Limited

Hofstede,G., (1968) *The game of budget control.* - London: Tavistock,

Howarth,R., & Gruen,A. (2005) *Financial Management in Health Services* Milton Keynes: OUP

McAlpine,T,S. (1976). - *The basic arts of budgeting.* - London: Business Books,

Mellett, H. J. (1993). - *Financial management in the NHS: a manager's guide.* London: Chapman & Hall,

NICE (2010) *Measuring effectiveness and cost effectiveness: the QALY* London: National Institute for Health and Clinical Excellence (NICE).

NICE (2014) *https://www.nice.org.uk/glossary?letter=q*

Pyhrr,P.A. (1978) *Zero-base budgeting : a practical management tool for evaluating expenses.* - London: Wiley

Rivett (2014) *timeline@nuffieldtrust.org.uk*

Sloman (2006) *Economics* London: Prentice Hall

Weetman *Financial and Management Accounting: an introduction* London: Prentice Hall

Wheeler,N. (1992), The Principals and Methods of Capital Charging and Their Value to the Functional Manager, *British Journal of Occupational Therapy* 54 (12) 444 - 8

Marketing

Introduction

Marketing may be defined as succeeding in business by providing goods and services that best satisfy the demands of customers. This involves the four components of the Marketing Mix (Kotler & Keller 2009) (Chapman & Cowdell 1998).

The Marketing Mix (Product, Place, Price, Promotion)
1) identifying from and with future customers the goods/service that will best satisfy them;
2) creating, packaging and delivering these services/goods to the best location for the customers;
3) ensuring the best price;
4) advertising the fact that they are available and describing their qualities; *and then*
5) return to customer to discuss product enhancements, etc

The Marketing Mix, is an iterative exercise. A marketer does not go through the process once and then consider the task complete. Rather he/she cycles around the loop throughout the product or services' life cycle. All stages are under constant consideration, with sequencing in which one aspect of the mix clearly informs the next, in a continuous loop.

The marketing function has an important place in health and care industries, in achieving all of the above four targets and without which the organisation would exist in isolation from an essential understanding of consumer aspirations. The critical role in marketing health care is performed by the clinician who has access to consumers and is in a position to make decisions for them far beyond anything achievable by managers. This is discussed at length in this chapter.

Customers and Consumers

The notions of customers and consumers are important in marketing. It may appear that these are foreign notions in health and social care, where patients and clients are the normal language (Kotler & Keller 2009). However, it is important to distinguish between customer (who pays for the service) and consumer (who receives the service), and use this framework to better conceptualise and understand how to help patients/clients. To be successful in the market place, of course, the organisation must please both customer and consumer simultaneously. If there is a conflict between the aspirations of these two bodies, then it may be the responsibility of the service provider to act as intermediary and develop a service to the satisfaction of both. If only one party is satisfied, then the product/service will not succeed. Dog food will not sell unless the customer (dog owner) thinks it is good value and quality and the consumer (dog – hopefully!) will eat it. Children's shoes must satisfy the parent and the child. Thus, we see hard-wearing leather that comes in six width fittings and has a star on the sole that might grant wishes. Similarly, if the GP did not think out-patient S&L Therapy locally is good value, he/she would not commission it, but if it is purchased being excellent value but patients refuse to attend because it is in the wrong location, then the GP will not purchase it again. Marketing health care must satisfy the demand of purchasing Health Authorities/Primary Care Groups, referrers and patients/clients/carers.

When customers and consumers choose a product, they do so on their perceptions of the information and services available. Therefore it is not sufficient to have an excellent service. That will not assure custom. The service must be perceived to be excellent. That requires marketing effort by all involved. Additionally, benefits appreciated by one customer may not be appreciated by another. The best advice is that the more benefits there are the more customers and consumers will perceive the service to be desirable.

The history of getting goods onto the market

The marketing of goods and services may be seen as having passed through a number of distinct phases (Kotler & Keller 2009). It is helpful see former stages as developmentally transcended rather than simply discarded. Early developmental stages have been subsumed into new stages and associated behaviours or values remain active, but enhanced by developments. The way in which goods have been marketed in the past gives insight into current practice. It is helpful, therefore, to know the historical progression in understanding current practice.

The Product orientated approach

"Build a better Mousetrap and the world will beat a path to your door."

In the 18th Century and 19th century, a great emphasis was placed upon engineering innovation, with a creative elite developing better products and an intelligent consumer, also from an elite minority, naturally buying that product in preference to an inferior product from another source.

The Production orientated approach

As the 19th Century progressed and industrialisation created a far wider consumer class, the notion of mass production emerged in the 20th century, most famously but not exclusively, from Henry Ford. This approach sought to minimise production costs by efficient production and thereby make goods available to a far deeper consumer constituency. Production became possible by a less skilled workforce and consumption became possible for a far less elite consumer group. Mass production by production-line organisation did not replace the drive for ever better products, but introduced greater cost awareness and accepted a degree of trade-off between the two considerations of excellence and price. In actuality, mass production has resulted in increased quality and reduced prices in many manufacturing areas.

This period of manufacturing history is often retrospectively described as the Fordist era. That era has been associated with "Modernist" thinking, and provides a focus for discussion of a "Post-modernist" approach to industrial and economic thinking.

The Sales orientated approach

With the advent of high quality mass communications accessible to all of the franchised population, the era of sales focused marketing emerged in the mid-20th Century. The power of communications to persuade the consumer that a product was the best one at the best price became more important that the drive to achieve the reality of both, or either. The era emerged as a result of accessible communications on paper and TV, but was supplemented by a significant increase in face to face sales staff, both in retail outlets and on the doorstep.

The Marketing approach

As a result of progressively sophisticated consumer behaviour the industry focus has moved from the importance and ascendance of the supplier to that of the consumer. It remains essential to have the best product at the best price and to advertise that fact to potential consumers, but it has become necessary to see those definitions from the perspective of the consumer. The discipline of market research has gained ascendance in this period. The easiest way to make consumers want a product is to develop the product that consumers said they wanted in the first place. Many models emerged to define products from a progressively wide perspective always viewed from the consumer's standpoint. The Marketing Mix, introduced above, is described below.

The Holistic (Green) and Post-modern approach

In the 1980s two new perspectives began to emerge.

Firstly, consumers started to make demands about the product that went beyond its direct function. They began to view products holistically. Washing powder had not just to be effective and inexpensive, but also had to perform without causing harm to the environment. Eggs had to be free range in the interest of chickens. This has gained momentum in the 1990s with lead-free petrol, recycled paper and timber from sustainable forests.

Secondly, there has been a rejection of the consequence of mass production. The Post-Fordist era has consumers wanting not to "Keep up with the Jones' " but to differentiate themselves from the Jones'. Thus a large proportion of motor car sales involve sales of mass-produced models disguised as individual by offering an unusual combination of extras and calling them "Limited Editions" or "Specials".

All of the above phases are evident in current marketing practice and in a health and social care industry, regulated in part by market forces, they can be clearly seen at work. The clinician and service manager have a duty to use marketing practice to ensure that patients and clients enjoy the very best service affordable. This chapter sets out to equip the reader with insights and abilities necessary to perform to an optimum level.

The Theoretical Framework

Strategic and operational Marketing

Marketing practice is often divided into strategic and operational marketing (Kotler & Keller 2009). Strategic marketing involves making long-term plans for the organisation based upon macro analysis of the marketplace and the position of the organisation therein. Operational marketing involves looking in detail at individual goods or services and ensuring that they gain the best possible market share. It may be argued that these functions are stages of the same process and that to divide them is artificial. To see the items as separate is untenable and to see them as linear is misleading. Although strategy informs operational plans, it is also the case that operational marketing collects information that is necessary for strategic analysis to take place. It is helpful to see the relationship as an iterative process in which strategy and operations are continually informing each other. Although this is a persuasive argument, it is convenient to conceptualise the functions separately for explanatory purposes, provided that the practitioner recognises the interdependence that exists.

Strategic marketing:

Analysis and planning

Marketing planning involves a number of stages (Kotler & Keller 2009):

1) Market audit
2) Market Analysis
3) Making Assumptions
4) Generating Strategy
5) Implementation Plan

This planning process is conducted in close association with business planning. See the management of financial resources.

Market Audit

Market analysis and planning are intertwined practices. The first stage in devising a market plan is to conduct an audit of the organisation and the market place. This involves collecting information external and internal to the organisation. External information includes information about:

- *Growth, reduction or redirection of the market,*
- *Influences on and interplay between consumers and customers*
- *The legal, economic and sociological environment,*
- *Competitors,*
- *Workforce supply,*
- *Other supplies, such as buildings equipment and materials,*
- *Technological advances.*

Each of the analysis areas is capable of generating threats and opportunities for consideration.

Internal information includes:

- *Reputation of the organisation in each product/service area.*
- *Market share,*
- *Qualities of Human resources*
- *Premises,*
- *Suppliers,*
- *Synergies between products/potential products*

Each of these areas is capable of producing strengths and weaknesses for consideration.

An audit may be carried out simply, by;

1) a brainstorm of key individuals in the organisation,
2) by including customers and other stakeholders in a brainstorming exercise, or
3) by having a formal audit conducted by internal or external consultants. The latter option would take the form of a research exercise and deliver very objective data.

Commonly, in the NHS and Social Services, data is collected by methods 1 or 2. This is inexpensive and has the advantage of easily gaining ownership of essential managers. However, it can result in a major strategic planning exercise being based upon unproven information. It might be the case that, as appears in HM Armed Forces Regulations, "Time spent on reconnaissance is seldom if ever wasted".

Market analysis

A number of analytical devices exist that help to order the data collected in an audit. The simplest and most commonly seen in public sector industries is the Strength Weakness Opportunity and Threat (SWOT) (Wheeler & Grice, 2000) analysis that sets out to order what is known for participant consideration. At worst, this is published in Business Plans with no obvious consequences, but at best, it becomes a focus for a divergent thinking exercise and changes the whole direction of the organisation. More complex analytical devices are available for employment in devising a market plan and these can reward the planner with strategic direction improvements based upon sound scientific analysis.

Strategy generation

Examination of the audit analysis will show up areas for development of strategic directions. These strategic directions are intentionally broad brush exercises stating the broad changes to activity that are to be achieved over a long period of time. For example, a NHS Trust may plan to reduce its investment in services to people with accidental injury and increase its investment in services to older people in response to its analysis of local industry decline and demographic trends. This strategic direction would be reflected in operational decisions in business and marketing plans. This route would incrementally implement the strategy. The reduction in accidents is an assumption, not a known event, and would need to be closely monitored.

Assumptions

In any plan, there will be areas where a factor is not known. Here the plan will be based upon assumptions. These assumptions are the best predictions that can be made, but must be distinguished from known fact. Above, an assumption was made about accident reduction. This assumption must be made explicit and a contingency plan created for implementation if the assumption proves false. I.e. if accidents continue to happen at the previous rate or above, how will the service move to ensure that services can be made available?

Case example

It was assumed in a marketing plan that legislation for individual Extra Contractual Referrals (ECRs) rom GP fund-holders would continue, and marketing effort was focused on making relationships with General Practitioners (GPs) accordingly. This appeared as an assumption on the marketing plan.

When the assumption was disproved and the white paper "The New NHS" (DoH 1997) abolished ECRs, the NHS Trust was immediately able to spot the change and implement the contingency plans associated with that assumption.

Implementation plan

Strategy is not directly implemented. One cannot simply drive to Scotland. The Southerner first drives to the nearest Motorway, then journeys along a link Motorway to access the M5, then travels North onto the M6, then joins the..., etc. Implementation is incremental through operational marketing and business planning practice. I.e. the service identifies short-term actions that will advance the drive towards the strategic objective. It is important that a strategy has milestones and time-scales and that progress is closely monitored. Therefore the plan will show an overall Aim and a number of Specific, Measurable, Achievable, Relevant and Timbound (SMART) Objectives.

Operational Marketing: The Marketing Mix

Developing a service or product in line with stated strategy might be addressed by application of the marketing mix. This involves attention to four main areas (Chapman & Cowdell 1998):

1) The product, along with any package building considerations,
2) The placing of the service, in space and time,
3) The price, seen in financial and other terms,
4) The promotion of the service.

Product

The product/service must be designed to best satisfy the demands of the customer and the consumer. This service design is done through market research where need is discussed, a new product is proposed and its acceptability thoroughly evaluated. This same approach is used to continually improve existing products. This should result in a constantly improving product/service base. If the organisation is to remain in operation in a dynamic environment its product/service offer must be constantly under review and constantly improved in line with customer and consumer aspirations.

Views about existing services, and services that customers and consumers yearn for, can be collected by a range of devices. These include: suggestion boxes, end of intervention questionnaires, focus group discussions, interviews, outcome evaluations, etc. The information collected should be through a variety of media: verbal and paper, formally and informally collected: questionnaires and over coffee when visiting a GP Surgery, group or individual. Time must be set aside to make the best use of this information rather than, as is too common, collecting masses of data and making reports but never really acting upon what is learned.

Price

The price to be paid by the customer and the consumer needs to be kept to a minimum in health and care services. In strict marketing parlance, price is "whatever the market will bear", and this cannot be ignored. If the price of a service exceeds that of another provider because of inefficiency or even excessive quality, then customers and consumers will prefer the other service and the other provider will take over the market. Customer loyalty and quality differentiation may in part mitigate this, but the problem of excessive price cannot be ignored for long. Marketing theory also says that the provider may price the service as high as the market will allow. This is the incentive that the marketplace offers to induce suppliers to enter sparsely served markets. However, in health and social care there is an ethical imperative not to charge more than necessary for a service, since to do so would take unnecessary resources out of the service thus diminishing the service as a whole. This is reinforced by DoH instruction that Price = Cost (DoH 1990). The financial price to customers must be as low as possible and certainly no higher than that of the competition.

The price to the consumer should also be considered. The claim that health care is free at the point of delivery is misleading and excessive "Price" to the patient/client is unethical. If the consumer is forced to pay a price that he/she considers unacceptable, then he/she will cease to use the service and the contract will decline. This imperative to minimise the price to the consumer in a paternalistic system has only recently been a matter for serious consideration.

The patient may not pay full fees for health services but there are many other costs to him/her. Among many, these include:

- *Financial costs in the form of lost earnings, paying for commercial child care, travelling/parking costs, co-payments, etc;*
- *Pain and discomfort as a result of assessment and treatment of illness. Who would not be willing to travel to access pain free dental care? Does this not also apply to Physiotherapy and Osteopathy?*
- *Intrusion into private areas;*
- *Inconvenience and distress in the form of stigma associated with some illnesses, long waits, difficult journeys poor circumstances, poor courtesy, etc;*
- *Difficulties in accessing services exacts a cost. E.g. a mother of twins pays a high price for care if it requires her to push a double buggy for two miles to access treatment.*

The service that minimises these costs to the patient maximises service uptake and shows greatest ethical respect for the individual.

Place

Where a service is placed, will have a significant impact on demand from customers and consumers. This has already been reflected in part in Price, above. The mother of two babies cannot easily get to a hospital that is three bus connections away, or to a clinic where there is no public transport service. Where clinics are placed will therefore effect the uptake.

The place a service is located can convey prestige. A service placed in a District General Hospital can assume an air of technical sophistication that is not possible when placed in a Health Centre. This may affect both the patient and his/her referring GP. There is always a queue of complementary practitioners keen to rent a room in a Health Centre, because of the implied approval conferred. Conversely, a service placed in a Village Hall, can achieve an air of informality and approachability, and this might increase referral and uptake of service.

It is also important to consider when a service is placed in terms of time. An evening clinic will more easily attract employed and self-employed patients, and their dependants. A clinic timed to coincide with the referrer's clinic will be likely to attract more referrals.

Case example

Occupational therapists and physiotherapists were vying for orthopaedic referrals following a Tuesday afternoon hand trauma clinic. The physiotherapists offered an excellent service on Monday afternoons, and the occupational therapists offered an equally good service on Tuesday afternoons. The consultant was faced with a choice of two good services. "I can get you seen by a Physiotherapist next Monday, if you will come back then, or I could send you to the Occupational Therapist who will see you later this afternoon and get your program started". Which service won the lion's share of the referrals?

Promotion

Once a service has been correctly defined, priced and placed in time & space, then it is necessary to let potential customers and consumers know that it is available and make sure that they realise how good it is. Thus, relevant individuals must be notified about the service. This notification must be adequately assertive to ensure that the audience comes to recognise the qualities offered. The promotion process is often also a good medium for collecting information about desired further improvements to the service. It should, therefore, be a two-way process. There is only a very limited place in health and social care for formal advertisement through leaflets and brochures, etc. The bulk of the work needs to be done through more-fortuitous routes. This involves widespread involvement of clinical staff.

Clinicians meet referring consultants and GPs at case conferences etc, and this is a good opportunity to ensure that they understand what is being offered, and comment on what they would like to see. Clinicians spend extended time with patients and clients, during which time they can ensure that patients understand the service provided and express any needs for changes.

Five stages of customer & consumer interest

In promoting a service, the marketer is seeking to move the consumer and/or customer through five stages leading from ignorance to demand (Kotler & Keller 2009). It is important to know where the customer is in this process because it is unlikely that desire will be achieved if the customer does not yet even know of the existence of a service. In good marketing the customer moves from: ignorance, to awareness and interest, to desire, to demand and ultimately to satisfaction.

Awareness: It is frequently necessary to begin by making the potential consumer or customer aware that a service exists. For nursing or social work, this is not necessary because everybody knows about them but for occupational therapy, it may be essential.

Interest. Alongside awareness, it is necessary to induce interest. Until these have been achieved, there is no benefit in striving to achieve service demand.

Desire: When a potential customer is aware of a service and interested, it becomes necessary to move them to a position of desiring the service. This is necessary for all health care professions, and is achieved by giving them information about the benefits available to them if they use the service.

Demand: A desiring customer will only demand a service when he/she is willing to pay the price. This is addressed by discussing and minimising the price, in all of its aspects, and demonstrating value in relation to the benefits.

Purchase: A customer making a demand needs to be facilitated to a "purchase". Many "Sales" are lost because the necessary assistance is not forthcoming to make the purchase at the appropriate moment. Just as in a shop, we may walk out because there is no assistant available, so a referring clinician may give up if the referral process is made too difficult, or the patient may not ask for a service if it is too difficult to access.

Satisfaction: After purchase, the customer and consumer should be aided through good aftercare to achieve satisfaction in order to achieve repeat and recommendation business. This involves the way in which clinicians make reports to referrers and follow up patients, etc.

It is easy to see clinicians and service managers operating on all of these areas. However, this is often random in nature. Marketeers need to assess exactly where the potential customer is on this progression and focus efforts to move them along.

Market Research

Defining the most appropriate service to offer in health and social care, as with all industries, involves asking consumers and customers what they want. In the past, paternalistic professional practice has preferred not to ask patients and clients. Rather they have relied upon their professional expertise to tell them what is needed. However, since the 1990 reforms "The NHS and Community Care Act" there has been a growing willingness to consult, and many service improvements have been achieved as a consequence. Clearly, health care services are not available from a shopping list, and there will be a need to temper demand with professional knowledge. However, good market research will be needed to define the service that funders, referrers and patients/clients want. The closer the provision can be to that ideal, the easier it will be to achieve high satisfaction rates and increasing demands for service provision. Market research delivers market intelligence (Kotler & Keller,2009).

Segmentation & Niches

Markets should not be seen as homogenous (Kotler & Keller 2009). Each customer and consumer group can be segmented. E.g. to see GPs as one group might be inappropriate. A GP in an inner city practice with high social deprivation factors will have a different opinion and be responsive to different messages from a GP in an affluent, rural practice. Thus, the opinions collected from one catchment will not be the same as those of another. This must be reflected in the market research approach adopted. It must also be reflected in the package of services offered. If there is one particular segment for whom the organisation has an ideal service, then it may be appropriate to focus energy on that area and aim for a very high share of that market. Alternatively, a service provider may wish to address all segments of a market, so the offer must reflect local conditions.

The theory of household behaviour

It is the case that in some settings parts of a community are disenfranchised concerning consumer choice (Lankaster, 1975). This is evident in a normal household. Consumers, such as children, are rarely able to exert their preferences over the choice of most household products. In this case marketing effort is aimed at the housewife assuming that she makes such decisions. This is evident from a short study of TV advertising. The parallels in terms of health care are clear. Many patients abdicate their right to make decisions to their GP, parents, adult children, carers, etc. marketing in this setting must take account of the phenomenon. However, to assume abdication can be dangerous as well. Children may be indifferent to choice of soap and towels, but many have a strong view about breakfast cereals. Marketers talk in terms of benefits for the consumer, but as might be perceived by the decision-maker, e.g. parents.

A taxonomy of need

Need and demand are central to health care delivery.

- A need is a deficit, affecting the individual, requiring a service or product.
- A perceived need, is a need, which the individual recognises. It may also be that an individual perceives a need that does not objectively exist.
- A demand is a perceived need for which the individual is willing to pay all aspects of the price to receive goods or services.

Health care is generally delivered in response to demand. I.e. the patient/client must perceive that he/she has a need and be willing to pay the price in cash, time, discomfort, etc. Only when these conditions are fulfilled does a demand for service emerge in the form of presentation at a health centre.

The NHS & Community Care Act (1990) confirmed that the services provided should be based upon a priority of need, and the subsequent growth of evidence based medicine has been a reflection of this requirement. Therefore for a service to be provided there must be a need, it must be perceived by the patient/client, he/she must be willing to pay the price of treatment and the referrer must be able to confirm that the proposed service will meet a genuine need. Marketing activity can be aimed at alerting needy patients/clients to their needs and giving them enough information to enable them to make a decision about their willingness to pay the price of treatment. This exercise is not simply "drumming up business". If providers do not make every effort to achieve this end, then the result is that the well-informed segments of the population benefit from services and the disadvantaged groups are missed out because they do not have enough information to demand services. This results in care going to the segments of the population that least need them.

Value added chains

The value of a service to a customer or consumer is an aggregate of all that has been done from the beginning to the end of the process (Kotler & Keller 2009). The maximum perceived benefit can be obtained by considering every stage of the process and ensuring that maximum perceived benefit is added at each one. To consider that benefit is only perceived at the treatment phase is misleading. The satisfaction a patient/client or referrer feels is effected by each stage. Careful consideration is needed at each stage. The marketer considers perceived as well as actual benefit. To perform as well as possible is an ethical imperative, but this excellence must also be perceived by influential players, if the service is to be appreciated and continue to be funded. In how people see a service, "Perception is all there is" (Peters 1989)

Referrer	Quality of interaction with referrer	➢	Knowledge that the matter is being professionally addressed	➢	Primary problems alleviated	➢	Maximise referrer appreciation	➢	
	Referral	➢	Assessment	➢	Treatment	➢	Report	➢	
Client/ Patient	Quality of Client/P't interaction	➢	Instil confidence, show consideration, assure professionalism	➢	Maximise benefit	➢	Maximise appreciation of benefit	➢	

The potential to add value to the service through every stage of the encounter, not just the treatment. This parallels the shopping experience in which customers chose supermarkets, not just for product and price, but also for isle space, checkout efficiency, layout, etc, etc.

Queuing and queuing theory

A standing waiting list implies that the number of treatments is the same as the number of new referrals. Therefore the queue is a result of some past event, and is diminishing quality and therefore the appeal of the service unnecessarily. A single initiative to clear waiting lists will increase the quality of all services thereafter. If the referral rate remains the same, then the same productivity will provide a service without delay. However, this will affect demand. If the queue is long, then referrers and patients/clients will not chose to use the service. When the list shortens, referrals will increase. On a hot day, we may wish to buy ice cream from a van. If, however the queue is very long we may not bother where when it is short, we may join it. Thus, the queue is in some part self-regulating. The size of a waiting list may therefore be a useful tool for demand control, if used consciously, but it is far too influential to be allowed to float out of control.

Occasionally, as with Morgan and Rolls Royce Motorcars, there is a paradoxical effect where the waiting time adds to the value customers perceive for a product. However, to attempt to use such a mechanism in health and care provision would be a dangerous strategy.

Requirements of a market economy

Under ideal conditions, the marketplace will ensure that all goods and services are available at a price and quality that is fair to supplier and customer (Rothbard, 2008). Competition prevents a supplier from charging too much for a product, because a competitor will charge a fairer price and take all of the customers. The price will not fall below an economic price, because there is no incentive for any supplier to operate at an economic loss. Were this to work in ideal conditions, then the consequence for health care would be excellent. However, for a perfect market, a number of requirements exist:

1) There must be perfect information. I.e. all suppliers and customers must have information about each other's products and prices. For this reason honest promotional activity will benefit health care generally;
2) There must be no externalities (desired benefits to parties other than supplier and customer/consumer). The health of one person affects that of another. For this reason, GPs are encouraged to make strenuous efforts to persuade parents to immunise children without waiting for demand from the parent. In addition, the service has the right to detain people with infectious diseases or dangerous mental health disorders regardless of their consent or any belief that detention will directly benefit the detainee. Otherwise, however, there are few externalities associated with health and social care provision.
3) There must be no predatory pricing, i.e. a willingness to sell at a loss for a period and thereby eliminate opposition. Legislation forbids cross-subsidisation, which is the only method by which a NHS Trust may sell

a service at less than cost The NHS and Community Care Act (1990). However, the apportionment of overhead costs will affect the price of some prized services, and therefore providers may seek to subtly cross subsidise services. Cross-subsidisation in the private sector is more common and more difficult to regulate.

4) There must be no cartels or monopolies. I.e service commissioners and providers may not collude and agree not to compete, thereby sustaining an unfair price. This is also outlawed by The NHS and Community Care Act (1990).

The Practice,

or How you might go about It

Marketing of health and care services is not carried out by extensive sales department. The marketing of your services, for the benefit of your patients/clients and of your NHS Trust, SS Department, etc is the responsibility of clinicians in your service, with some planning contributed by managers.

Market Audit

Market audit involves systematically identifying plusses and minuses in the internal organisation (strengths and weakness) and the external environment (opportunities and threats). These are most easily organised into a SWOT analysis, This exercise is best carried out by those near the point of service delivery, i.e. clinicians. The audit is often conducted as a brainstorming exercise. A large flip-chart with a SWOT grid, below, is posted and individuals place comments in boxes. Other participants build upon the comments made by colleagues and thus a comprehensive list is created.

This list will be more comprehensive if the participant list includes patients/clients, carers, family, colleagues and managers. When this is completed, a comprehensive list is obtained. Although, by definition, nothing is found that was not already known by somebody, the interaction between engaged people and the detailed attention always delivers far more that the group was aware of knowing and could therefore have been used in marketing planning.

This information can be supplemented by data collected from a variety of sources including

Suggestion boxes

These do collect "humorous" content, but these are easy to discard and much of value can be gained. Frequently, when consuming other services, you must have wished you could tell them just where they are going wrong, or occasionally right. A suggestion box, with pen & paper, will capture these thoughts in patients/clients, etc. they often have all too much time to make such contributions when in waiting rooms. The content might inform or supplement the SWOT analysis.

End of Intervention Interviews

Sitting down with a patient, perhaps while he/she waits for transport home is an ideal time to discuss how good the service is and how it could improve. This unpressured time delivers good information, and gives an air of consideration to patients who might otherwise thing that staff no longer value them, because they are finished with.

SWOT Analysis

This tool, created by the Boston Consulting Group, provides a useful brainstorming vehicle through which a team can collect share and plan with ideas (Adcock, Halborg, 2001). however, far too often it is an exercise without a product:

Hill and Westbrook (1997) found that SWOT often resulted in over-long lists of factors, general and often meaningless descriptions, a failure to prioritise issues and no attempt to verify any conclusions. Most importantly, they found that the outputs, once generated, were rarely used. Pickton and Wright (1998) argue that using SWOT to produce a simple listing output is inadequate or even dangerous, since a false sense of confidence can be generated by its use

It may be improved by moving to Heinz Weihrich's TOWS analysis, see below.

Strengths	**Opportunities**
▪ ▪ ▪	▪ ▪ ▪
Weaknesses	**Threats**
▪ ▪ ▪	▪ ▪ ▪

Focus groups

If individual patients/clients are too nice to say where improvement is needed, a small group together maybe far more forthcoming, by building on the comments of one another. "Nurse was lovely". "Oh yes she was. Mind you, I do wish that they wouldn't wake you so early". "Oh yes! And the way they serve tea in the morning. I can't manage it when I have just woken up". Etc, etc. This build-up of comment from one informant to another can deliver excellent information, for improving a service.

Questionnaires

Simple questionnaires for completion at discharge will answer questions on any predicted subject. However, they will not give you information you had not thought to ask. That is why they work well in conjunction with focus groups. Questionnaires should be filled in and handed back there and then. Any promise to do it later and post it, even with a pre-paid envelope will deliver very few results, and these cannot be deemed representative. Anonymity may be important, so allow respondents to put the form in an envelope and place it among a number of others. This will allow them to be more honest. Although some criticism may be uncomfortable to receive, it is essential to know, or you cannot improve.

Informal Opportunities

Many suggestions for changes or new services arise in conversation. You need to put yourself into situations where this can happen, and show colleagues that you are willing to hear these suggestions. This may be described as management by wandering about. If you can engineer to drop into a health centre around coffee time, you may hear many useful things from the staff there that you can use in marketing. It is important to capture these throwaway remarks, and to be seen to note them. This delivers much useful intelligence and is likely to result in repeat coffee invitations.

Market analysis

The information collected can be very great, and many NHS Trusts and Local Authority Social Services Departments (LASSDs) do not organise and use it. In some areas, it is collated into a report that is applauded and then used only to attract dust. Too rarely is this information integrated into hard plans.

The TOWS analysis (Weirich,1982) is a good tool for organising what is known and generating long-term plans to exploit that knowledge.

Above, the data was sorted into Strengths, Weaknesses, Opportunities and Threats. Applying Strengths to Opportunities shows where possibilities can be immediately exploited. The interaction of Strengths and Threats shows you how to move to prevent losses and mishaps. Where there is interaction of weakness and Opportunities, there is an urgent need to develop in order to take advantage of possibilities. Where there is interaction between Weaknesses and Threats, there is need for development or disengagement. You may recognise that a service loss will occur and your plan must show the replacement of this business.

A TOWS Analysis will generate a short list of strategic changes to the organisation and a further number of more immediate changes to make. This forms the basis of a strategic marketing plan.

TOWS Analysis Weihrich, (1982)	Strengths	Weaknesses
Opportunities	**Strategies relating Strengths to Opportunities**	**Strategies relating Weaknesses to Opportunities**
Threats	**Strategies relating Strengths to Threats**	**Strategies relating weaknesses to Threats**

PEST

Examining strengths and weaknesses is an 'internal analysis', because you are examining factors internal to your organisation. Examining opportunities and threats is an 'external analysis' because you are examining factors external to your organisation. Remembering this can help when you are unsure whether the demographic trends towards older people is a strength or opportunity. (It is an opportunity.)

The external analysis, opportunities and threats can be examined in greater depth, by breaking these up into Political O&Ts, Economic O&Ts, Social O&Ts and Technological O&Ts. Addressing each in turn, will ensure a more thoprough brainstorm. This gives you a PEST analysis. Some writers, go even further and advocate addressing Legal T&Os and Ethical P&Ts, resluting in a PESTLE analysis (Iles,2006). There seems to be no limit to this list and you should select the analysis that suits your situation. For this text we will be content with PEST.

Political	**Social**
Threats	Threats
Opportunities	Opportunities
Economic	**Technological**
Threats	Threats
Opportunities	Opportunities

Operational Marketing: The Marketing Mix

The marketing mix may be organised by service managers, but if it is to be achieved, its enactment must be primarily achieved by clinicians. There are four points to consider, Product, Place, Price and Promotion, as described below.

Product

Defining and continually improving your service is a result of market intelligence collected by clinicians as described above. This must be in line with the organisation's strategy and must closely meet the demand of customers and consumers. It is your job to be constantly in touch with the demands of patients/clients/carers and referring agencies. You are responsible for noticing where the match could be improved and working with your organisation to bring about continuous improvement. Where there is conflict between the demands of a) the referring "Customer", b) the referred "Consumer" and c) your own clinical expertise, it is your responsibility to bring about reconciliation. You must find a way forward that satisfies the patient/client/carer, referrer/funder and your clinical conscience. In the ultimate case, however, if conflict really is not soluble, your accountability requires that your clinical knowledge of what is right must take priority. You cannot behave in a way that you know is wrong, either on doctor's orders or the client's wishes. If you did so, then you could be brought to account. (See: The Management of People)

Price

There is a price paid for care by the consumer and the customer. You have the responsibility for minimising this price in all areas.

Minimising the consumer paid price

You must identify and reduce the price paid by your patient/client, carer etc. This may involve attention to a number of areas including:

1) **Financial price**. Consumers consume, where they consider that the price is satisfactory. You must ensure that costs incurred by travel, loss of earnings, child care, etc, are minimised as far as is reasonable, by choosing a location and timing of clinics that best accommodated most service users. Ensure that they have free access to hospital car parks and can reclaim us fares, wherever possible. This will reduce the number of clients who are put off by the financial cost of treatment. The old belief was that patients should be grateful for what they receive and not mind paying a bus fare. This paternal approach to medicine has only changed in very recent years.

2) **Inconvenience and distress**. If a service is inconvenient or distressing to access, then some patients/clients will not feel able to receive treatment. You must ensure that your clinic is sited where there is as little inconvenience as possible. E.g. where public transport access is good. Ensure that attendance attracts as little stigma as possible, e.g. for clients attending mental health services, and that there is suitable childcare assistance where needed.

3) **Pain & Discomfort**. Discomfort will make a client less likely to attend regularly for treatment. You must ensure that any discomfort associated with treatment is minimised. This may involve a number of actions, such as selecting the least painful treatment media, careful pacing of treatment, suggesting that the patient takes any PRN analgesia prior to a session, removing anxiety by ensuring that the patient understands the treatment, maximising privacy, etc.

Place

The location of a treatment in space and time is crucial to ensuring high referrals and attendance. This is referred to in price. Discover, in conversation, whether referrers favour a clinic in the surgery or the hospital. Examine records to see whether patients/clients prefer one to the other. This may be indicated by data such as the Did Not Attend (DNA) rate for each setting. The clinician is in the best place to know which location will best attract referrals, attendance and funding. There may be management action needed to move a clinic location, but the initiative and drive should come from the clinician.

Inconvenient placing may be erroneously used as a discrete form of rationing for an oversubscribed service. "If it is made difficult, then only those who really need it will come." In reality, a difficult service to access will favour the middle-class, middle-aged patient, who has access to private transport and communication skills sufficient to overcome poor information. The section of the community described in health care as "Socially Deprived" will be disadvantaged by an inaccessible service, although it is known that this population needs health & social care most (Townsend and Davidson, 1982).

Promotion

The promotion of a service involves making sure that all audiences know what is available and know just how good it is/could be.

This promotion is often carried out by managers visiting important audiences and telling them about service possibilities. However, audiences, such as GPs are very experienced at dealing with representatives, through their relationship with pharmaceutical companies, and are very sceptical about what they hear. A high percentage of leaflets and brochures are "binned" unopened. The best advertisement for a service is the clinician who is in contact with the referrer talking about live clients/patients.

There is no message or medium that will meet the need for all parts of the audience. Therefore, you should adopt a strategy for each target area. Much of the work can be a by-product of work happening already, such as case conference reports, if you alter the way in which you perceive these opportunities. Where extra effort is needed for promotional activities, then if the audience is seen in segments, energy can be focused on the most influential area at any given time.

Promoting your service to the Consultant

Consultants and Junior Doctors are key to nurses and PAMs gaining referrals and contracts. Frequently, they do not understand the support the professions make available to them, and therefore do not make appropriate referrals provide adequate resources. Your immediate response might be to "Go and tell them". However, although being on an induction programme is helpful, there is little that medical colleagues will learn from a lecture, either in terms of new knowledge or change of attitude. Leaflets and brochures are also very unlikely to gain much attention, although they have value for reference once attention has been gained.

The best route for promoting a service to a medical colleague is through a case conference or ward round. You could use this as a time to state the minimum about a patient/client, and therefore do your job, or you could use it as a forum to show just what you can do with a patient/client and thereby promote your service as well as conveying the facts.

> **Case Example**
>
> One occupational therapist in a department routinely says at case conference the like of, "The patient can go home on Friday". Another routinely says: "When I examined the patient I found that he/she could not manage transfers, could not wash and dress and the bedroom facilities at home were no longer safe. I have conducted a home assessment, worked on the transfers, arranged for handrails to be fitted, and arranged for a home carer to call daily. He can now go home on Friday". Which of the above OTs works on a ward where OT is understood and appreciated?
>
> You may feel that a succinct answer is appreciated by any meeting, and rightly so. However, you have a number of reasons to be at the meeting, and you can pursue your professional agenda, to the good of patients generally, as well as satisfying that of the meeting. The caveat is, however, that you should not overdo this so that it is obvious what you are up to and so that your long-winded contributions become an annoyance.

Promoting your service to the GP

As with the Consultant, the best approach, to this sector will be through live patients. There is some opportunity for case conferences, and these should be maximised, but far more frequently, you can reach a GP through letters about individual patients. Letters are normally written at the beginning and the end of an intervention. However, if your client group stays with you for a longer time, then you might consider regular reports at three or six month intervals. The important thing is that the report tells the reader about the service, rather than a minimalist comment that you are, or are not involved.

> **Case example**
>
> **One physiotherapist courteously writes**
>
> "I have been working with the above patient for three weeks and I have achieved as much as I can with his/her back problem. She reports some improvement.
>
> Please refer again if the problem recurs, or if there are similar cases."
>
> **Another writes**
>
> "Thank you for referring the above patient. On examination, I found that he/she has a disorder of..., which meant that he/she could not ..., therefore he/she was not able to attend work. I have treated him/her with... and the pain is reduced by 80% as measured by the Chicago Pain Scale. He/She can now perform all normal activities and feels able to return to work.
>
> Please refer the patient back the case of relapse, and I would be pleased to see any other patients in pain whose functional impairment is troublesome.
>
> The second physiotherapist was more successful in attracting referrals than the first.

Promoting your service to the Patient/Client

The least well understood profession is occupational therapy (OT). Or, so say the OTs. OTs solve problems for GPs they never knew they had. It is little surprise, then, that they gain little credit. Patients may report benefit to the doctor saying, "The lady from the welfare was a great help". This advantages OT very little and in this situation, patients cannot ask for more OT because they do not understand that it was an OT that worked so well before or helped their neighbour. Therefore, when working with patients/clients, it is essential that each professional ensure that patients/clients know what profession they are, and what is the point of what they are doing. Patients/clients, carers, etc. can watch a clinician going through the motions of treatment, but if it is not explained, they will not have the opportunity to recognise the scientific method behind the activities they see. Without this explanation, many carefully prescribed treatments can seem trivial. Leaving the patient and carer ignorant of the point of what was done prevents them from asking for more treatment in the future or recommending the service to friends and their doctor.

Promoting your service to the commissioner

Clinical Commissioning Groups and NHS Trusts decide what health care services are provided in their catchment area. It is therefore essential that they know what your service is and how well it helps their patients/clients. Senior managers will, occasionally, be invited to address the Boards of each authority, and it is essential that a succinct, but thorough explanation is available, with AVA accompaniment and comprehensive yet brief hand-out material. Multi-channel communication is known to convey more material to an audience that any single medium alone. Authorities have Lay Members (Non-Executive Directors) who are keen to come to understand the services provided. When approached by lay members you should recognise this as an excellent opportunity to become understood, rather than a threatening scrutiny. Many departments will be proactive and approach new CCG members to offer a visit and therefore give them the opportunity to understand better the business of health care from the sharp end. This also allows the service to promote themselves.

CCGs are under pressure to focus resources on treatments that are proven through research to have therapeutic benefit (evidence-based practice). You therefore have a duty to know the evidence in support of your treatment and to explain how it informs the work that you carry out. It is frequently bemoaned that there is insufficient evidence, and all clinicians should be supporting research, in order to continue to be supported. This is correct, but there is also a wealth of evidence available that clinicians do not access and do not therefore bring to the attention of service commissioners. Your duty, therefore is to ensure that every opportunity for contact with commissioners is exploited, that you know the evidence for your efficacy and efficiency, and that you present yourself in a focused, succinct and comprehensive way.

Promoting your service to the General Public

Public opinion influences commissioning and referring practice. All clinicians have a part to play in helping the public to understand the profession and what it can offer. Newspaper advertising and poster campaigns are the domain of the professional bodies, and are of limited value if attempted by departments. However, offering to collaborate on an article describing your profession is of considerable value. These often take the form of "A day in the life of…" You could also contribute by speaking to the WI, Church groups, Men's/Women's fellowships, etc who are always hungry for different topics, and find health/social care of permanent interest.

Schools are important means of influencing children and parents. They welcome occasional lectures from professionals for career education reasons, but you might add a little education for the benefit of the profession. It may be possible to attach one member of your profession to each of the local schools, and over time build a string of valuable relationships.

Open-days in departments are useful for fostering public understanding of a service, and if timed carefully can be used to accommodate those children who ask for a careers visit, rather than allowing each child to disrupt services by asking for an individual visit.

Promoting your service to Colleague Professions

Other professions may by contacted through case conferences etc. Additionally, you can influence other professionals through being transparent in your working when collaborating over a client/patient. Journal clubs and similar meetings where research may be shared across professions offer a good opportunity for promotion of a service. Taking part in the training or induction of other professions allows you to be present when individuals are at their most receptive.

When promoting a service to a colleague profession you are seeking to gain referrals and, ultimately, business contracts. If this is seen as competition, then a colleague profession cannot be expected to help you. However, if you are operating a win/win approach to your collaboration you can talk in terms of developments that will allow your professions to benefit together. If occupational therapists seek to outperform physiotherapist, and vice-versa, then both will fail over time. If however they work together to advance the case of occupational therapy and physiotherapy collectively, than both will steadily gain. Therefore, emphasise the ways in which you can both benefit through collaborative action.

Marketing yourself

All of the devices and practices described above for marketing an organisation or service can equally be applied to marketing yourself. You can market yourself in order to be seen to perform well in your present job, or to gain promotion, or a new job. You could also market yourself in your community and gain places on committees, etc, or even market a good diet to your children.

Self-Market Audit

Conduct an audit of your strengths and weaknesses, and analyse your environment to identify opportunities and threats. This audit should be led by yourself, but you might collect information from colleagues, etc either individually or collectively in a brainstorm. You might consider a 360^0 audit in which you consult your manager, one or more peers and a number of subordinate staff. You might also include the views of patients/clients and those who know you in other settings such as at home or in any society you may join.

When this information is collated, verified and sorted into a SWOT format, use a TOWS analysis to interact factors and devise strategies to advance yourself in any or all of the settings above. This should allow you to devise some long-term strategic directions so that your life goes where you want it to and at the same time some short-term tactics to move you in the right direction. This picture will change rapidly, so you may want to reaffirm your strategic direction and tactics at least annually.

Deciding on your strategic direction is the most difficult part of this exercise. Many people simply make incremental advances, each logical in the context of the last, but none calculated with a long-term intent to make your life meaningful seen as a whole. You climb the ladder one step at a time. However, are you sure that it is leaning against the wall you really want to go up? One device is to consider what might be said in your obituary, or in marketing headlines, on your headstone. If you continue as you are, what will be said, and is that OK? If it is not enough, then what would you like said. That points to your strategic plan. Alternatively, what will be your greatest regret on your deathbed? Few people will say, "I wish I had spent longer in the office, or I wish I had made more money", so why do we seek so hard to do that now? Most of us will say, "I wish I had made more time for family or church" or I wish I had bothered with people more", or "Just stopped to smell the flowers" So, why not add that to your strategic direction now. Check that the ladder you are on is going up a wall that you would like to be atop.

Avoid being seduced by the idea that more money or more importance is always positive. These are bought at the expense of something else, usually family, leisure, and art. The added income will certainly deliver increased Quality of Life (QoL). However, the loss of family time etc reduces QoL. You might consider QoL as the base currency with which you make decisions. Will a promotion giving more "Money QoL", but costing "Family time QoL" deliver a net gain, or a net loss. Do not assume that all promotion delivers a net QoL gain for you or your family. It may, but it may not, so the sums should be examined carefully. Of course, you cannot devise a strict mathematical formula to carry out these calculations but this does not invalidate the notion. Think in general terms about the gains and loss in any possible change, and decide whether they seem to you to aggregate to a gain or a loss. The answer will be different for different people. A promotion to Head Office involving daily commuting to London may result in a net loss to anyone who dislikes trains and the underground railway system. However, it may be a net gain to anyone who can spend many hours per week travelling with equanimity and will not miss the extra time away from home.

Assumptions

Your life-plan will be based on assumptions, such as "The NHS will remain a growth area", or "We expect to remain healthy into old age". If an assumption proves wrong, it is essential to notice and review your plans accordingly. Be explicit with yourself about the assumptions that you make. Notice when one proves erroneous and take swift action to alter your plans accordingly. If your health, or that of somebody close to you, deteriorates then your high-flying plans may no longer be in your best interest.

Implementation plan

Your TOWS analysis will have delivered tactics and pointed to plans. It will also show areas where you want to undergo development. Convert these into a long-term plan. If there is a MSc in there and counselling training as well as a long holiday to Australia, do not hold on to them in a vague way, because that way they will not happen. Draw up a long-term plan showing where each will fit. Then draw up a year-plan showing where this year's components will fit. Know that you will realise these dreams and know when. This plan should be shared with your manager and other significant people in your life. Ensure that your partner has a plan, and that it is compatible with yours. The plan should show how it is to be funded, what consents are required, and how they will be obtained, what the assumptions are, etc.

The pan needs to be reviewed for success and modified to allow for failures or changes to circumstances.

Operationally Marketing Yourself:

The Marketing Mix

Your Product

So, what are the "products" that you are offering? And to whom? This is based upon your audit and analysis. These products must be the ones that best advance your strategy. Think in terms of services beyond your core function. You may have a main service based on your nursing skills, doing that aspect of nursing that you are especially good at and that your colleagues most value. However, you may also offer services such as mediating disputes, writing reports for the board, or giving public lectures.

Your service list should be that calculated to get you the best reputation possible in the chosen and desired setting.

Price

Everybody pays a price for your co-operation and help. How difficult do you make this? If your contribution is at meetings, are you also a pleasant colleague to be at a meeting with. If the "price" of your eloquence at a meeting is having to listen to your views on every other agenda item, then you may not get invited again. If you can minimise the "price" paid by others for your services, then you will maximise the appreciation you gain.

Place

Where is the best place and time for your contribution? Careful timing and placing can make that value of what you do far greater. If you propose to make a virtue of your management report writing skills, what is the best venue to offer and deliver these? Chose venues where the value will be greatest for the minimum input.

Promotion

How you let others know what you could offer is crucial. Self-promotion is essential but can be counter-productive if it is too obvious. Too little, and you will go unrecognised, and too much and you will be blocked. Ideal promotion is by good word of mouth. This can be achieved by asking colleagues who recognised a good piece of work to bring it to the attention of influential others. If you promote a colleague in his/her presence, it is likely that he/she will reciprocate. If you promote everybody in his or her presence, you might get them all at it! There is no harm in joining mutual admiration societies.

If you produce a good piece of work, ensure that your name is discretely, but noticeably at the foot of each page. Wear a name badge and ensure that everybody knows whom he or she is talking to on the telephone. Always speak from the audience at meetings, and write papers on activities that go well. Do not claim all of the praise for yourself, be willing to share authorship with colleagues, and encourage them to reciprocate. Where you have a well-established colleague, work in tandem with them and benefit from their experience. A paper that you cannot get into print because you are a newcomer may well be printed if you collaborate with an established name and offer a joint publication. Later you can get onto the other end of this equation.

Value added chains

Consider all aspects of each service that you offer and add value to each. Writing a paper is not the whole service. There are several stages to any process and you should seek to add value at each one.

In, for example, writing your paper, there are a number of stages: consultation, writing, proof reading, attribution, launch, follow-up.

Consider how you enhance your reputation when you are consulting on content. The more people you consult, the more people will have ownership of the product, even if you do not really need the help. Consult on drafts, again this will widen the ownership. In particular, ask influential names to look it over before the final print. Acknowledge influential individuals, prominently in the paper, and they will ensure that it gets the best circulation. When the paper is released give advance copies as a favour. Get it a powerful launch, with good AVA support and, perhaps, a senior person to act as sponsor, introducing you to the meeting and getting you a good audience. Seek responses to your work and always thank respondents for their comments.

Conclusion

Marketing can appear aggressive and irrelevant in health and social care. However, ensuring that you are giving clients/patients what they really want, at the lowest "price" to them, where they want it and when and then ensuring that they understand the opportunities, is entirely appropriate. Marketing is best conducted by clinicians and others with direct contact and co-ordinated by managers. Good marketing ensures good services and maximised benefit. It is therefore within the duty of every clinician and manager to market services.

To market yourself is to ensure that you are the best that the organisation and the patient/client could want. To ensure that everyone understands just how good you are is part of your duty to yourself. Active marketing can make you the driver of your career rather than the passenger.

References

Adcock,D & Halborg,A (2001) *Marketing: Principles and Practice* London: Prentice Hall.

Chapman,D & Cowdell,T (1998) *New Public Sector Marketing* London: Prentice Hall

Frain, J. (1999) *An Introduction to marketing* London: International Thomson Business

Iles,V (2006) *Really Managing Healthcare.* Maidenhead: OUP

Kotler,P & Keller,K (2009)*Marketing Management* London: Prentice Hall

Lancaster,G,A (1999) *Introduction to marketing : a step-by-step guide to all the tools.* - London : Kogan Page

Lankaster,K (1975) The Theory of Household Behaviour *Annals of economic and social measurement* 4 (1) p5.
http://www.nber.org/chapters/c10216

Proctor,R,A. (1982) *Structured and creative approaches to strategy formulation* Management Research news 15 (1) 13 - 18

Rothbard, M N. (2008). *Free Market* In David R. Henderson (ed.). *Concise Encyclopaedia of Economics* (2nd ed.). Indianapolis: Library of Economics and Liberty.

Sheaff, R. (1991) *Marketing for health services: a framework for communications.* Milton Keynes Open University Press,

Townsend,P & Davidson, (1982) *The Health Divide* London: HMSO

Weihrich,H. (1982) The TOWS Matrix *Long Range Planning* 15 (2) 54 - 66.

Wheeler,N & Proctor,T.(1993) *Strategy Analysis in the Health Service Journal of Marketing Management* 9 (3) 287 - 300

Wheeler,N & Grice,D (2000) *Management in Healthcare.* Cheltenham: Nelson Thornes

CONTRIBUTORS
The publishing team are grateful to the following for their valuable contributions:
Brian Donnelly
Emma-Jane Lane
Julia Foster-Turner
Outi Pickering

This text is offered on the inventive new 'Createspace' Publishing platform for two reasons:

3) The costs to the reader are far lower than traditional publishing houses.
4) It is easy to update and improve the work; the text is continually under review. To this end the readers and the authors form a community to develop the work. As a reader, you are invited to email suggestions to *nwheeler@brookes.ac.uk*
These may be simple 'typo' alerts, additional references, new areas to cover, etc, etc.

Index

And personal notes:

Absenteeism and staff availability	69
Accountability	75
Alliances	296
Alphabetical data storage	368
Analysis and planning	430
Appointing staff	103
Apportionment of overheads	391
Arbitration	125
Art Therapists	80
Audit of accounts	396
Auditing standards	170
Back it up	373
Bed Occupancy	359
Biorhythms	48
Blake and Mouton's Managerial Grid	254
Break up tasks into manageable slices.	42
Budgetary control	402
Bulletin boards	239
Business Case	412
Business Plan	412
Capital and Revenue	392
Capital Charges	392
Career breaks	72
Case Examples	43
Category - Sub-category Storage	369
Chair	121
Changing	233
Chronological Storage	369
Clinical Governance	161
Clinical Psychologists	80
Collaboration	293
Communication and feedback	238
Communication systems	222
Company Worker	121
Completer finisher	122
Conditioning and Gestalt	194
Consultation meetings	166
Contacts Directory	371
Co-operation	295
Cost effectiveness analysis	398
Cost/benefit analysis	399
Costing no more that it must	156
Costings: Staff & Non-staff	405
Curriculum Vitae	140
Customers and Consumers	426
Databases	374
Deadlines	15
Delegation	39
Demand > Supply	54
Diary example	24
Dieticians	81

Direct & Indirect Costs	388
Disabled Persons (Employment) Acts (1944 & 1958)	59
Disciplinary Procedure	114
Dismissal	73
Disputes Procedure	113
DoH (2010) Business Planning Sourcebook -	423
Duty of confidentiality	355
Economic analysis	399
Economic appraisal	398
Efficiency	13
Encode: Transmit: Receive: Decipher.	361
Equal Opportunities	99
Ethical considerations	381
Evidence for Job interviews	134
Federations,	297
Feidler's Contingency Leadership Model	257
Financial Business Planning	412
Fixed and Variable Costs	398
Focus groups	166
Full and Marginal Costs	390
General Managers	81
General Medical Practitioners	82
Goal Alignment	67
Government information collection	356
Great Man Theories	251
Grievance Procedure	112
Group interviews	379
Handle paper only once	41
Health Improvement Programs (HIMPs)	288
Hertzberg's health and hygiene	262
Immediacy	362
Income and Expenditure	387
Independence	296
Individual Performance Reviews (IPR)	67
Induction	106
Industrial relations	68
Interruptions	44
Interview Planners	373
Interviewing	99
IPR & PDPs	108
Job hunting	136
Job Specification	136
Jobs for today	34
Leadership and Trust	208
Leadership	249
Lead-time	63
Lean thinking	336
Length of Stay	359
Make maximum use of breaks.	44
Making effort count twice	46
Management by wandering about (MBWA)	240

Managing a diary	22
Managing Change	188
Managing Financial resources	384
Managing Information	345
Managing Oneself	127
Managing People	51
Managing Quality	151
Managing supply and demand	53
Managing Time	13
Market analysis	432
Market Audit	431
Marketing yourself	461
Marketing	425
Maslow's theory of motivation	260
Medical Laboratory Scientific Officers (MLSO)	82
Meetings	45
Midnight Bed State	359
Midwives	83
Minimising the consumer paid price	454
Models of change management: Forcefield analysis	230
Models of change management	212
Monitor Evaluator	122
Month thirteen	404
Negotiating teams	124
Negotiation	123
Networking	294
Newsletter	238
NHS reorganisation Act (1970)	281
Nurses	83
Objective Setting & the Personal Development Plan (PDP)	66
Observation	375
Occupational Therapists	84
One and two way communication	361
One comprehensive organiser	374
Operational Goals (Objectives)	36
Operational Marketing: The Marketing Mix	434
Operationally Marketing Yourself:	464
Option Appraisal	325
Organization	335
Outsourcing and Tendering	52
Parkinson's Law	19
Participant observation	380
Participative leadership and Involvement of employees	196
Personal & Professional Development: Portfolios and Profiles	129
Personal Organisers	371
Personality types	301
PEST	451
Pharmacists	84
Physicians	85
Physiotherapists	86
Podiatrists (formerly Chiropodists)	87

Portfolio	132
Power and Politics	263
Primary Care Groups (PCGs)	285
Primary/Secondary/Tertiary	280
Prioritising	29
Probation	104
Probity Audit	398
Promoting your service	461
Psychological Behaviourist Theories	253
Psychometric testing	98
Public Health Physicians	86
Quality Adjusted Life Year (QALY)	394
Quality and efficiency management	287
Quality Assurance & Total Quality Management	162
Quality Assurance	157
Quality Circles	177
Quality Control	157
Quality	152
Questionnaires	164
Queuing Theory	16
Race Relations Act (1976)	61
Reactive or Proactive?	17
Reciprocity	363
Record Keeping	117
Recording patient/client information	349
Recruitment & Selection	56
Redundancy & re-deployment	73
Rehabilitation of Offenders Act (1974)	60
Resource Investigator	122
Resource requirement	134
Retirement	74
Role Blurring	90
Self-evaluation	133
Setting standards	47
Sex Discrimination Act (1984)	61
Shaper	122
Short listing	98
Situational and contingency Leadership	255
Skill mix analysis	64
Social Workers	88
Speech & Language Therapists	87
Staff Development & Performance Management	106
Stakeholder analysis	324
Strategic and operational Marketing	430
Stress	127
Subsidiarity	223
Suggestion boxes	163
Suggestion schemes	239
Surgeons	88
SWOT Analysis	447
Team Briefing	238

Team considerations	301
Team life cycles	302
Team Roles	120
Team types	301
Team Worker	122
Team-working	117
Terminating contracts	70
The Disability Discrimination Act (1995)	59
The Employment Lifecycle	56
The Equality Act (2010)	60
The Hersey-Blanchard Situational Leadership Model	255
The Human Resource (Personnel) Department	555
The New NHS - Modern and Dependable (1997)	284
The NHS and Community Care Act (1990)	282
The theory of household behaviour	441
The Vacancy Factor	406
The White Paper, *Equity and excellence:* (2012)	290
Theory X and Theory Y	253
Time & motion analysis	46
Time Log	27
Time Sampling	28
Time use analysis	26
Time	127
Total Quality Management	159
Trait Theories	252
Transactional and Transformational Leadership Theory	258
Tribalism	89
Turnover Interval	360
Urgency/importance	33
Value added chains	442
Value for Money Audit	398
Virement	403
Waiting lists/Waiting times	16
Wastage rates	63
Workforce Planning (Manpower Planning)	62
Zero based Budgeting	404

Printed in Great Britain
by Amazon